When You Get Older,

WHERE WILL YOU LIVE?

A Practical & Creative Guide

ELLEN F. RUBENSON

author of *When Aging Parents Can't Live Alone*

Disclaimer:

This book includes links to information on external websites. While effort has been made to include resources and links to the most accurate information available as of this publication, the information will ineveitably change over time. Further, referencing or linking to external sites does not imply endorsement of views and advice on the website by the author or publisher of this book. Always verify accuracy and currency of information before relying on it.

Please visit whenyougetolder.com for more resources, information and updates.

When You Get Older, Where Will You Live?

A Practical and Creative Guide

Single-family homes, apartment living, over 55 mobile and manufactured home communities, cooperative and shared housing, sustainable alternative housing, recreational vehicles, houseboats and other floating homes, overseas living, retirement and theme communities, assisted living, adult care homes, nursing and rehabilitation facilities, finding medical care, in-home services, employment opportunities and more...

Ellen F. Rubenson

Special thanks to Lisa for all her time, energy, and support.

"Life would be infinitely happier if we could be born at the age of eighty and gradually approach eighteen."

-- Mark Twain

Table of Contents

Introduction

"To retire: to withdraw, as for rest or seclusion; to go to bed; to withdraw from one's occupation, business, or office stop working; to fall back or retreat, as from battle; to move back or away; recede."

-- The Free Dictionary.com

On my 50th birthday, I received a flyer in the mail from the American Association of Retired Persons (AARP.) I was amused by the idea that I was considered mature enough to qualify for their membership services. After glancing at the information, I added the mailer to my pile of recycled papers. Now, years later, I watch my baby boomer friends celebrate their 60 plus-year birthdays and think that being a "retired" person is not so far away.

Most people want to believe that they can 'retire' wherever and whenever they choose. We look ahead to the times when we can decide how to spend our future years. But do we plan how we will transition from work to retirement? How do we wind down our careers? What will our circumstances be? Will we count the years until we are eligible for Social Security income and Medicare benefits? Will our children leave home, leaving us to be empty nesters? Or will they live with us as they attend college or vocational classes, search for employment, or try to figure out what they want or need to do? Will our parents, members of the Greatest Generation, be living independently in their own homes, renting houses or apartments, living with family or others, moving to be near family, or residing in standard or continuing care retirement communities, assisted living facilities or in adult foster care homes. Will we need to provide them with financial and /or caregiver support and assistance? How will that affect our plans for retirement? What do we want to do when we have the time to do whatever we want?

Retirement is upon the baby boomer generation, but only in relation to an expectation set by the previous generation. The fact is that remaining employed in a struggling economy is essential to retain healthcare benefits, pay our monthly rent or home mortgages, and to support our family. When asked, "When do you plan to retire?" we still shake our heads and reply, "I don't know" or exclaim, "I don't think I'll ever be able to retire," Yet the idea of being retired and being able to enjoy our family time, hobbies, travel, or doing whatever we want, lingers. Some common reasons we view our retirement prospects as doubtful include:

- changes in our employment status sometimes resulting in reduced income, reduced hours, underemployment, or unemployment;

- up's and downs of financial markets;

- depleted retirement and savings accounts;

- increased daily living expenses with rising costs for gas, utilities, food, and consumer goods;

- loss of home equity;

- soaring healthcare costs;

- waiting to be eligible for Social Security and Medicare benefits;

- potential caregiving and financial responsibilities for our children and/or parents.

We know the phase of 'retirement' is approaching, waiting for us to decide when, where, and how we wish to shape it. Yet we postpone retirement and continue working, pushed by the need to retain our healthcare coverage and wait for a stronger economy so we can rebuild our retirement nest egg. What steps can we take to enter retirement while still leading active and healthy lives? What is within our control so we greet retirement as a positive period in life, an opportunity to explore fresh alternative housing and living options? Do we want to stay in our homes, move to another home, age in place, receiving help wherever we are living, or seek an adventure or living experience that is new and exciting?

Meet the Baby Boomers

*"Wisdom doesn't necessarily come with age.
Sometimes age just shows up all by itself."*

-- Tom Wilson

Enter the baby boomer generation, an explosion of post-World War II births from 1946 -1964. The boomer generation seeks to identify itself in ways different from previous generations. Most notable are our numbers: 80 million people, all coming of age during a struggling economy in which our 401 (k) retirement savings have plummeted by 18% (Hewitt Research) and our healthcare systems do not cover the medical needs for millions of Americans. We hear that healthcare reform is on its way but it may be several years before we feel its full impact.

We are a generation raised without a World War, but with the legacy of the Vietnam Conflict that persisted from 1959 until its end on April 30, 1975. As the war escalated in the early 60's, many early baby boomers found themselves sent overseas to Vietnam, Cambodia, and Laos. Others marched in protest against the war and questioned its rationale; some became conscientious objectors.

The 60's and the 70's were a time for self-discovery and change. We are a generation that experienced the assassinations of John F. Kennedy, Bobby Kennedy, Martin Luther King, and John Lennon. In the wake of its devastation, the AID's virus was discovered and laws were passed that barred discrimination against those who were infected. We lived through the Space Shuttle Challenger disaster, listened to the raw guitar of Jimi Hendrix, the raw and sweet voices of Janis Joplin, and then felt disbelief over the news of their heroin overdoses. We sang the lyrics of Bob Dylan, danced the pony, the monkey, the swim and twisted to the Beatle's lyrics of *Twist and Shout*. We danced through the era of rock n' roll and segued right into disco. When introduced to Star Trek, we formed our fingers into the Vulcan sign and became Trekkies. This popular science fiction television series with messages of social responsibility was first viewed in 1966. It spawned its television and theater successors in the form of Star Trek: The Next Generation, and a series of films. Some baby boomers embraced an alternative lifestyle as Hippies; others, beginning in the late 60's, became Young Urban Professionals or Yuppies. As we rejected or modified many of our parent's beliefs, some viewed the boomer generation as greedy, spoiled, self-centered, and self-absorbed. However, the baby boomer generation helped end segregation, pushed for women's rights, and supported equal rights for minorities.

Boomers pride themselves on feeling younger and are sometimes critiqued for acting younger than their actual age. Even though I use the "'-boomer-'" term to describe this generation, boomers do not like being called 'baby boomers' or having the words,

"'-aging-'", "'-old-'", "'-elderly-'", "'-golden agers-'", "'-geezers-'", "'-senior-'" or "'-retiree-'" associated with themselves. We feel young at heart but the reality is that both our minds and bodies are maturing. We expect to live 20–25 years post-retirement, leading healthy, productive, and financially solvent lives. Engaging in an active lifestyle is considered a necessity, not a luxury. We count on attending fitness centers and exercise classes, becoming involved in community projects, attending Elderhostel programs or university classes, or traveling to other parts of the world.

As a group, boomers have not prepared for retirement. We are leery about the future and recognize that future Social Security payments may be inadequate to sustain our current lifestyle. Before the Social Security Act of 1935, most people worked until they experienced health concerns or reached a specific age at which they were removed or removed themselves from the employment force. Now, people who have worked and paid into the Social Security system are eligible to collect early retirement benefits beginning at age 62. However, by delaying the collection of Social Security benefits until age 70, we can maximize our monthly benefits. We do not expect the government to take care of us, yet we look forward to collecting Social Security and Medicare benefits. The cost of healthcare remains a top concern. Insurance premiums, co-payments, and deductibles continue to rise and the number of insurance companies that deny insurance because of pre-existing conditions continues to be a problem. *(These problems are currently being addressed by the new Healthcare Reform Bill, passed by the United States Congress and signed into law on March 2010.)*

We expect to live longer than our parent's generations yet have not saved enough for retirement. This could be due to many reasons including higher education costs, loss of home equity, changes in the financial market, unforeseen and soaring healthcare costs, procrastination or poor savings habits, and early job termination. In recent times, we have seen our employment income and retirement savings decline or evaporate during the 2008 financial crisis, making it likely that many boomers will feel forced to postpone retirement.

Age to Receive Full Social Security Benefits

Year of birth	Full retirement age
1943-1954	66
1955	66 and 2 months
1956	66 and 4 months
1957	66 and 6 months
1958	66 and 8 months
1959	66 and 10 months
1960 and later	67

Note: People who were born on January 1 of any year should refer to the previous year.
--Source: http://www.socialsecurity.gov

Are the Baby Boomers Prepared for their Retirement Years?

Boomers are now entering their 'retirement' years. Although our older family members and our children may continue to need our support, we look forward to the days when we can explore all the traditional, non-traditional, and creative choices available to us. One of these choices will involve where we will live. As we consider our choices, some boomers will look at luxurious life-care (also called continuing care) complexes that guarantee care for life; others will choose to stay in their homes and age in place or move to be closer to children and grandchildren. Some will choose new and innovative living options.

As we begin to look at the baby boomers entering their retirement years, we should remember that every boomer has different life circumstances. With 80 million boomers, there is a wide variance in our individual situations. We can be:

- employed, self-employed, under-employed, or unemployed;

- professionals or non-professionals;

- married, single, divorced, or widowed;

- living with a spouse or partner;

- living with a family, children, parents, a relative, or others;

- living in a home we own or rent;

- living near our children and parents or living far from family members;

- with healthcare insurance or without healthcare insurance;

- active and in good health or in fair or poor health with chronic health conditions;

- financially secure, with moderate or livable income, or living near the Federal poverty limit. (See *Appendix for Federal Poverty Income Guidelines*)

Let's meet three single baby boomers and two baby boomer couples.

Melanie is in her late 50's, a single mother with a child in her first year of college. She rents her two-bedroom home. Although she works three jobs, her employers do not provide health insurance benefits. As she cannot afford to purchase healthcare insurance, she relies on community health clinics for medical care and uses a pharmaceutical financial assistance program to purchase essential medications. During the recession, she saw her hard-earned saving depleted. Quitting her jobs so she can 'retire' is not something she can afford to contemplate.

Susie is mid-50, divorced, with one child completing graduate school and another entering her first year of college. She rents her third floor one-bedroom apartment. She works full-time and attends university classes part-time to work on her Master's degree. Her employer provides both healthcare insurance and college tuition benefits. She is actively involved as a community volunteer. Retirement is not on her radar at this time as she anticipates a new career, being an empty nester, and beginning to save for her retirement nest egg.

Paul is in his late 60's, self-employed as a carpenter/contractor, and owns and lives in the home that he built many years ago. His income fluctuates each month, dependent on the economy that affects the construction of new homes. For retirement, he hopes he can age in place in his home, but struggles to meet his mortgage payments and fears that he will lose his home to foreclosure. He cannot afford to buy health insurance and recently signed on with the Department of Veteran's Affairs for outpatient healthcare benefits. His children are grown, self-supporting, and live in another state. However, they cannot help him financially.

Sam and Vanessa are in their late 50's and early 60's. They are both employed retain retirement savings, and own their own home. Both receive healthcare benefits from their employers. Their two adult children are employed and live independently. Their 21-year old child did not have healthcare insurance and through the recent *Affordable Care Act,* her parents' insurance now provide healthcare benefits When Sam unexpectedly lost his job through downsizing, he found that buying healthcare insurance took a sizable chunk from his monthly unemployment check. With high healthcare premiums, co-pays, and deductibles, the health insurance coverage provided benefits in case of a catastrophic event. For every day medical care, the insurance benefits were very limited. As Sam and Vanessa look forward to their 'retirement,' they wonder what healthcare insurance they will be able to afford. Without employment, Sam can no longer continue to build his nest egg, an investment that he had anticipated adding to for five more years.

David and Sharon are in their late 50's and early 60's. Sharon is a full-time employee; David is self-employed. Sharon receives healthcare benefits through her employer; David must buy his own healthcare insurance. They own their home, as well as a rental property that brings in additional income. They have two adult children, one employed and living independently and one living at home, working and attending college. David's mother lives in a separate apartment on the property and requires daily assistance. While David and Sharon look forward to 'retiring', David's health has limited his ability to work and Sharon is not feeling secure in her job. They anticipate increased care needs for David's mother. Both recognize the need to work for another five years or so and hope that their health and jobs will last until then.

These five living situations are not unique. Every day, boomers are laid off from their jobs, underemployed, self-employed and without health insurance, or working long hours at numerous jobs without healthcare benefits. All have watched their hard-earned retirement savings plummet and their income remain stagnant. Yet, they continue to support their children and parents, both financially and as caregivers, offering necessary care and help. All worry about the future and hope that someday they can join the ranks of people enjoying their retirement years.

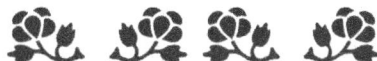

The Greatest Generation:
Retired and Entering their Twilight Years

"You know you are getting old when the candles cost more than the cake."

-- Bob Hope

Although this book focuses on the baby boomer generation, it would be remiss to over-look members of our parent's generation, those now in their 80's and 90's. We look at our parent's generation and their options of where to live. We see the daily health and living challenges faced by our "'oldest old'". We see them struggle to remain independent and re-tain control of their lives. After 60-plus years of self-determination, it is no wonder that they resist any changes that threaten their autonomy.

The Greatest Generation, a term coined by journalist, Tom Brokaw, includes people born between 1901–1924, who grew up during the Great Depression and lived through World War II. They are also referred to as, *'The Veteran's'*. They came of age during post-World War II and helped rebuild our country. This generation, the boomer's buffer, is almost gone.

Meet four couples who are members of The Greatest Generation. Two couples are educated professionals living in their own homes with ample finances to choose where they want to live. One couple faces unexpected health issues and challenges as they cope with progressive Alzheimer's disease. Another couple lives in their own home, but with a low-income, close to the Federal poverty income guidelines. *(See Appendix)*

Martin, an engineer and intellectual property lawyer, reluctantly retired from his law firm at age 82. Within a week, he began volunteer work at the local *American Association of Retired Persons (AARP)* office, learning Washington D.C. housing law and handling landlord-tenant issues. His wife, Sarah, a retired psychotherapist also in her 80's, had retired several years earlier and volunteered at a local community shelter for at-risk adolescents. Together, they take classes at a local university, attend theater, play bridge, and enjoy an active and social lifestyle. Health problems have slowed them down yet both retain their ability to think and problem solve. They continue to drive and are able to walk independently. Although they visit the doctor more than they go to the movies, they consider themselves the "healthy" ones in their group of peers.

Nick and Carol are in their late 80's and early 90's. Carol is extremely active, pursuing her career as a ceramic artist by offering classes, hosting pottery exhibits, and participating in gallery shows. With part-time hired hands, she continues to run their working ranch, harvesting an apple and pear orchard. And, she is the caregiver for her spouse of 60 years.

Nick remains active but in a much slower way. His limitation is his mobility and balance and over the years, after several falls resulting in broken bones and a fractured hip, it is increasingly difficult for him to walk distances. He uses a walker around the home and when traveling, resorts to utilizing either a wheelchair or, most recently, a power scooter. While his thought processing has slowed down, he still tells good jokes, participates in managing the household finances and helps run the family ranch.

World travel is an important part of their life. Since retiring in their mid-60's they have journeyed to the jungles of Papua, New Guinea, trekked on jungle safaris in Africa, and traveled across the European continent and to the high mountains of South America. While this love of travel never died, their ability to travel independently became increasingly difficult. Enter their boomer generation children. With their children providing the driving and the muscle, they have been able to visit France, the National Parks of Wyoming and Montana, New Zealand, France and Northern Spain.

Both couples have grown children and grandchildren living nearby who are available to help with basic home maintenance and transportation and are available if there is a medical crisis.

Both couples chose to remain in their own homes. One home has difficult access with steep stairs to the front door; another has four low steps with a rail. Both homes have yards that require mowing and yard maintenance. Simple home repairs, such as changing a light bulb, are dangerous if changing the light bulb involves climbing a stepladder. Cleaning the gutters on the roof is hazardous. Shopping for food involves driving and carrying heavy grocery bags. Falling becomes a daily fear. When driving a car presents a danger to them and others on the road, both couples say they may consider moving to an apartment or a retirement community. Until that time, both couples plan to age in place in their homes. There really is no place like home and both have no immediate plans to move.

Lydia and Samuel are both in their mid-80's and have lived in their own home for over 40 years. Although they have grown children living near-by, they are estranged and do not see them. Although Samuel worked most of his life, they did not accrue a significant savings account. Lydia raised their family, tutored children, and volunteered in their community. Lydia never learned to drive and walked or rode her bicycle everywhere in town. Living on Samuel's income enabled them to live an active and often frugal life. When Samuel passed away, Lydia found her income reduced to her Social Security widow's benefits. Unable to pay the monthly costs for her home or perform home maintenance, she began to take in boarders to help pay her day-to-day living expenses. Lydia received rent payments from her boarders and assistance with her yard work and house maintenance. Without the extra boarders, Lydia could not safely remain in her home.

Paul and Phoebe are both mid-80 and have been married for over 50 years. They lived in their own home and cared for each other. Both were in good health. In their early 80's, Phoebe began to show symptoms of progressive Alzheimer's disease. Paul embraced his role as caregiver and helped his wife every day with her activities of daily life, helping her get dressed and groomed, perform her toileting, feeding her at mealtime, and walking with her every day. Both expected that as Phoebe's Alzheimer's disease progressed and she became increasingly dependent on Paul, that he would always be there to take care of her. Unexpectedly, Paul had a heart attack and passed away. It was difficult for Phoebe to live with her grown children as both worked full-time jobs and were unable to provide her with the 24/7 care and supervision she required. Unable to live alone or care for herself, Phoebe's children located a memory care facility nearby. Luckily, Paul and Phoebe had substantial savings and were able to private pay for her care in the memory care home. Over the years, as her condition deteriorated, she did not recognize her own children and became unable to dress, groom, toilet, or feed herself without assistance. As her finances depleted, with help from the facility, her family applied for Medicaid assistance to pay for her continued memory care.

> "These couples are considered, by the U.S. Census Bureau to be the "oldest old," those ages 85 and over and now the most rapidly growing senior age group. For the "oldest old", women are more likely to outnumber and outlive the men. By age 85 and over, the ratio is 5:2. While "oldest old" non-institutionalized men are more likely to be married and living with their spouse, the "oldest old" women are more than 3 times likely to be widowed. While most elderly men have a spouse when their health fails, most elderly women do not. In 1990-1991, over 50 percent of people in the 85 years and older group needed personal assistance with their activities of daily life." (May 1995: Economics and Statistics Administration, U.S. Department of Commerce)

While all these couples prefer to live in their own homes without daily support from family or the community, they recognize they no longer have the abilities of their youth to manage all aspects of their lives. Many steps to enter the home will eventually become a major accessibility issue. Driving a car may be a necessity for grocery shopping, medical care, and more. When driving is no longer possible, it may precipitate the need to move to a more convenient location. Finances may play a major role in the decision to move to a smaller home, retirement or assisted living community, choose a long-term residence for a loved one or share a home with others.

Members of the Greatest Generation may choose to age in place in their own homes, with or without supportive community services and assistance from family and friends.

Alternatively, they may choose to age in place at a retirement or assisted living community, receiving help with meals and care needs. Moving in with family is often an excellent choice; it can also be a difficult one if family members are working full-time, caring for small children, and have the added responsibility of being caregivers to their aging parents.

Often the cost of care is the ultimate decision-maker. People with adequate financial resources can choose to live in a retirement or assisted living community as private pay residents or can hire help in their home. But, for those living on their monthly Social Security income payments and maybe a small pension, the cost of living in a retirement community or assisted facility, or even in their own home with hired caregiver support, may be beyond their financial means. *(Note: Some states offer services/financial support for low-income persons to live in assisted living facilities and adult foster care homes, or receive limited caregiver support in the home.)*

Home is Where You Choose to Live

"A house is made with walls and beams.
A home is made with love and dreams."

--Anonymous

In my last book, *When Aging Parents Can't Live Alone,* I focused on caring for and finding appropriate housing for your parents and relatives as they aged. In this book, I focus on you, or, including myself, on us. We are the boomer generation and we are the ones now aging, now contemplating retirement. Specifically, this book tackles head on and with creativity, the issue, the choice, of where you, where we, the boomers, will live. There are many influences on this decision of where to live and when and how to make the move or whether to remain where we are. Similarly, this decision will affect other aspects of our lives. We must take an honest assessment of our current situation, looking at what is important to us, and what our future resources are likely to be.

An abundance of living choices is available for people entering their retirement years. Some options have been around for many years while others are newer and a bit outside the box. Although many people will choose to stay in their own home, others will seek alternative living situations. Some housing alternatives include:

- independent living in your own home;
- downsizing to a smaller home;
- condominium/townhouse/duplex communities;

- apartment living;

- renting;

- bringing in services to "age in place";

- living with family;

- living with others in shared and cooperative housing;

- creative housing such as living in a recreational vehicle, on a houseboat or yacht, in a tiny house, eco-cottage, or yurt;

- overseas living;

- adventure living;

- standard /continuing care retirement communities;

- assisted living facilities;

- adult care homes;

- memory care homes.

Eventually most boomers will retire. Being able to choose your home environment while retaining a good quality of life becomes an important part of the retirement process. We can sell our homes and move to be near our children or parents. We can rent or buy an apartment/ house/condo. We can move to a theme-based retirement community near a university, equestrian center, golf course, or other community that caters to our interests. We can purchase/rent/lease a recreational vehicle (RV) and take to the road, traveling the United States, Canada, and Central America. We can ship our RV overseas or rent one in another country. We can buy/rent/lease a houseboat, floating home, eco-sea cottage, or live-aboard yacht on a quiet bay or lake, or in a marina. We can seek adventure at sea by traveling on a working freighter. We can move to a foreign country and live overseas. Moreover, in many of these settings, we can find jobs that fit with our lifestyle. The possibilities are endless.

Alternatively, we can choose to age in place with necessary services and help brought into our homes, provided by family, friends, religious organizations, and community and government programs. We can also age in place in a completely new and unique living arrangement that offers different levels of care, ranging from independent living to assisted living with caregiving assistance to receiving medical care in a healthcare facility.

The Employment Factor

"The Age Discrimination in Employment Act of 1967 (ADEA) protects individuals who are 40 years of age or older from employment discrimination based on age. The ADEA's protections apply to both employees and job applicants. Under the ADEA, it is unlawful to discriminate against a person because of his/her age with respect to any term, condition, or privilege of employment, including hiring, firing, promotion, layoff, compensation, benefits, job assignments, and training."

-- U.S. Equal Employment Opportunity Commission

While some professions mandate retirement at a specific age, most professions do not. We will retire or leave the workforce at different ages, some in our 50's or 60's, and others in their 70's, 80's or even 90's. Although age discrimination is unlawful in the United States, there are some businesses and professions considered dangerous or demanding a high level of physical and/or mental aptitude such as military service, federal police agencies, air traffic controllers, and airline pilots. These professions can have a mandatory age for retirement.

The financial, physical, spiritual or emotional need or desire to work, unexpected job termination, or changes in health can influence the length of employment. We may continue to work to bring in income to pay our living expenses and retain healthcare benefits. We may decide to resign from a steady job or continue working at the same job with reduced hours, reduced income, and/or different responsibilities. To pay our bills and maintain our lifestyle, we may work several jobs. We may be underemployed, working part-time while seeking full-time employment. We may be the early termination casualties of business competition and economic downturns. Some will be offered early retirement and embrace the chance to stop working; others will try to remain so they can receive necessary income and healthcare insurance until age 65, the age that Medicare benefits kick in. Those who can afford to stop working may view being retired as an opportunity to develop new careers or hobbies, volunteer at a non-profit organization, move closer to family, travel, or do all the activities there was never time to do.

An *American Association of Retirement Persons (AARP)* study showed that 20% of people, aged 55-64, will choose to postpone retirement due to low investment returns and high healthcare costs. A study by the *National Institute of Aging: The Health and Retirement Study: Growing Older in America* shows that 25% of women and 20% of men, ages 55-64, have health problems that may limit their ability to work and be active. Of these, 1/5 with health limitations will still choose to work. A new phenomenon called "phased" retirement encourages older workers who would normally be retired to continue working reduced hours or during peak times. It is a way for would-be retirees to supplement income and remain active employees.

> *"Institutional changes in pension plans, health insurance, and Social Security give older workers more reason to keep their jobs longer."*
>
> *-- Congressional Budget Office, March 22, 2011*

Considering Financial Matters

Financial issues will play a crucial role if we decide to make changes in how we live our lives. As the United States economy recovers, we, in contrast, have lost significant amounts of our hard-earned savings and pension plans. We have paid into Social Security and are calculating our future monthly income. Our reduced retirement funds mean more years working and later retirement. A study by the *GE Center for Financial Learning* shows that 70% of the baby boomers feel they will not have pensions and retirement benefits from their place of employment. They fear they will need to rely on monthly Social Security payments and their significantly reduced financial nest egg for retirement and long-term care needs.

To those on the verge of retiring, this savings reduction substantially limits retirement choices. Thoughts of living the American dream are now reconsidered in light of a weak economy, job insecurity, reduced employment income, depleted savings and pension plan funds, and increased daily living costs.

How much income and assets will you have at retirement? To estimate your potential income at retirement, answer the questions below. We will calculate our current monthly income and compare it to our estimated retirement income, the sum of monthly Social Security checks, pension payouts, investment income, and savings.

- If you are working, what is your monthly income from your job?

- How much will you receive from Social Security payments? *You can get your Social Security statement online of your retirement, disability, and lifetime benefits at:* http://www.socialsecurity.gov/mystatement/

- Are you eligible for Veteran's retirement benefits? *You can get information about Veterans' benefits , check your claim status, apply for benefits on-line, view a benefits summary at* http://www.vba.va.gov/VBA/

- What does your retirement nest egg look like? *How much do you have in IRA's, Roth's, money markets, savings, 401K, 403B, and other cash accounts that might be available at retirement? Do you have non-liquid assets such as property, homes, vehicles, artwork, musical instruments, or other items to sell or otherwise exchange for cash, as needed?*

- From your retirement nest egg, how much are you permitted to withdraw each month without incurring a penalty? *Talking with a tax advisor is recommended. The IRS website offers advice on tax on early distribution from retirement Plans, other than IRA's at* http://www.irs.gov/taxtopics/tc558.html

- What additional income can you expect each month from pensions and investments?

- Have you saved enough for your retirement years?

- Is your monthly income, savings and investment accounts sufficient to allow you to change your current living situation?

- Can you afford to pay to live in a retirement, assisted living or memory care community?

- Should you consider a home option that would be less expensive than what you are currently spending?

- If you feel that your future income will not support your current lifestyle, what living options are available?

In addition, calculate your monthly expenses for rent or mortgage payments, utility costs, healthcare premiums, insurance premiums, gas and transportation costs, and any other monthly expenditure. Some will find the combination of monthly Social Security payments, pension payments, and investments more than adequate to retire comfortably. Many will feel the need to continue working as long as possible to rebuild their nest egg and retain valuable healthcare benefits. For those with low Social Security payments, minimal or no pension, and limited or no investments, any changes to your living situation will be difficult. As some state assistance programs can supplement housing and in-home services, for more information contact the **United States Department of Housing and Urban Development (HUD**) at http://portal.hud.gov/hudportal/HUD?src=/program offices/housing/sfh/fharesourcectr

Family Matters: Our Children and Parents

Family issues can also influence our decisions about the future. Most boomers entering their retirement years have grown children entering or graduating college or vocational schools or actively looking for work in a tough job market. Our children may be independent and able to support themselves or they may rely on us for financial support, healthcare insurance, and housing.

In addition, many boomers have aging parents in their 80's and 90's. Our parents may live independently in their own home, with family members, or in a residence, that offers caregiving support and services. We may encourage our parents to move nearby in case of emergencies or so we can help them with daily activities. On the other hand, we may choose to move so we can be caregivers to our parents and/or babysitters to our grandchildren. Certainly, caring for our family can play an important role in where we choose to live.

If our parents live far away, we may need to travel to visit them or to help during an illness. If there are other concerns, such as financial management, safety, or a need for more assistance, these can be difficult to manage from a distance. Hiring a geriatric care manager to assess care needs or introducing local community agencies to our parents may become necessary.

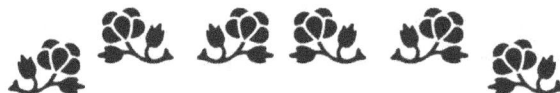

Most of the Starr family lives in northern California. At 75 years of age, Grandma Maude, decided to leave her family and the cold weather to settle in the warmth of coastal Florida, close to several elderly friends. Over the years, due to changes in her health, Maude's care and homemaking needs increased, until it became difficult for her to live safely in her condominium. Despite several trips to Florida by her family, concern about her safety and the handling of her routine finances persisted. Her family worried about her fear of falling at home and felt guilty that they were unable to help her. On one of their visits, they hired a geriatric care manager (GCM) to assess her daily care needs, handle financial issues, and monitor her current living situation. When Maude eventually required more care, the GCM helped her visit facilities and facilitated her move to a more suitable living arrangement that provided care and assistance. Throughout the transition from independent to more dependent living, the GCM provided Maude with emotional support. The GCM kept in contact with her family by telephone, reassuring them that Grandma Maude was now in a safer environment with caregiving assistance.

Healthcare Issues

Healthcare issues include both personal health and healthcare insurance. When we retire, we expect to live independently, perform activities of daily life (ADL's) that include walking, eating, dressing, grooming, bathing, toileting, and personal care. We expect to remain vital, active, and in good health. If we have excellent to good health, we enter our retirement years with many possibilities. We can choose to stay where we are, move somewhere else, or try a new and different lifestyle.

If we have health issues that limit our ability to perform basic activities of life and require assistance to live independently, we may need to look at alternate living possibilities. Consider the following:

- How significant a role will healthcare issues, either yours or a family member play in determining where you live?

- How important is it to live near your current physicians, clinics, or hospitals?

Consider your activity level. When you reflect on a normal day, are you working, staying at home, watching television, working on your computer, or reading a book? Or are you taking the dog for a walk, gardening, golfing, fishing, hiking, running, biking, skiing, going to exercise classes or working out at the gym, attending lectures or taking community or university classes? People who have active lifestyles often choose to continue this lifestyle when they retire. Think about the following questions:

- Do enjoy staying busy and active in your daily life?
- Do you exercise or walk on a daily basis?
- Do you go to the gym or take an exercise class on a regular basis?
- Is an active lifestyle important to you?
- Do you prefer a more sedentary lifestyle?

We plan to enter our retirement years in excellent to good health. We do not want unexpected or chronic health issues that require significant medical care to determine how we spend our retirement years. Worse, we do not want someone else making these choices for us. Think about the following questions.

- Are you concerned about any chronic health issues?
- Do you visit your primary care physician or a specialist on a regular basis? i.e. annually or more often?
- Have you recently been hospitalized for an injury, accident, or outpatient surgeries?
- Do you have trouble with hearing or vision?
- Have you abused drugs and/or alcohol on a regular basis?
- Have you received treatment for drug and/or alcohol abuse?
- Can you easily remember information?
- Can you follow directions easily and accurately?
- Are you more confused at night?
- Have you felt sad, quiet, withdrawn or low on energy more than usual?
- Do you sleep more than usual, especially during the day?
- If you needed assistance, could you call for help?
- If you needed assistance, would you call for help?
- Do you depend on others for daily care?
- Do you use a cane, walker or wheelchair for mobility?
- Is your activity level limited by medical problems?

Healthcare insurance, something you may consider as essential to retirement can be very expensive to purchase on your own, without help from an employer. It is common for people to work past their preferred retirement date in order to continue healthcare coverage until they are eligible for Medicare benefits. We prioritize the retention of health insurance benefits, either through an employer or as a self-employed person. We know that our medical care needs will play an instrumental role in the decisions we make in our retirement years. If you are without healthcare insurance because your employer does not offer it, you are self-employed and cannot afford it, or you are unemployed and cannot afford it, changes in our current healthcare system through the *Affordable Care Act* may make healthcare more accessible in the future.

For additional information on **Medicare basics**,
Go to http://www.medicare.gov/navigation/medicare-basics/medicare-basics-overview.aspx

---

It is possible to subscribe to several insurance policies that work together. For example, you can participate in Medicare and a private supplemental insurance policy to pay the Medicare co-payments and deductibles. Alternatively, you may enroll in Medicare and the state Medicaid insurance program (or a low-income assistance program) to help pay the amounts that Medicare does not cover.

In this book, insurance benefits pertain to specific living options. For example, Medicare does *not* pay for care in a retirement community, assisted living facility or adult foster care home. Medicare *does* pay for care in a skilled nursing facility, hospital, or a rehabilitation center, if your care meets specific Medicare requirements. Review your private insurance policy benefits. Like Medicare, private insurance policies do not have benefits for care in a retirement community, assisted living facility or adult foster care home. The benefits for care in a skilled nursing facility, hospital, or a rehabilitation center will vary with each policy. Medical care through the Veteran's programs is dependent on the veteran's service-connected status and the proximity of the nearest VA facility.

What we decide in our retirement years will depend in large part on our medical needs. For those who decide to age in place in their homes or in another setting, accessing medical services and community programs and services could be the difference between living in a safe or dangerous environment. Healthcare insurance for medical care can determine where you choose to live. Here is a general review of current healthcare insurance.

- If you are **over the age of 65 or disabled**, you are eligible for either *original Medicare or a managed-care Medicare Plan. (If you are still working and receiving private insurance, you can keep this insurance as your primary insurance.)*

- If you are **under the age of 65**, in good health, employed by another or self-employed, you may either have insurance benefits through your employer or purchase *private* insurance.

- If you are **under 65 years and disabled**, with a **low-income** near the poverty level, you may be eligible for insurance through the state *Medicaid* program. If you have been disabled 2 years or have End Stage Kidney Disease (permanent kidney failure requiring dialysis or transplant), Railroad Retirement Benefits, or Lou Gehrig's disease (ALS), you may be eligible to receive early Medicare benefits.

- If you are a **Veteran,** you may receive medical care through the *United States Department of Veteran's Affairs.* If you are over 65, you may also obtain *Medicare* benefits. You can also purchase private insurance to supplement your Medicare. If you have a low-income near the poverty level, you may also be eligible for the state *Medicaid* program.

To review and apply for **Veteran benefits** through the United States Department of Veteran Affairs, go to http://www.va.gov/healthbenefits/

Signed into law on March 23, 2010, the **Affordable Care Act's** goal is to decrease the number of uninsured Americans, reduce the overall costs of healthcare, streamline the delivery of healthcare services, strengthen Medicare, and require insurance companies to cover all applicants at the same rate regardless of pre-existing conditions or gender. Here are some highlights.

- Lower cost prescription drugs;

- Free preventive services for seniors including flu shots, cancer, diabetes, blood pressure screenings, and a free annual wellness visit;

- Fight against fraud with tougher screening procedures, stronger penalties, and new technology;

- Improve Care Coordination and Quality to reduce costs and strengthen the quality of healthcare;

- Provide healthcare choices while lowering costs;

- Coverage for young adults through age 26 on their parent's healthcare plan;

- Coverage for Americans with pre-existing conditions. In 2014, insurance discriminating against anyone with a pre-existing condition will be illegal;

- Affordable Insurance where consumers can choose a private health insurance plan that fits their health needs. Starting in 2014, they will offer to the public the same kinds of insurance choices members of Congress will have. (Data excerpted from the website: Go to http://www.whitehouse.gov/healthreform)

A Personal Worksheet: Getting To Know You

"Of middle age the best that can be said is that a middle-aged person has likely learned how to have a little fun in spite of his troubles."

-- Don Marquis

Making important decisions about your future is a difficult task. Numerous factors, especially finances, family, employment, and health can affect how you transition from a working career to a retirement pace. For some, there may not be a noticeable difference; for others, retirement can open new doors, opportunities, and challenges.

Your **financial portfolio** can dictate your choices. If your income and assets are substantial and permit you to live very comfortably, you may choose to consider luxurious living accommodations. If finances are not a concern, you can reflect on what is important to you, and match your home and lifestyle accordingly. Depending on the degree to which finances are a concern, you would weigh your options more carefully. If your financial situation is dire, don't despair as there are still reasonable ways to enjoy your retirement years.

Your **physical health** is an important factor on your retirement decision. If you are in excellent physical condition, your choices are many; if you have some limitations, you will need to weigh these carefully before you choose a different home and lifestyle. As an extreme example, traveling the world on a freighter is difficult for a person with mobility issues.

Your **mental health** needs to be sound and sharp enough to process information, use critical thinking and problem-solve, enabling you to arrive at reasonable and informed decisions.

Family is an important consideration. Will you live near your family or are you comfortable contacting them by telephone or e-mail and visiting during the year?

If you are **working,** do you plan on continuing to work, reducing your hours, or finding a new job that fits your new lifestyle?

Complete the following worksheet to assess and compare the factors that affect your current living situation and future options. Personal information is requested so that you will have all the necessary information you need when applying to homes or services. Gather your personal, financial, medical, and insurance information. Medical information is included as health matters often determine where you live.

To print a hard copy of this form, go to www.whenyougetolder.com and click "Forms" at the top of the page. Complete the questionnaire and make a copy for yourself and your family member. Keep this worksheet with your important papers.

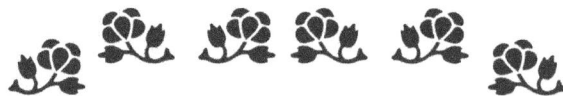

A Personal Worksheet: Getting to Know You

Personal information

Name: _____

Age: _____Birth date: _____

Address: _____

_____

_____

Telephone: Home :_____ Cell: _____

Marital status: _____Social Security #:_____

Name of spouse, significant other, partner: _____

_____

Social Security #:_____ Age: _____Birth date: _____

Emergency contact: _____ Telephone #: _____

Current Living Situation

I live with my:

- ☐ spouse
- ☐ significant other/partner
- ☐ friend

- ☐ roommate(s)
- ☐ alone
- ☐ other _____

I live in a:

- private single home, owner occupied
- townhome, duplex, or condominium, owner occupied
- apartment, owner occupied
- apartment, rental
- other rental property
- with family
- with others
- housesitting situation
- trailer on family property
- mobile home park
- recreational vehicle
- campground
- houseboat or other floating home
- retirement community
- assisted living facility
- adult care home
- memory care home
- other_____
- other_____

Please answer if you own your home:

- I pay a monthly mortgage
- I am experiencing difficulty meeting my mortgage payments
- I plan to remain in my home so I can age in place
- I plan to remain in my home, but may consider a move at a later date
- If I were to move I would consider keeping my house, but not living there
- If I were to move I would consider keeping my house and renting it
- I would consider selling my house and using the profits to move somewhere else
- I would consider arranging a paid or free house sitter to live there while I live somewhere else
- other_____

When I retire, I would like to:

- stay where I am move near my children
- live with my children
- move near my parents
- live with my parents
- continue living my life as I always have
- try living somewhere that is new and different
- continue working
- find a new job
- travel
- other _____

What is most important to you?

- family
- friends
- physical health
- mental health
- financial security

- adventure
- travel
- continuing to work
- continuing education
- other _____

Financial Information

I am:

- employed full-time
- employed part-time
- unemployed

- retired
- volunteering
- other_____

My Sources and Amounts of Monthly Income:

- wages_____
- Social Security _____
- Supplemental Security Income (SSI) _____
- Social Security Disability Income (SSDI)_____

- unemployment compensation_____
- veteran's benefits_____
- pension benefits_____
- food stamps_____
- other _____

Additional Assets and their Values:

- bank accounts_____
- IRA_____
- ROTH_____
- CD's _____
- stocks_____
- bonds_____

- business _____
- real estate_____
- rental property_____
- investments_____
- other_____

Outstanding debts:
- medical bills_____
- loans_____
  (personal, education, car, mortgage, home equity, other)
- credit cards_____
- other_____

My Total Monthly Income: _____

My spouse/significant other/partner is:
- employed full-time
- employed part-time
- unemployed
- retired
- volunteering
- other_____

Sources and Amounts of Monthly Income:
- wages_____
- Social Security _____
- Supplemental Security Income (SSI) other _____
- Social Security Disability Income (SSDI)other _____
- unemployment compensation___
- veteran's benefits_____
- pension benefits_____
- food stamps_____
- other _____

Additional Assets and their values:
- bank accounts_____
- IRA_____
- ROTH_____
- CD's _____
- stocks_____
- bonds_____
- business _____
- real estate_____
- rental property_____
- investments_____
- other_____

Outstanding debts:
- Medical bills_____
- Loans_____

- Credit cards_____
- Other_____
  (personal, education, car, mortgage, home equity, other)

Spouse/Significant Other/Partner Total Monthly income: _____

Medical information

My primary care physician is:

Name: _____

Address and telephone #:
_____
_____

Other physicians I visit at least annually:

Name	Specialty	Telephone #
_____	_____	_____
_____	_____	_____
_____	_____	_____
_____	_____	_____

List any medical conditions for which you are actively receiving treatment. (i. e. diabetes, thyroid condition, heart, cancer, other): _____
_____
_____
_____
_____

List each allergy and your reaction (i.e. penicillin – reaction is hives):

_____

_____

_____

List any medications you are currently taking. Include the dosages, the number of times per day, and any special instructions. *(po means by mouth or pill form, sub-q means by injection, IV means with an intravenous line.)*

Medication	Dosage	How dosage is taken	Special Instructions
i.e. Amoxil	*250 mg* po	*3x/day for 10 days*	take with food
_____	_____	_____	_____
_____	_____	_____	_____
_____	_____	_____	_____
_____	_____	_____	_____

Health Insurance Information

Please note: Due to HIPAA, the Health Insurance Portability and Accountability Act of 1996, your medical information is private and confidential and cannot be released to anyone including family members without your permission. This can create problems when family is involved in making healthcare decisions. Please contact your physician's office or your insurance company for a *Medical Release of Information Form* and send it to your healthcare providers.

My health coverage is provided through:

- Private insurance
- Medicare
- Medicaid
- Supplemental insurance
- Long-term care insurance
- Catastrophic insurance

- Veteran's insurance
- COBRA (Consolidated Omnibus Budget Reconciliation Act)
- I do not own health insurance
- Other_____

Insurance company, policy # and telephone #:

_____

_____

Insurance company policy # and telephone #:

_____

_____

Insurance company, policy # and telephone #:

_____

_____

If you are an independent and active person looking for a change in your current living situation, read _Part 1- Entering Your Retirement Years - Traditional , Non-traditional, and Creative Living Options._

If you are _content_ living where you are, are looking for more help in the home, considering assisted living or living with your family read _Part 2 - Aging in Place: Make it Work for You, and Part 3 - Preserving Your Independence with a Little Bit of Help._

If you are _undecided_ about where you want to live, read _Part 1- Entering Your Retirement Years: Traditional, Non-traditional, and Creative Living Options, Part 2 - Aging in Place: Make it Work for You,_ and _Part 3 - Preserving Your Independence with a Little Bit of Help._

If you have recently been in the hospital and/or are concerned about healthcare, read _Part 4 - Finding Medical Care in Your Community and at Home._

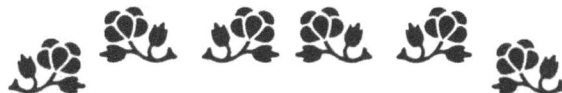

Part 1

Entering Your Retirement Years

Traditional, Non-Traditional, and Creative Living Options

Single-family homes, townhouses and condominiums, communities with homeowner associations, apartment living, cottages and bungalows, over 55 mobile and manufactured home communities, shared and cooperative housing, sustainable alternative housing, recreational vehicles, houseboats and other floating homes, ships and world-traveling freighters, overseas living, employment and volunteer opportunities

Independent Living:
Finding a Place to Call Home

*"We don't stop playing because we grow old;
we grow old because we stop playing."*

-- *George Bernard Shaw*

When the *Civil Rights Act of 1968* enacted the *Fair Housing Act* prohibiting discrimination based on race, religion, gender, family status, or handicap, 'independent living' was a term used primarily for the disabled. The *Free Dictionary* defined an independent living arrangement as one that "maximizes independence and self-determination, especially of disabled persons living in a community instead of in a medical facility." Not so long ago, 'independent living' also defined living situations for *The Greatest Generation*, our aging parents now in their 80's and 90's. Both groups struggled to maintain their individual autonomy by living in their own familiar dwelling, making decisions on their own behalf, driving to medical appointments and shopping, and performing their basic activities of daily life – such as bathing, dressing, grooming, toileting, and self-care with or without community and family support. Only when these daily tasks became difficult did people consider moving from an independent setting to a more supervised and assisted environment. Typically, these assisted environments included living with or near family, in retirement communities, assisted living facilities, adult care homes, or nursing facilities.

Independent living is no longer primarily associated with aging or the disabled; it now encompasses numerous living situations for our parents and for the upcoming generation of baby boomers and retirees. To broaden the definition, it now includes any living situation in which a person or persons live in their own home. Home is more than a building that shelters you from weather and provides security. It is a sanctuary where you can cook your meals, sleep in comfort, personalize your surroundings, and socialize with family and friends.

As boomers approach the retirement years, we have collectively decided that we need more living choices. What worked for our parents may not necessarily work for the 80-million boomers. Boomers plan on living active retirements, whether we are staying close to our current homes, moving to new locations or choosing to travel. As many boomers delay their retirement dates due to recent economic fluctuations and the loss to retirement nest eggs, it is an excellent time to think outside the box when we consider what we want to do and where we want to live.

Most boomers, in their late 40's to early 60's, and older boomers in their late 60's and 70's, have a place to live that they call home. Some live in a single-family dwelling they own, others in a rental house or an apartment. Some live with their parents, a relative, or with friends. The homeless people from this generation live on the streets or under a highway bridge, in parks, at community and church shelters, in missions, or in a Veteran domiciliary.

The "we're getting older, but we don't feel older" boomer generation spans a wide range of personal characteristics. Many find themselves financially solvent even in these difficult economic times and have the funds to consider options in retirement housing that require financial stability.

The boomers and greatest generation who face financial stressors to meet mortgage payments or pay monthly rental and utility fees often find themselves choosing between making house payments, placing food on the table and deciding which prescription medications to purchase. They will have fewer options and can find themselves more dependent on state and federal housing programs such as HUD, living in shared or cooperative housing, residing in an over 55 pre-fabricated mobile and manufactured home trailer parks or communities, taking to the road in a recreational vehicle, or utilizing local community services to remain in an independent living environment. Retirement and assisted living communities also offer some independence to those seeking increased help with their activities of daily life.

The Mission Statement for The U.S. Department of Housing and Urban Development (HUD) states, "HUD's mission is to create strong, sustainable, inclusive communities and quality affordable homes for all. HUD is working to strengthen the housing market to bolster the economy and protect consumers; meet the need for quality affordable rental homes; utilize housing as a platform for improving quality of life; build inclusive and sustainable communities free from discrimination; and transform the way HUD does business." Go to http://portal.hud.gov/portal/page/portal/HUD

Looking Outside the Box

"The walls, with the windows and doors attached to them, form the house, but it is the empty space within that creates the essence of the house. This is the rule: the material harbors usefulness and the immaterial impart the true essence."

--*Lao Tse*

Many boomers see retirement as a continuation of a chosen lifestyle. We may want to stop working at 58 or 62 or 65 but many of us do not have the financial means or savings to retire. We do not feel like seniors, yet AARP is knocking on the door and retirement looms on the horizon. We do not feel like seniors, but our hair is grayer, our waists a bit wider. We wear reading glasses, have slower reflexes and don't recover as quickly from injuries. Our lower backaches and pains are more frequent and the genetics inherited from our parents are catching up with us. Still, we also want to enhance our lifestyle, not cut back on it. As we look to the future, we are more likely to look outside the box of traditional solutions.

We look at the Greatest Generation and wonder what living alternatives will be available to us when we reach their age. Compared to living options available to our parent's generation, there are more creative and non-traditional living alternatives available to the boomer generation seeking an active lifestyle. There are now theme-based retirement communities that cater to the specific interests of many groups: equestrian enthusiasts, university and college-oriented individuals, golf and beach–based fans, arts-based individuals, and military home environments for military personnel and retired civic government employees.

Traditional living choices, some which offer support and assistance, are also available – retirement communities, over 55 pre-fabricated mobile and manufactured home parks, assisted living facilities, and adult care homes and nursing facilities for those needing 24/7 nursing care.

As boomers, we have grown up with connectivity of Net Gen, the Internet Generation. It is easy to turn on a computer and use a search engine to gather data on just about anything we wish to know. With a stroke of the keyboard, we can access websites on cooperative housing, relocation, retirement communities in other states, caregiving support, and healthcare. This brings the world of retirement options closer to us, making it easier to research new ideas and ways to live.

Living in a Traditional-Style Home

(single-family homes, townhouses and condominiums, communities with home-owner associations, apartment living, cottages and bungalows, over 55 mobile and manufactured home communities)

Many boomers and members of The Greatest Generation live in established communities and neighborhoods that support independent living. Many will choose to stay in their current home; others will look at moving into a smaller home or relocating closer to family. Some will rent; others will own the home they live in. Homes can take the form of a single-family home in a neighborhood, an attached unit such as a duplex, townhouse, or condominium, an apartment or self-contained rooms in part of a building, a pre-fabricated mobile or manufactured home community, or a small unattached or stand-alone unit placed on a person's property. In some instances, the community will have a homeowners association to help manage and govern the community. We will start by looking at the more traditional type of living arrangements.

Single–Family Homes

In the past, a freestanding single-family home typically had a single family living in it. Times have changed. Many boomers residing in single family homes live alone, with their spouse or partner, their children, their elderly parents and sometimes, young grand-children. Members of the Greatest Generation may still live in their own homes but find they need more help and support from family, friends, live-in or part-time caregivers, and community agencies. Owner-occupied homes offer privacy from neighbors and the ability to make renovations to the property, such as adding square footage to the existing dwelling or placing a small stand-alone unit on the property. A garage or carport can be attached to the house or be installed as a freestanding structure to park a car, store household treasures and appliances, camping gear and miscellaneous items, or set-up a functional wood shop. Sometimes the garage structure will include a separate furnished and fully functional apartment or "mother-in-law" suite.

Many basic single-family homes are designed with an eat-in kitchen, a living room, a bedroom or place to sleep, and a full bathroom with a sink, tub or shower, and a toilet. Some homes have an extra half-bath that does not have shower facilities. In larger homes, extra rooms can include a front room, a dining room for eating, a formal living room for entertaining, a study for working at home, a casual family room for watching television, playing games, or reading, a laundry room with a washer and dryer, and an extra area for storage. Luxury homes can house a library, wine cellar, a game room, an entertainment room for large screen televisions and a stereo system, and extra rooms for anything else.

Costs associated with living and owning a single-family home can include maintenance, repairs, landscaping, and lawn care. In addition, you will have to pay property taxes each year. Unless the house is in a community with a homeowner association, there are no management fees such as those often associated with townhouses and condominiums. Sometimes maintaining a single-family home necessitates taking in renters to share the financial obligations, maintenance and repair work. If you are renting the single-family home, it may be difficult to renovate and make changes in the home without permission from the owner.

Sophia, age 78, recently lost her spouse of many years to a long illness. Although she is able to perform her basic activities of life, she is unable to maintain her property – mowing the lawn, doing basic home repairs – or meet her monthly house expenses. Through her church, she found a renter / handyman to share her monthly house and utility payments and to help with home repairs and maintenance.

Townhouses and Condominiums

Used interchangeably, the terms townhouse and condominium describe a 1-3 story home attached to another home, sharing common walls. Each townhouse shares walls with their neighbors, but not a ceiling or floor. These buildings can be duplexes, triplexes or part of a large complex of similar homes. Townhouses, also called row houses, are attached rows of homes with shared walls that include individual ownership of the land. Condominiums or condos, are similar to townhouses as they are also attached homes. You can change or renovate the interior of the building, but not the exterior. However, when buying a condo you don't own anything outside your unit, including the land it sits on.

Homes built within a townhouse/condominium complex share a similar and uniform architectural style. Homeowner Associations (HOA's) and Covenants, Conditions and Restrictions (CC and R's) bylaws enforce shared neighborhood values. It is important to know what these "shared" values are before purchasing any property with an HOA. Although this type of housing is usually associated with large complexes, some townhouses are independent small units that share common walls.

Years ago, I lived in Pittsburgh, Pennsylvania in an old, renovated 3-story yellow brick townhouse with a finished basement. It was a center unit attached to three other units. It was narrow and long, running 12 feet wide by 100 feet in length. Two units were owner occupied: two units were rentals. All had postage-stamp size yards and alley parking. The owner or renter maintained the townhouses. There were no management companies, homeowner associations, or maintenance fees.

By comparison, friends living in larger townhouse complexes paid association fees to pay for maintenance of the complex. This included landscaping, security, open areas, shared buildings, and other amenities. Some were content with their services; others disliked the rules and restrictions placed on them by the homeowners association. This living arrangement is not for everyone, in part, because these complexes often have considerable restrictions and rules.

Advantages to Townhouse or Condominium Living

(less expensive, maintenance–free, homeowner association, amenities)

There are advantages to ownership in a townhouse or condominium. They tend to be less expensive than freestanding single-family homes. While they are not freestanding, they have the look and feel of a single-family home. This opens up the possibility of moving to a more expensive neighborhood for less money. Built with shared walls, the homes in the middle with two shared walls can have lower heating costs. End units have the advantage of more windows and light. No one lives above or below you. The yard is often small and easy to care for or is non-existent. Outside maintenance and repairs of your home - roofing, painting and landscaping in the yard - are the responsibility of the homeowner association. Upkeep of the surrounding property and common areas of the complex are important for resale. If the grounds are unkempt, the value of the townhouse / condominium may depreciate. Often these complexes include amenities such as tennis courts, a pool, clubhouse, and common landscaped open space.

Disadvantages to Townhouse or Condominium Living

(less privacy, more noise potential, difficulty retaining value, homeowner association fees and bylaws)

As townhouses are attached units, it increases the likelihood that you will have less privacy and are more likely to hear your neighbors' noise. The middle units have less light as only two walls are outside walls to bring light into the rooms. The resident living in a corner unit has three walls with access to outside light. There can be a common stairwell. While the homeowner association covers maintenance, the owner can have limited input and choices regarding home design, exterior paint colors, or landscaping. Parking can be located in a common area instead of directly in front of the home.

These homes are less expensive to purchase and most affected by changes in the housing market. In a depressed housing market, townhouses and condominiums may not retain their value as well as the single family home.

These shared homes are often part of a large complex, managed by an elected Board of Directors that in turn, hires a professional management company or a homeowner association to run the complex. Homeowner associations can charge significant fees for management services, landscaping the common areas, maintaining and repairing buildings, providing security and a gatekeeper, and paying any legal services that arise and more. Governed by CC and R's (Covenants, Conditions and Restrictions) – these bylaws for the community are usually strictly enforced. For example, the HOA can restrict the paint color of the exterior of your town home to a few choices.

Despite these disadvantages, many people enjoy townhouse living and like the well-maintained common areas and the close proximity to neighbors. They are pleased that they are not responsible for property upkeep and find this well worth paying HOA fees.

Living in a Community with a Homeowner Association (HOA)

A homeowners association is a legal entity or corporation created with formal bylaws called Covenants, Conditions, and Restrictions (CC and R's) which are issued to home-owners as a way to maintain the quality and value of the properties. A governing board of directors, elected by owner-members is responsible for hiring a property management company to direct and enforce community maintenance and general upkeep of common areas, recreation facilities, street services, and security and gate maintenance. It is responsible for setting design standards such as acceptable paint colors for homes or yard landscape designs.

Homeowner associations are not limited to townhomes and condominiums. Complexes with single-family homes, apartment buildings, mobile home and trailer parks, patio homes, cluster homes, and other living arrangements may also require contracts with a homeowners association.

In the artist community of Ashland, Oregon, Dillon McCord, age 15, painted an award winning rain forest mural on his garage door to enter a Cricket Magazine art contest. A neighbor complained to the developer that the mural violated the CC and R's of the subdivision and devalued neighborhood property. The developer notified Dillon's family they would need to paint over the mural as it violated subdivision rules and offered to replace the garage door if Dillon would donate half his sale price of the mural to charity. Dillon's mural became local front-page news, precipitating a flood of purchase offers from locals in the art community. The owners of the A Street Arts Building bought the mural and now display it in the city's First Friday Art Walk. Happily, Dillon won the Cricket Magazine contest and then donated his earnings to the Macaw Landing Foundation, a Portland, Oregon organization that helps preserve the rare tropical parrot, the macaw, prominently featured in his mural. (Ashland Daily Tidings, August 5, 2006)

With over 50 million Americans living in communities with HOA's, the CC and R bylaws differ from community to community. Some communities prefer adults only and install an over 55-age requirement allowing them to align available services with the age of the residents.

As membership in the HOA is mandated for all owner-members, it is important to understand and be comfortable with the philosophy and values of the HOA. Usually there is a Board of Directors comprised of owner-members, elected by other owner-members. The board, in turn, can choose to hire a property management company to handle day-to-day operations. Owner-members should expect to pay mandatory monthly fees for upkeep of their property and the common shared areas within the community. These monthly dues pay for professional management fees, landscaping and gardeners, maintenance and upkeep of common areas, insurance for the community, security, gate maintenance, trash pick-up, sewer services, roads, sidewalks, water, cable television, correspondence and newsletter charges. They support the community amenities such as a pool, clubhouse, tennis courts, trails, gymnasium, basketball court, or playground. Monthly assessment fees encompass a wide range and may increase over time. These fees are mandatory and payment strictly enforced by threat, levying fines, or even legal action. (*Please note that some HOA's do not have common areas, but will charge for other services such as exterior structure repairs, roofing, yard maintenance, security, and other amenities.*)

Advantages to Living in a Homeowners Association Community

(shared values, conformity, uniformity, maintenance-free, community involvement)

There are advantages associated with living in a large complex governed by a homeowner association. To many, the benefits will outweigh the disadvantages. Owner-members can live with neighbors that share their values. Or, they may appreciate conformity and uniformity with building structures. They can expect that residents will not paint their homes within the community a garish color and that yards or landscaping will not become an eyesore. By having the HOA responsible for maintenance and upkeep of common areas, residents are able to relinquish some of the typical homeowner responsibilities for maintaining their home. By electing a board of directors and attending monthly or quarterly meetings, property owner-members feel they have a say in how the community operates.

Zogby International an American market research company known for non-partisan opinion polling surveyed 709 persons who were owner-members of a homeowner association. They found that for every owner-member who rated the experience as negative, 10 persons felt the experience was positive. The majority of persons surveyed lived in single-family homes. While the poll surveyed a wide range of ages, I focused on the results of seniors – age 65 and older - and boomers - age 50-64 years. People over age 65 were most satisfied with their overall living experience. Seniors and boomers were more likely to attend board meetings and have contact with the board at least five times a year. Seniors were more likely to think that the board represented the best interests of the owner-members; boomers were close behind. Seniors and boomers felt that the management provided value and support to residents and the community while boomers were more likely than seniors to interact with the managers. (Zogby International, November 2007.)

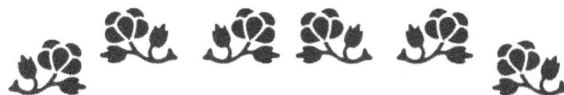

Disadvantages to Living
in a Homeowners Association Community

(restrictive, limited diversity, rules and regulations, fees, less homeowner autonomy)

Some people considering living in a community with an homeowner association and CC and R's can find them oppressive or restrictive. They may not like conformity and uniformity but rather relish diversity and a bit of a rebellious attitude. They may not embrace the rules and regulations about how they should conduct themselves and use their property. They may prefer to make changes to their property without oversight by a board of directors and their neighbors. They may be uncomfortable with the monthly dues that can be raised to pay for services. They can feel that living in a managed community diminishes their autonomy as a homeowner. Some communities have strict over 55 age restrictions for residents. This can create some difficulty when it is necessary to have younger family members assisting with care. Check with the HOA regarding their policy on having family members stay with older residents on an extended basis.

Is Living in a Homeowners
Association Community Right for You?

Before deciding to live in a community with a Homeowner's Association and CC and R's, do your homework. Prior to closing escrow read the CC and R's so you are familiar with the bylaws, rules, conditions, and restrictions. Be aware that these can change. Look at the current dues and then at the dues history. Look at the CC and R's to note trends toward more or less restrictions. Compare the homeowner association fees with other communities in the areas. Here are some questions to ask.

- What are the current monthly and/or annual dues?
- How often have dues been raised in the last five years?
- What is the consequence (s) if you do not pay your dues?
- Can the HOA evict, fine or force you to sell your property?
- Are there special assessments planned to address deferred maintenance?
- What rights do owner-members have if they have issues with the quality or frequency of maintenance?
- Does the current board of directors have term limits?

- Have board members attended management-training classes?
- Is there board governance training?
- Does the HOA have litigation or other legal issues pending?
- Does the HOA have adequate cash reserves for capital improvements or unexpected projects?
- Are there pet restrictions such as size, type, and/or number of pets? Is there a designated pet area?
- Is there a pet fee?
- Is there an age requirement for living in the community?
- Is there a mental or physical health standard for remaining in the community?
- Who manages the property?
- How many units are rented versus owned?
- How long is the standard lease?
- What is the turnover rate? What are the reasons?
- What are the rules regarding rentals?
- How quiet is the neighborhood?
- Are there plans for construction in the community? Is there anything else that could affect value? Is it in or near an area with natural gas deposits that might be developed?
- How is the community and surrounding area zoned?
- Is there any ongoing litigation? Is there a recent history of litigation?
- Do the shared walls have adequate soundproofing?
- Is there a charge for key replacement or guest parking?
- How secure is the community?
- How accessible is the community to guests?
- Is there a community newsletter that discusses legal issues, community events, contains local business resources?
- Read the CC and R's and be sure that it does not prohibit sales to people based on gender, race, or belief.

Robert and Vera live in a gated community in Florida. To enter the community, Robert had to notify the gatekeeper that they expected a visitor. When the visitor arrived, her name was on the visitors list, giving her admission to the senior housing community. The visitor found an immaculate landscaped community with common areas, a pool, spa, and a clubhouse. There were paved paths for walking. It was easy to get lost, as every home looked identical to the other homes – same paint color, same style of architecture. A community newsletter provided articles and information about all the community events. There was also an important notice about the spa. It warned that the spa was for soaking only and that whoever was shaving their legs in the spa should stop that behavior or face paying a fine. The newsletter provided the community board of directors with a way to communicate with the owner-members.

Communities with HOA's are not for everyone. Ascertain whether the values of the community are shared values that you can abide by. If you are considering living in one, be sure to read the Covenants, Conditions, and Restrictions before purchasing property. Talk with potential neighbors and spend a day walking around the community to get a feel for living there. For persons with physical disabilities, be sure there is accessibility for a walker, wheelchair and electric scooter or power wheelchair on the grounds and in the home. Be sure you can upgrade the home, if needed, with a ramp and safety devices such as grab bars and other durable medical equipment.

Apartment Living

Apartment living is residential living in a building or house that is divided into individual units. They may be rented or owner occupied. Apartments may be located in a large or small complex or a hi-rise, a low-rise garden apartment, an older home with separate entrances and individual facilities, or a mixed-use building that houses a commercial use or business on the first floor with residences on the upper levels or part of a cooperative. Some apartments are part of a cooperative with owners sharing part of the corporation that owns the building. The size varies from one-room studio, efficiency or bachelor apartments to larger one, two, and three + bedroom units. Studios include a kitchen and small private bathroom housed in a small room off the main living area. Larger units - one, two, and three bedroom apartments - provide more living space and separate areas for sleeping, dining, and relaxing. Bathrooms are larger and may include a bathtub and shower.

In a hi-rise apartment, the doors usually open to a shared hallway. Elevators transport residents to a main lobby, the parking area and outside areas. In a garden apartment, the units are arranged around an outside landscaped area. In an older home, the apartment space may be an entire floor, again with individual facilities for cooking, sleeping and bathroom. A separate entrance may lead to the individual apartment units.

People rent apartments by the month or the year or they can own the apartment. The apartment can be furnished or unfurnished. Depending on the operation of the apartment, some will provide necessary services such as a laundry room, security, parking spaces, and trash removal. Pets are welcome in some apartment units. Others may have rules prohibiting pets in the apartment, may place restrictions on the size of the animal or the number of pets allowed, or may charge a fee or require a deposit to pay for any pet caused damage to the unit.

Cottages, Bungalows, and Over 55 Mobile/ Manufactured Home Communities

A cottage or a bungalow is a freestanding dwelling with the basic features and physical layout of a smaller home. A cottage is small and cozy. Often used as a rental property, a bungalow is usually a single story building with no stair steps between rooms. If it is wide enough to accommodate a walker or wheelchair, it can be an excellent option for a disabled person or a senior wishing to downsize their living space. Some bungalows have an extra half story or a loft, additional space that is available to a person able to climb stairs.

Over 55 Mobile and Manufactured Homes are pre-fabricated single-family long-term residences. Manufactured homes are factory built, transported to a permanent home-site and then installed with connections to utilities. They are usually inexpensive and rarely moved. Owners sometimes trade them in order to upgrade or sell to new owners. Built to strict construction and performance codes established in 1976 by the *Housing and Urban Development* (HUD), these homes differ from mobile homes. A mobile home is *"a dwelling unit manufactured in a factory and designed to be transported to a site and semi permanently attached."*(Barron's Real Estate Dictionary.)

Found throughout the United States, over 55 mobile and manufactured home communities are affordable relative to a single family home and retain a neighborhood setting. An individual can own her own mobile or manufactured home, but the land it sits on is usually a leased home-site. As these homes tend to be on small lots, your neighbor can live very close to you. Many of these communities enforce community rules such as requiring reasonable property and lawn maintenance, restrictions on yard debris and non-running cars. An age limit for residents over 55 or over 62 years of age may be strictly enforced.

MobileHomeParkStore.com has an extensive listing on Mobile Home Parks throughout the United States. Information at this website includes the number of units, which parks are designated Over 55+, and contact information. For more information go to: http://www.mobilehomeparkstore. com/directory/listoregon.htm

Living in a Non-Traditional-style Home

(shared and cooperative housing, sustainable alternative housing, recreational ve-hicles, houseboats and other floating homes, ships and world-traveling freighters, overseas living, employment and volunteer opportunities)

There are alternatives to living in a single-family home that can help contain costs, in-crease socialization, provide help with daily tasks and responsibilities, and offer assistance and supervision for those needing more support. Ranging from shared or self-governing cooperative housing to multi-family dwellings to temporary structures and sustainable al-ternative living, these choices may be more affordable.

Shared and Cooperative Housing (COSH or Co-op)

"An autonomous association of persons united voluntarily to meet their common economic, social, and cultural needs and aspirations through a jointly-owned and democratically-controlled Enterprise." --Source: International Cooperative Alliance

A cooperative is a democratic voluntary organization open to all, regardless of gender, race, social, racial, political, or religious discrimination. Co-ops are likely to attract more di-versity than other housing arrangements. Each member of the cooperative brings their own skills and personality to the group in addition different backgrounds, cultures, and income brackets, creating a stimulating atmosphere.

As boomers look to the future, cooperative living is becoming increasingly popular in many states. Although most cooperative living facilities at this time are located in the Midwest states of Minnesota, Wisconsin, Missouri, and Iowa, the concept of cooperative living is catching on in other communities across the country. Designed for people seeking a democratic way of life with self-determination and responsibility, openness, and caring for others, cooperatives are intended to offer interdependence and cooperation from other members. As a democracy, all residents have membership in the cooperative, vote, elect a board of directors (often other shareholders), and purchase a share of the cooperative which entitles them to occupancy rights or the right to live in the cooperative housing unit. The board of directors is responsible for making business decisions regarding maintenance and membership, and maintaining the financial stability and sustainability of the cooperative.

Many factors can persuade a person to seek out a cooperative as a new living situation. A survey on *Rural Cooperative Housing for Older Adults* (The Journal of Extension, April 2001, Volume 39, #2) found that major factors influencing a person considering a move to a cooperative environment are the desire for an easier maintained home and the need to remain in or near their community.

Secondary factors include the need for a handicapped accessible home, a better financial investment, the ability to participate in decisions affecting their house, and accessibility to supportive services. Difficulty with mobility in their home, feelings of isolation, or the desire to live closer to town did not influence most people surveyed. Members of the cooperatives in this study appreciated the ease of maintaining their home, the ability to live independently, feelings of personal safety, increased life satisfaction, easy access to activities and entertainment, feelings of happiness, the amount of contact with friends, personal privacy, and better physical health. The members surveyed were primarily white females (68 % female to 32% male), ages 65- 85, most married, widowed, or divorced with high school and post-secondary education and moderate to low-income.

Types of Cooperative Housing

Cooperatives include multi-family homes, town homes, single-family homes, garden apartments, high-rises, or mobile homes. While the median age of residents is in the 70's, there is an increasing number of "empty nesters" in their mid-late 50's and early 60's selling their single family homes and using the equity from the sale to move a short distance to a cooperative housing project. They seek affordable housing with good quality of life.

This type of housing has proven to be less expensive than assisted living and continuing care retirement communities (CCRC's), a cost difference because the assisted living facilities and CCRC's provide different levels of personal care and supervision as part of their fee structure. Members in a co-op can independently hire individuals to provide these personal services or collectively decide to care for each other.

I recently met three women, all widowed, who decided many years before to care for one another as they aged. When Claire, age 83 was diagnosed with Alzheimer's disease and needed 24/7 supervision and care, Sophie, age 75, and Anne, age 82, became her caregivers. While Anne remained active, a brief hospitalization reduced her ability to help caring for Claire, leaving the task of caregiving exclusively to Sophie. The cooperative they set up was informal yet they shared the cost of housing, utilities, food, and hiring caregiver assistance. They made decisions together, although Claire became less involved as her disease progressed.

Affordability of Cooperative Living

The economic advantage of cooperative living begins with affordability. These facilities are non-profit corporations. The cooperative association pays costs. Members benefit by saving costs for housing, services and items purchased on behalf of the cooperative. Members purchase and then own a share in the cooperative. By signing an occupancy agreement, also called a proprietary lease, the members have the legal and exclusive right to live in the housing unit according to the cooperative agreement.

Cooperatives structured as a market-rate housing cooperative permits members to sell their shares in the cooperative just as they might sell other residential property. As members contribute equitably to the co-op, they also retain control over the capital and how it is used on behalf of the co-op community This capital can be used to benefit all members of the community by supporting activities, setting up a rainy day reserve, marketing the cooperative, or developing their community.

Housing cooperatives offer lower down payments, lower closing costs, economies of scale or lower average costs per unit, and longer mortgage terms closing costs, making them more financially affordable compared to other owned housing. When living in a cooperative, the cost of living in terms of monthly charges usually remains reasonable. Costs can increase if there is an increase in taxes or operating expenses.

Each cooperative member is an owner with a share in the cooperative housing. As homeowners, they can deduct their share of real estate taxes and mortgage interest paid by the cooperative on their tax returns. Market–rate co-ops allow members to sell their share at resale market prices, maintaining equity in their share. When a shareholder decides to move out or passes away, their share sells at whatever the market bears at that time.

Although this is similar to owning and selling a condominium, the difference is that the cooperative carries the mortgage. When a new member moves in, he finances the out-going member's equity. This transfer of shares can include some settlement costs. This means that the purchase price of the co-op share is lower than buying into a condominium. Co-ops however, can have a higher monthly fee. All financial benefits accrue to the senior owners, including return of equity upon resale. Tax deductibility of mortgage interest and real estate taxes, identical to single-family homeownership, applies to cooperative ownership.

Another more affordable option is a limited equity structure that allows members to purchase a portion of the cooperative, and accordingly, limits the sale price to their membership share. With limited equity, members may elect to pass their traditional share cost or down payment to another member or an estate in the event that they move or pass away.

Limited equity co-ops place limitations on equity but allow for long-term affordability for members. Members are not liable for the co-op mortgage loans. This enables individuals with limited means to qualify for a limited equity share in the co-op; an advantage to people without adequate financial resources to qualify for an individual mortgage. The economy of scale can help save costs for each co-op member.

Living in a Self-governing Community

As members of a self-governing community share ownership of the cooperative, they have the opportunity to actively participate in decision-making and maintain greater control over their living environment then they might if they were renting an apartment or house. They retain more control over how long they choose to live in the co-op whereas in a rental, housing and rental fees it may be at the discretion of a landlord. Members are obligated to meet their co-op responsibilities and to abide by the bylaws, rules and regulations.

Each cooperative elects a board of directors composed of cooperative members. It is the responsibility of the board to keep its members fully advised of events within their community. Newsletters, an information bulletin board, and co-op meetings enhance communication between members. Open communication and accountability is essential to successful cooperative living.

Living in a democratic community enables members to provide supportive services to other residents. These supportive services can include credit unions, the purchase of large quantities of supplies or food, the provision of healthcare support such as caregivers or a trained medical professional and more.

Many people believe that the most difficult aspects of maintaining a home are the routine repairs and maintenance. Under the co-op, members have only limited responsibility for maintenance. The cooperative association pays for major repairs, insurance, replacement of old equipment, and upkeep of the common grounds and buildings. As members own equity in the co-op property, they share responsibility in protecting the premises from vandalism and property destruction by providing excellent security.

In Ashland, Oregon, there is a sustainable cooperative with 36 financially independent residents living in 13 small townhouses. The homes have passive solar, superior insulation, and radiant heat. Each townhouse has one to four bedrooms, and a small private yard. Co-op members acted as their own developer. They have a 1775 common house and a community garden. Shared meals are once a week. There is a no smoking policy. There are no common spiritual practices. Each resident participates in governance by consensus and contributes ten hours a month of labor. All pay joining fees, monthly fees, and homeowner association dues. -- Source: CoHousing.com

The Senior Cooperative Foundation website offers a housing list, resources, education programs, and more for those interested in learning about living in a senior cooperative.
Go to http://www.seniorcoops.org/index.php

CoHousing, building a better society, one neighbor at a time, maintains a directory to help you locate cohousing in the United States.
Go to http://www.cohousing.org/directory/view/6355

Other Types of Shared Housing

(multi-family, cluster housing, congregate housing, accessory apartments, ECHO housing and granny flats)

- **Multi-Family Housing** describes any building – duplexes, triplexes, four-plexus, condominiums, townhouses and apartment-type structures – with two or more family homes within the same attached structure.

- **Cluster housing** is a subdivision or land divided into homebuilding lots, where detached homes are close together with shared common areas that may include open space, recreational facilities, kitchen and laundry areas, parking, and more.

- **Congregate Housing** residents live independently in their own apartments but share at least one meal each day in a central dining area. Services for heavy housekeeping, as well as social and recreational activities are usually included. For information about these housing options, contact your local State Area Agency on Aging or Senior and Disabled Services Office.

- **Accessory apartments** are self-contained units located in a house in which other people live such as family, friends, or an unrelated person. It allows you to live independently without living alone, perhaps in a neighborhood close to friends and family. Another advantage is that there is usually little to no maintenance required such as lawn care and repairs. If this is a rental situation, it can be advantageous for both parties. The income received helps the homeowner with her expenses, and the rent amount paid for the unit is likely to be more economical than that of an entire home. To live in an accessory apartment, you should be fairly independent and self-sufficient. You will need to care for yourself, shop for groceries, cook your own meals, and clean your apartment without assistance. If you are unable to care for yourself, you and the homeowners may find several disadvantages to this arrangement.

- **ECHO Housing**, also known as Elder Cottage Housing Opportunity, are small, barrier-free self-contained units. They are for seniors and disabled people who are unable to maintain their homes due to physical restrictions or limited financial resources. Started in Australia in the 1970's as Granny Flats, they became an inexpensive housing option for older people in the United States in the 1980's.

These units - a separate structure, a garage apartment, a mobile or modular home or a pre-fabricated home - are placed in the back or side yard or sometimes above a garage of a single-family home. Each unit includes all the amenities of a single-family home – a kitchen, bedroom, bathroom and a living room. Easily moved, this often-temporary structure can be removed when it is no longer needed. Or depending on zoning laws, it can be reused or rented to another individual. The cost for erecting temporary ECHO housing is reasonable, ranging from $25,000 for a 500–700 square foot home to over $100,000 for a high-end unit. There may be extra costs if you need to lay a foundation.

The **Senior Resources** website provides information and referral services. Resources include information on housing choices, aging in place, finance, insurance, a legal help center, resources by states, a free monthly E-zine magazine, and more.
Go to http://www.seniorresource.com/

There are multiple benefits of ECHO housing to you and your family. By living on your family's property, you have additional support from people who love you, yet you are able to maintain your independence. Family members will not need to travel great distances to provide any needed care. Some families – from the adult children to the youngest generation – form stronger bonds due to the close proximity. For vulnerable seniors, who often fall prey to con artists, ECHO housing brings more safety and security. Financial security strengthens as living expenses decrease. If family members decide to charge a fair market rate for their rental, the extra income becomes available to your family. Before consulting with a licensed contractor, consider the factors involved with living in close proximity to your family.

- What are your physical or mental capabilities?
- Will the unit be comfortable for a single person or a couple?
- Will you need an accessible and/or a private entrance?
- What size unit would meet your needs – a studio or a one or two bedroom unit?
- Do you want to build in full or partial kitchen facilities for your daily meal preparation?
- If it is an attached unit, will you share bathroom facilities?
- If it is an attached unit, will you be expected to participate in household responsibilities?

There can be obstacles or challenges to ECHO housing. Foremost are the zoning laws that differ in each locale. By contacting the local zoning authority, you can gather information about their requirements and restrictions. Some may stipulate that only a family member or relative can live in the ECHO housing can rent the property. Others may allow non-family tenants. Some zoning laws can require a high quality of construction so the dwelling will compliment other existing structures in the neighborhood. A special use permit may be required. Other considerations include the following:

- Do the dimensions and features of your property allow for installation of a temporary dwelling with utility hook-ups?

- What is the approval process for construction?

- Are there county or state restrictions regarding construction?

- Are there high development fees involved in construction?

- Is there a minimum or maximum unit size?

- Does the unit require you need a specific clearance distance between the unit and the neighboring property? If so, how much clearance is needed?

- Are there setback or building restrictions that determine where the unit lies in relation to the property next door, the street, or other natural boundaries such as rivers or wetlands?

- Can the unit face a busy street?

- If the building is a manufactured home, will it increase or decrease property values for you or your neighbors?

- Are there roofline – the shape or style of the roof - or height requirements?

- Will the unit be easy to remove when you no longer require it?

- Are there local services that you can hire to remove the structure?

- How will your neighbors react to you building an ECHO housing unit?

- Are there age restrictions for renters of ECHO housing?

Even though you can remove these homes, they should comply with zoning laws and regulations. A building permit may be required. These laws protect your neighborhood by preserving property values. Before proceeding, be sure to contact your local city or county zoning department for specific permit information.

Sustainable Alternative Housing

(eco-cottages, tiny houses, small homes, and yurts)

For people interested in building a small "green" cottage or house, there are several companies that offer quality crafted, easily assembled, and energy efficient small homes made from recycled materials.

- **Eco-cottages** are small, economical, energy efficient, and often, sustainable footprint cottages, used as additional elder housing, rentals, studios or offices or as an expanded family unit. These units range from 250 square feet to over 500 square feet of completely "green" homes that meet or exceed the Leadership in Energy and Environmental Design (LEED) building codes in all 50 states. These independent units link to a larger home, expanding the home size, yet allowing privacy and independent living. The difference between these cottage units and the ECHO housing is in the connection to the main dwelling and the degree of integrated environmental conservation and sustainability. The units qualify for Energy Tax Credits. An eco-cottage team can assemble these custom-built homes on-site in less than 3-weeks. The property owner, however, must secure all the building permits and prepare the site including the installation post and beam and sub-structure framing. An on-line website and telephone support is available from the eco-cottage help desk as is a Do-It-Yourself package

---

For information on **Energy Tax Credits**
go to http://www.irs.gov/uac/Energy-Incentives-for-Individuals-in-the-American-Recovery-and-Reinvestment-Act

---

If you are considering building in an area off the grid, eco-cottages offer a wilderness package with solar panels, water collection cisterns, propane tanks, an eco-John waterless incinerator toilet and other off-the-grid features. The cost for the eco-cottage package structure with installation is about $46,000. Custom options are available. In addition, there are now eco-sea cottages or cottages built on the hull of a catamaran for those interested in living on the water.

Eco-sea cottages are discussed later in this chapter under, *At Home on the Water.*

Nationwide-Homes Eco-Cottages:
Go to http://www.nationwide-homes.com/ecocottages/main.
cfm?pagename=ecoMain
Tele: 1-800-216-7001

- **Tiny Houses** are tiny and small houses ranging in size from 65 to 837 square feet. The tiny houses are on wheels and require no assembly. They can be towed to the home site by a standard truck or car with a trailer hitch and brake controller. Or for a fee ranging from $1000 to just under $4000, they can be shipped and delivered to the home site. They are ready to live in. The tiny houses are equipped with basic appliances – 2-burner stove, under counter refrigerator, bar sink, hot water heater, compost or green toilet systems. They plumb to public water services or to a portable tank. No building permit is required for the Tiny Houses and Do-It-Yourself plans are available.

Tumbleweed Tiny House Company:
Go to http://www.tumbleweedhouses.com/

Tiny Green Cabins:
Go to http://www.tinygreencabins.com/

Small Homes Oregon:
Download plans for building your small home.
Go to http://www.smallhomeoregon.net/

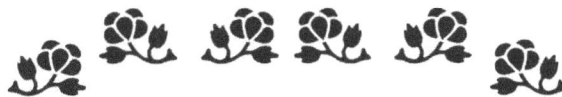

- **Small homes** range in size from 251-square feet to a 2-3 bedroom home of 837- square feet. These houses are not on wheels and require a permanent foundation. Plans are available for purchase and meet the international building codes. The approximate cost is $100-$200 per square foot.

- **Yurts,** adapted from the nomads of Central Asia, have gained popularity in the United States as vacation homes, lodging in park campgrounds, temporary homes, and appealing permanent residences. A simple yurt is a dome–shaped fabric covered structure built on a wooden framework. It sits on a platform or floor and is portable, self-supporting, and eco-friendly. Yurt's are lightweight, low cost and built with plumbing and electric.

There is a feeling of spaciousness when you stand inside a yurt. Diameters can range from about 16 feet or 200 square feet to 30 feet or 708 square feet. Wall heights can be as low as 7 feet and as high as 13 feet. By utilizing connecting breezeways between two yurts or another wooden structure, you can expand the yurt size. For the handy person, yurts are relatively easy to set-up with telephone support. Alternatively, you can hire a contractor. Building a yurt takes 1-3 days. Prices range from around $4500 - $10,000. You can also order custom yurts with special windows, awnings, French doors, and a variety of wall panel and roof cover colors. Be sure to check the building permit requirements as they vary from state to state and community to community.

Pacific Yurts Inc.:
Go to http://www.yurts.com/
Tele: 800-944-0240

Blue Ridge Yurts:
Go to http://www.blueridgeyurts.com/index.php

Yurtinfo.org:
Go to http://www.yurtinfo.org/companies.php

Creative Living Options

*"I suppose real old age begins when
one looks backward rather than forward."*

--Mary Sarton, Excerpts from a Life

Most boomers resist thinking too far into the future. Questions such as, "Where will I live when I need more help?" seem absurd when we feel healthy, are physically active, and retain our ability to make decisions and engage in a career or job. Our personal desires vary. We may choose to move near our children, to age in place in our own homes, to live some place with a high quality of life, to travel or decide on something original.

Creative living options have emerged as the 80 million boomers enter their retirement years. For many years, stories circulated on the Internet about an elderly woman living aboard a Princess Cruise Line, receiving a small room to live in, gourmet meals, healthcare services, access to activity programs, and travel benefits. Another story floating through the Internet describes a person choosing to live in Holiday Inn Hotels. When senior discounts, AARP membership discounts, and frequent traveler and long – term residence discounts apply, the cost was similar to living in an assisted living facility. *(Snopes.com, an Internet verification website confirms that some people have avoided retirement centers in favor of living on a cruise ship or in a hotel.)*

For the more adventurous and active person, here are some of creative living options you can explore as you approach retirement.

- **Recreational vehicles (RV's):** There is a large contingent of boomers and the Greatest Generation living in their RV's, traveling the United States, Canada, and even Central America. Boomers and the Greatest Generation members who still drive and love to travel often become *Snowbirds,* driving south for the winter in recreational vehicles and returning north in the spring when the weather warms. *Sunbirds* live in a warm climate and follow the sunshine in the winter to even warmer climates. Some camp in their RV in established campgrounds; others live in RV parks designed for short-term or long-term stays. By living in their home on wheels, these individuals bring all the conveniences of home with them wherever they go.

- **Floating Homes:** You can now live aboard a floating home such as a houseboat, an eco-sea cottage or a live-aboard yacht or power cruiser, a world traveling freighter, or a passenger cruise ship or luxury residential cruise ship. Houseboats, live-aboard yachts and eco- sea cottages are for those interested in community living on the water;

- **Passenger Ships and Luxury Residential Ocean Liners**: Many people think of a cruise ship only for short vacations such as cruising to the Caribbean or to southern Mexico. However, there are also opportunities to travel for longer periods, receiving room and board and many amenities. Passenger cruise ships can be booked back-to-back and range from affordable to extreme luxury.

- **World-traveling Freighters:** Travel on freighters is for the daring voyagers in good physical condition who are also flexible, not stuck on a schedule, and yearning for a true world adventure.

- **Overseas Living:** For the retiree who always wanted experience another culture, there are many opportunities to live in another country. You can ship your RV to another country, travel the world by air, ship, car, bicycle, foot, or other means, or live overseas as an expatriate.

- **Employment Opportunities:** For the more adventurous, work and living opportunities include campground-hosting, caretaking in the United States and abroad, staffing a fire tower lookouts during the summer months and scores of other job opportunities for people over 50 years of age.

Taking to the Road in
Your Recreational Vehicle

"Hang up the keys, give up"

(RV motto)

While many retirees in their 50's and 60's decide to stay in their current homes or down-size and move to a smaller home within the same locale, other retirees take to the road in pursuit of travel and adventure. Being on the road becomes their "retired" lifestyle. As most people prefer a familiar place to return to and call home (a home-base), some retirees rent their primary dwelling instead of selling their home. Others take to the road as full-timers, living in their RV homes 365 days a year. They may sell their home and place their belongings in storage, making their home wherever they park their recreational vehicle (RV.)

Many RVer's sell their home and use the home sale assets to purchase an RV equipped for all their daily needs. It is their home on wheels and with it comes the freedom of the road. Called full-timers, they travel 365 days a year, often heading south in the cold of winter and, like the migrating birds, returning north to the warmer climates in the summer. It is not a lonely journey as many like-minded people congregate at RV encampments and camp grounds, year after year, creating a social network among other people on the move.

RV Dreams.com: For information about rallies, campground reviews, a community forum, live chat room, financial information, and more, go to http://www.rv-dreams.com/

RVers Online: This website includes links for RV travel and destinations, clubs and organizations, general interest sites, commercial and manufacturing sites, and on-line owners' clubs. Go to http://www.rversonline.org/RV6.html

Active Full-timers on the Road

Planning to hit the road as a full-timer means that you will need to decide where you want to travel. A flexible pre-determined travel route allows for visits to remarkable side trips and spontaneous adventures. Are you interested in traveling to areas where other RVer's tend to travel and often stay for extended periods? Alternatively, do you prefer a quieter place, off the beaten path, where you can find some solitude? Think about your comfort zone. Do you want to travel within the United States or Canada, travel south to Central American countries, or fly overseas and rent an RV in another country? Do you prefer to ship your RV overseas? Depending on where you decide to travel, the daily cost of living will differ. Traveling and living in Central America is less expensive than in the United States, Canada, or Europe.

If you decide to stay in the USA, you will not need a passport or visa. If you travel outside the USA, a passport is required. You will also need to check whether the visas are required in the countries to which you plan to travel.

On the road, your vehicle is your home. It is where you will sit, hour after hour alone or next to your partner, plotting your route on highway maps, listening to the radio, and/ or engaging in conversation. If you are making the trip alone, be prepared for periods of quiet and even loneliness. Long road trips, solitary or with a companion, are not for everyone.

For information on **Passports**,
look at the **United States Department of State** website.
Go to http://www.travel.state.gov/

Advantages to Traveling
in a Home on Wheels

"You meet very interesting people here. Spend your summers up North and your winters down south." -- Advice from Joan, owner/manager, Snake River RV Park and Campground, Idaho Falls, Idaho

There are many advantages to living in an RV. Like a turtle, everywhere you go, your home is with you. It is affordable, flexible, convenient, and, if you desire, social.

- **It is affordable:** Living in your recreational vehicle can save you money. Since you live in your RV, you will not have the expense of staying in hotels. Your main cost will be campground fees and fuel. You can cook in your RV that saves on dining out costs. You can bring kayaks, canoes, rafts, or bicycles, saving on the rental cost for outdoor gear. If your RV is your primary residence, you do not have to pay property taxes.

- **It is convenient:** You have your home and all your necessary possessions with you. Many RV's are equipped with a bathroom, bedroom, kitchen with refrigerator and stove, and sitting area. Smaller RV's, offer the convenience of sleeping quarters and a small kitchen. You can hookup a TV or DVD player. You can bring your pet cat or dog with you instead of housing it in a pet care facility. Many RV parks provide pancake breakfasts, activities, laundry facilities, showers, stores, restrooms, and more.

- **You can be flexible:** You can be spontaneous and go whenever and wherever you decide to travel. You do not need to have a set schedule or destination and if you are comfortable with no itinerary, you can plan your trip as you travel.

- **Travel wherever you want:** In your RV, you can travel across the United States, north to Canada, south to Central America and even overseas. In the United States, you can visit the National Parks and camp in RV campgrounds and parks, on Forest Service and Bureau of Land Management (BLM) land and at privately run campgrounds. If you decide to travel outside the U.S., be sure to bring your passport and necessary visas.

- **It is social.** Along the road, you will meet interesting people who have also chosen life on the road. Attend rallies, join live chat rooms and forums, and eat with other RVer's at campground pancake breakfasts. Many RVer's form close-knit communities and return annually to the same locations and rallies.

Disadvantages to Traveling in a Home on Wheels

Traveling the road in an RV is not for everyone. To some, the disadvantages of taking to the road in an RV will outweigh the advantages. Here are some drawbacks you may want to consider before embarking on a road trip.

- **Too small a living space:** Living in a confined space day-after-day can make some people feel cramped. As you will need to downsize your possessions, you may feel that you are unable to bring items that you would normally use in your primary residence. Although it is possible to rent a storage unit for many possessions, you still will not have all the comforts of home with you as you travel. Some people will rent their home base (so they will have a home to return to) and leave their possessions in a secure locked room.

- **It is inconvenient:** You may not be able to travel on some roads due to the size of your RV. For electricity, you may need an established campground or RV park with a plug-in.

- **There is no privacy:** Living in any small space limits your amount of privacy. As the bathroom, bedroom, and sitting areas are all close together, be sure you are comfortable living in close proximity to another person. At many campsites and RV parks, you may find that your neighbors are camped just outside your door.

- **Too much noise:** Camping at campgrounds and RV parks can place you near to your neighbors. If they have noisy children, a loud barking dog, play loud music, or have raucous parties, you may find RV camping stressful. Many campgrounds and RV parks have noise regulations, ushering in a quiet time after 10 pm.

- **Gas and repairs are expensive**. If your RV needs repairs, you may need to stay in a hotel and dine out while the RV receives repairs. With the price of gas continuing to rise, you may decide to stay or base your RV in a short-term or long-term campground to minimize your fuel costs.

- **Too much driving:** If you do not like to drive a large vehicle, you may want to take a practice drive in an RV before purchasing one and thereby committing to a life on wheels. Sometimes the idea of an RV overpowers your actual preferences. If you do not enjoy driving long distances or driving a large bulky vehicle, traveling in an RV may not be the right choice for you.

- **Parking** a large RV or backing up into a small narrow space can be difficult if you have not had experience maneuvering an outsized bulky vehicle. Finding a space long enough to accommodate your RV when you stop for rest breaks might be a challenge.

- **It is too cold to travel in the winter. Cold weather preparation** is necessary if you plan to travel in the winter. Many camper walls have poor insulation that contributes to higher heating bills, frozen water pipes and drains, and burned out furnaces. Some septic tank disposal facilities close in the winter.

If you choose to live the nomadic life of the RVer, the advantages should outweigh the disadvantages. You should enjoy the social interaction at campgrounds; take pleasure in cooking homemade meals and sleeping in a familiar bed at night. You may opt to bring a pet. You should appreciate the flexibility of not adhering to a set schedule. Before you set out on the road in your RV, be sure to prepare for your road trip, both in terms of needed supplies and expectations of daily like in a confined space.

What Activities Do You
Find Enjoyable or Disagreeable?

If driving a vehicle for a long distance trip is pleasurable and comfortable, you are half-way there. If you have a backache or need to stretch your legs every few hours, take the time to get out of the RV to go for a walk. Caring for pet is always a great reason for stopping, giving you a break from the road and your dog exercise time. Pace yourself and develop a daily routine that allows relaxation, sightseeing, and a reasonable amount of driving each day.

- **Sit down with a piece of paper and a pencil or your iPad or tablet**. Discuss your plans with your traveling partner and think about how you would like to spend your time on the road. If you are traveling alone, think about what you want to do.

- **Be sure you are compatible with your driving companion**. Even if you are on the road with your spouse of 40 years, being together 24-hours a day, seven days a week, can create tension. Discuss your travel plans and be prepared to compromise or change your plans. Take each day as it comes and even if you do not accomplish the distance you planned, enjoy the activities that you are able to do. Occasionally take some "alone" time to run an errand or shop, allowing you and your companion some private space.

Think about the following when considering a life on the road.
- Is a year of travel too long? Is three months? Is six months?
- What is your comfort zone for being away from your current home?
- Are you planning to maintain your primary residence so you can return to it whenever you choose?
- Are you planning to sell your home and use the money for your trip?
- Are you planning to rent your home so you can later return to it?
- What type and size vehicle will you be comfortable in for an extensive trip?
- Do you plan to keep moving or to drive to a specific destination and stay for an extended period?
- Do you want to incorporate your travel with visits to family and friends?
- How long are you comfortable being away from family?

- Do you have an easy way for family and friends to communicate with you?

Preparing for life on the road can help smooth the way. A little bit of research using maps, publications that highlight destinations for RV's and campers, and a listing of National Park and Forest Service or BLM campgrounds and parks, can guide you to areas that cater to people on the move.

Many snowbirds or retirees heading south for the winter months end up in Quartzite, Arizona. Located by the intersection of Interstate 10 and Highway 95, this desert region attracts over 1.5 million visitors in January and February. Drawn to the area by the warm weather, RVer's partake of an annual RV show, flea markets, unique geology and history. This RV friendly spot offers secluded camping areas and inexpensive camping on government land ($40 for 14 consecutive days / $180 for seven months on designated BLM land*.) Look for non-fee parking for up to 14-consecutive days in a 28-day period, and private RV camping ($135 per month plus electric, $80 per week, $20 overnight*.) Amenities may include clubhouses, swimming pools and even storage for a small fee. Access to medical care is an easy drive from Quartzsite. *Rates may change.

Preparing a Road Trip Budget

"I believe the second half of one's life is meant to be better than the first half. The first half is finding out how you do it. And the second half is enjoying it." -- Frances Lear

With the recent downturn in the economy and most people looking at reduced retirement savings, it is necessary to consider carefully your budget for the time you are on the road. Look at your current income and savings accounts and the set costs for maintaining your primary home and/or RV. Calculate whether you will need to find temporary work while you travel or whether you can live off your monthly income and financial nest egg.

To locate your **State Department of Motor Vehicles office**, go to http://www.dmvlocator.com/

Once you have decided where you plan to travel and for how long, prepare a budget. Include:

- **the cost of maintaining your primary dwelling or rental.** (unless you plan on selling your primary residence) What are the monthly costs for your mortgage, utilities, insurance, telephone or cell service, routine maintenance, and property taxes? If you arrange a house sitter, what is the cost for this service?

- **calculation for the cost of purchasing an RV**, mobile home, or travel trailer. Depending on the type of RV, the cost can range from a few thousand dollars to over one million dollars.

- **calculation for the cost of fuel and routine vehicle maintenance.** Allow for unexpected emergency repairs and temporary housing while you have your vehicle repaired.

- **preparation of a daily budget for RV travel that includes activities,** food, fuel, campground and RV park fees, insurance, cell phone and wireless costs and private P.O. Box services that will hold or forward mail.

For **Tax information,**
check with an accountant or on-line at http://www.irs.gov/

Buying a Vehicle

(basic camper van, travel trailer, large RV or motor home, luxury motor coach)

Let us get started by buying the type of vehicle that meets your traveling needs. Some people will purchase a non-towed rear engine, fuel-efficient passenger or camper vehicle without many amenities, such as a **basic camper van** like a VW Vanagon. It provides a small space for sleeping and cooking, maybe with a small refrigerator and efficient storage.

Others purchase a **travel trailer** with a bumper or frame hitch that is towed by a car, van, or pick-up and includes a place to sleep, cook, and relax. Consider a very small RV such as a pop-up and tent trailer, microlite or teardrop. Built as a weekend camper, a compact car can pull these lightweight vehicles. They are so small you can move them by hand. They are easily detached enabling you to use your vehicle for driving. The compact interior of a very small RV can house a camping kitchen, built-in storage, refrigerator and entertainment center, power outlets, and up to a queen-size bed. A used travel trailer can cost between $7500 to over $50,000. The cost is dependent upon the condition and age of the trailer, the number of miles traveled, amenities, add-ons and re-sale potential.

Larger RV's or motor homes range from 21 feet to 45 feet in length; they can use either diesel or gas fuel. Some sit over a RV chassis while others are built with a driver compartment similar to a van with a sleeping area above the cab. A towed fifth- wheel RV can detach from your pick-up and offers lots of room and comfort. Consider the size of your motorhome and the size of your vehicle that will tow it.

It is hard to miss the **luxury motor coach RV's** lumbering down the highway, the driver sitting above the traffic, looking down on all the smaller vehicles. These deluxe RV's can offer all the amenities of a quality home – kitchen with granite countertops, microwave, cook top, refrigerator and dishwasher, living room with sofa, dining room, bedrooms that accommodate a queen size bed, full baths, air conditioning, remote controls for windows and television, smoke detectors, and more.

The purchase cost for a luxury RV can range from $100,000 to over $700,000. This depends on the condition, model year, size and luxury of the RV as well as the featured amenities. As these vehicles feature large gas tanks, each fuel fill-up is expensive. The average fuel mileage for a gas-powered vehicle is 5-10 miles per gallon; for diesel, it is 9-14 miles per gallon.

Long-distance driving in a vehicle this size, regardless of the features, is tiring. Parking is difficult unless the parking space is designated for RV's and semis. Many people will tow a smaller vehicle behind for easier transportation once the RV is parked.

For a family, a luxury RV provides space, comfort, and extras like television, stereos, and DVD players to entertain the family. However, if you are traveling with your partner – that's 2 people –think about whether an RV of this size is necessary for comfort. A luxury RV does have limitations. It may not be as conducive as a smaller RV or trailer to rustic camping or city driving.

If you can claim a motor home as a primary or secondary home, the interest paid on a loan may be tax deductible. Consult your accountant or an attorney for updated tax information.

Recreational Vehicle Clubs

Many RV clubs offer services geared toward RVer's. By subscribing for a nominal fee, you receive access to the immense network of RV services: mail forwarding services, free ID/ theft protection, pharmacy drug programs, emergency air ambulance and road services, discount RV parking and fees, and magazines and newsletters directed at the RV communities.

RV Clubs and Insurance Programs

CampClub USA offers a 30% discount when you camp in a CampClub campground. Go to http://www.campclubusa.com/

Good Sam VIP Insurance is an RV loan finance company. Go to http://www.goodsamvip.com/

Family Motor Coach Association offers helpful services including trip routing, mail forwarding, MEDEX PLUS, emergency medical evacuation program, emergency road service and technical assistance and the Family Motor Coach Magazine. Go to http://www.fmca.com/

Escapees RV Club is a total support network which includes many services for RVer's . It also sponsors CARE program – Continuing Assistance for Recuperating Escapees. Go to http://www.escapees.com

---

The **Escapee RV Club** recognizes that many full-time RVer's live by the motto, *Hang up the keys, give up.* These RVer's do not want to give up their community of RV friends or the independence and freedom they have discovered cruising down the road. Some vow they will never reside in a nursing facility. The club offers a variety of services including educational seminars as well as an RV boot camp for novice RV drivers.

Where do older RVer's with decreasing vision, progressive arthritis, and other disabilities retire when driving their motor home becomes too difficult or begins to present a road hazard to others? The Escapee RV Club offers a unique program in Livingston, Texas called CARE - *Continuing Assistance for Recuperating Escapees.* Set up in 1976 as a 501(c) (3) non-profit retirement center for American RV Escapees, it offers an abundance of assistance programs for RVer's whose travels are temporarily or permanently disrupted due to illness, surgery, accident, or deteriorating health.

In addition to providing a space to park the RV, CARE offers personal care services to RVer's less able to care for themselves. Trained staff is on duty Monday-Friday, at night and on weekends; trained volunteers also assist residents. CARE can accommodate 35 RV's at a time. The cost for one person is $849/month; for two persons, it is $1273/month.* A nurse meets residents on the premises 8-hours per day. Staff members assist with scheduling and arranging transportation to medical appointments, feeding residents three meals daily, performing laundry and housekeeping services, planning activity programs, carrying out security and well-checks, and providing adult day care, 24/7 call assistance, individualized care plans and caregiving assistance for anyone needing help with the basic activities of daily life – bathing, dressing, grooming, and toileting. Local home healthcare agencies offer physical and occupational therapies and skilled nursing care in the RV. RVer's continue to live independently in their recreational vehicle instead of moving to a facility, receiving needed assistance.

Escapees Care, Inc. offers an **adult day care program** to support RVer's afflicted with Alzheimer's disease. Designed in a secure setting to prevent dementia residents from wandering and getting lost, it provides nursing supervision, medication management, a sensory stimulation program, and help with the activities of daily life, including assistance with feeding at mealtimes.

At **Pearl's Place**, an overnight and weekend cottage separate from the CARE day care program, the caregivers of CARE residents can receive a break or respite time from caregiving. Available for $40* per night, it gives caregivers the opportunity to relax and recharge their energy. Caregivers are responsible for hiring a sitter when using Pearl's Place. Still, at least in the short-term, it is a less expensive alternative to placing a family member with dementia in a nursing facility. *Rates may change.*

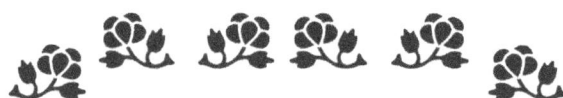

Mary and Gus, both in their mid-70's, sold their single-family home in 2000 and moved into a moderately-sized recreational vehicle. Over the next years, they traveled around across the United States, camping in the National Parks and National Forest campgrounds and occasionally at a RV Park. In the National Parks, they enjoyed hiking and fishing. At the RV parks they met other full-time RVer's and established a close network of friends. Last year, both suffered a series of health problems. Gus's cataracts and a progressive crippling arthritis made it difficult for him to drive. Mary's mild dementia became worse and twice she wandered from their RV and became lost. Recognizing their limitations, they discussed their alternatives – sell the RV and move into an assisted living facility, move in with their family, or move to an RV assisted park. After careful reflection, they decided to continue living in their recreational vehicle for as long as possible as it had been their home for 10 years. They leased a long-term RV site with full hook-ups, a shed for storage, and a patio. Services provided through the RV Park helped them continue to be independent while living in their RV.

Escapees CARE, Inc. (Continuing Assistance for Recuperating Escapees) offers older RVer's with permanent or temporary health problems an affordable safe haven. Go to http://www.escapeescare.org/ or e-mail: careinc@escapees.com / Tele: 936-327-4256

International Homes on Wheels

For the more adventurous, taking your RV on a road trip to another country, perhaps in Central America, Europe, or New Zealand opens an array of opportunities. To make a trip of this sort will take time and preparation, but the benefits of seeing the world in the comfort of your home on wheels is immeasurable. By utilizing campgrounds instead of hotels and cooking your own meals instead of eating out every day, even the most expensive country can become more affordable.

For Travel in another country,
Go to http://www.travel.state.gov
for information about passports, visas, immunizations, and other helpful material.

Renting a Recreational Vehicle Overseas

While some people choose to rent an RV in their country of choice, others may decide to ship their RV to another country. Certainly, it is easier to rent a RV when you arrive at your destination, just as you would rent a car in a foreign country. In this way, you are able to re-serve the type of RV you want and have it waiting for you when you arrive. Be sure to bring:

- a driver's license;
- visa (*some countries will require a Visa*);
- international driver's license *(if required)*;
- up-to-date passport *(expiration date should be more than 6 months away)*;
- credit card for payment;
- insurance information *(additional insurance may be mandatory.)*

Check to see if there is a minimal time for the rental. Check the number of miles included in the rental. Are miles unlimited or do you get a set amount of miles and then have a mileage fee added? Check for extra fees. For example, there may be an extra driver fee. Drop-charges can apply to one-way rentals. For added amenities, such as a GPS, picnic table and chairs, satellite phone, or an electric adaptor, there may be a daily or one-time fee. Discounts may also be available for seniors. While you may find the basic travel costs reasonable, think about all the costs that you can encounter including:

- air fare;
- RV shipping costs *(if you decide to ship your RV)*;
- shipping fees for personal belongings;
- gas;
- RV rental fee;
- food;
- campground fees;
- insurance fees;
- passport and visa fees;
- international driving permit fee;
- customs fees;
- unexpected expenses.

If you are interested in renting a vehicle overseas, rates in Europe range from approximately $100 USD per day to over $200 USD per day depending on when you rent: - low, off-shoulder, or peak seasons - your pick-up location, the type of vehicle, and the length of time you will be renting. In countries where the dollar is worth more than the local currency, the exchange rate can be much lower.

Senior Motor Home Rental in Australia offers 2-6 berth motor homes with manual or automatic transmission, gas cooker and grill, refrigerator, microwave, television, shower, toilet, starting at AUD $35 per day* for a 2-berth budget camper van to AUD $122 per day for a 6-berth motor home rented for an extensive travel trip. For more information on renting an RV in Australia or other countries, go to www.seniormotorhomerental.com.au * *(In 2013, the exchange rate is close to the dollar.)*

Shipping Your Recreational Vehicle

For RVer's thinking about shipping their RV overseas, shipping agencies require specific information about the RV. The shipping agencies will need to know:

- year, make, and model of vehicle;
- vehicle condition;
- pick-up location;
- destination;
- weight;

- accurate measurements *(length x width x height)*;
- insurance coverage;
- your name and contact information.

There are many shipping companies that offer licensed and bonded relocation services such as packing, organizing logistics for the move, setting up storage services, arranging transportation between ports, providing necessary documentation, and handling customs clearance. In addition to shipping your RV, they can help you ship your personal belongings.

Motor Home International: For renting an RV overseas in Canada, Europe, New Zealand, Australia, and South Africa. Go to http://www.motorhome-international.com/

Cruise America: For renting an RV overseas in British Columbia, Nova Scotia, Ontario, Quebec, Yukon, and Alberta, in addition to other parts of North America. Go to http://www.cruiseamerica.com/

USA RV Rental: For renting an RV in the United States, either one-way or round-trip, this website offers online RV rental quotes and a reservation system. Go to http://www.usarvrentals.com/

Preparing Your Recreational Vehicle for Shipping

You will need to prepare your vehicle for shipping. The gas tank should be less than 1/8 full. No personal items should be placed in the RV. Only permanent fixtures, installed items, and original equipment such as spare tires, and auto tool kits should be stored in the vehicle. Vehicle size, pick-up specifics, and the final destination determine the price. The vehicle can be transported by RO-RO (Roll on-Roll Off), where the vehicle is driven on and off the ship. Alternatively, the vehicle can be transported on a flat-track or in containerized shipping. Be prepared for country sales taxes, port handling fees at destination ports, and customs clearance paperwork and fees.

As it is relatively easy to rent a motor home for an extended time, you may want to compare costs of shipping to the cost of renting an RV at your chosen destination.

Shipping and Transport Services

Direct Express: Offers international relocation services.
Go to http://www.shipdei.com/householdgoodshipping.html

DAS Car Shipping and Auto Transport Services:
Go to http://www.dasautoshippers.com/

USAC International Shipping:
Go to http://www.usacintl.com/
Tele: 888-950-4454

FreightCenter.com: offers a free freight calculator to help you estimate your freight costs.
Go to http://www.freightcenter.com/landing/shipping_costs/landing/shipping_cost.aspx?gclid=CKvly43nuLMCFUdxQgod1isAuw

USA International Shipping:
Go to http://www.usainternationalshipping.org/
Tele: 1-702-714-0227

Driving Licenses and Permits

To drive a large RV in the United States, it is necessary to check with your state Department of Motor Vehicles to determine if you will need a commercial driver's license. *Changin' Gears, Trading City Lights for the RV Lifestyle,* a website devoted to the RV lifestyle, has compiled a summary of RV Driver's License Requirements from official driver's license websites in all 50 states and Washington D.C. For information, go to http://changingears.com/rv-sec-state-rv-license.shtml

An **International Driving Permit (IDP)**, booklet issued to you by your home country or state used with your valid driver's license and accepted in 175 countries, is required by some major car rental agencies overseas. Used in conjunction with your driving permit it is not a substitute for your current driver's license when you drive in another country. You must also bring your current driver's license. *Please note: The IDP cannot be issued more than 6 months prior to your departure.*

There are only two organizations authorized by the State Department to issue the IDP, the **American Automobile Association (AAA)** and the **National Automobile Club (NAC.)** You can easily download an application at their websites and take it to a local AAA office or mail it to the NAC. In addition to the application, you will need:

- a valid driver's license *(2-sides if you copy and mail it)*;
- (2) Traditional passport type photos;
- $15-fee.

Allow 4-6 weeks for delivery if you apply by mail.

International Driver Permit Applications

American Automobile Association (AAA):
Go to http://www.aaa.com/vacation/idpf.html

National Automobile Club:
Go to http://www.thenac.com/idp_faqs.htm

Finding Employment on the Road

(caretaking positions, seasonal volunteer and paid camp ground hosting)

Caretaking positions involve, "being responsible for taking care of a property for trade or financial compensation, and sometimes in exchange for rent-free living accommodations."

-- Wikipedia Free Dictionary

For the many retirees on the road who are passionate about travel opportunities, there are some excellent resources geared toward helping you find work on the road or in a unique location. Some RVer's find they can live on their assets and maintain a primary residence to return to when they no longer wish to travel. Others will be self-employed, taking their work with them on the road or they will look for employment to supplement their income as they travel. They will discover a world of volunteer and paid job opportunities on the road. For some volunteer positions retirees must provide their own RV or mobile home; other positions provide free on-site housing or camping and utilities in exchange for light services. Some jobs provide the above with wages and greater work responsibilities. There are several websites and magazines designed to help retirees and people who love to travel find part-time and full-time jobs, nationally and internationally.

The Caretaker Gazette, first published in 1983, lists caretaking opportunities all over the world ranging from volunteer park hosts positions, such as caretaking at a 70-acre ranch in Arizona, a cattle station in Australia, or at a resort on Vancouver Island, Canada. Other opportunities might include working as a property manager in Minnesota, or as a house-sitter on the island of Rhodes in Greece. Some of these positions offer a place to stay; others require you to provide your own portable home. Some positions last a few weeks; others continue several months to a year. Additional opportunities include apprenticeships or internships where you can learn to run an inn or an organic farm. Some of the caretaking positions can become the adventure of a lifetime. For those wishing to travel within the states, campground hosting can offer benefits to the volunteer host and to those paid to host at private campgrounds.

What types of responsibilities come with these jobs? Depending on the position, you can expect to work from 10 hours per week to 40 hours per week. Be prepared for a range of activities from landscaping and gardening, to feeding and watering animals, property maintenance and construction, basic housekeeping, snow removal, management services, and hosting.

One of the more unusual listings in The Caretaker Gazette *is an ad for a house sitter / cat sitter position on a converted 100-year old whaling ship berthed at a golf resort up the Santi River in the Malaysian jungle. Daily duties included checking the boat for leaks when it rains and monitoring the crew, in addition to watering plants and caring for the ship's cat.*

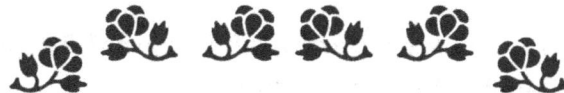

In WorkingCouples.com, an ad for an Estate Gardner/Housekeeper Couple reads:

A professional estate gardener needed for the management of a large, country property in Orange, Virginia. The property consists of an historic home and gardens, open fields and woods nestled along the Blue Ridge Mountains. Within the garden, there is an herb garden, terraced beds, foundation plantings, naturalized bulb plantings, vegetable garden, cut flower beds and a small orchard. Duties will include seasonal management of garden beds as well as scheduling day-to-day projects. These tasks include fruit and vegetable production, pruning of small trees and shrubs, pest and disease management, weeding, mulching, trimming, lawn care and flower arranging for the main house. Some experience in all of these areas is essential. Head gardener is also responsible for finding plants and supplies for seasonal plantings as well as new gardening beds. Must act as working supervisor to seasonal employees as well as coordinate and oversee work done on property by outside contractors. Competitive salary based on experience and paid vacation. Housing available. There is also an excellent opportunity for a couple to hold this position. In addition to the head gardener position, a housekeeper is needed to care of the main house.

Jobs for RVer's on the Move

- **Workampers**, a clearinghouse for jobs for RVers.
  Go to http://www.workamper.com/

- **Caretakers Gazette,** a clearinghouse for national and international jobs.
  Go to http://www.caretaker.org

- **Working Couples,** a website geared toward couples looking for job opportunities together.
  Go to http://www.WorkingCouples.com

- **National Park Service Temporary and Seasonal Employment**
  Go to http://www.nps.gov/personnel/seasonal.htm

- For a **listing of volunteer job opportunities in the National Parks,**
  Go to http://www.nps.gov/search/index.htm?page=1andquery=campground+ho st+jobs

- **Bureau of Land Management Seasonal Employment**
  Go to http://www.blm.gov/wo/st/en/res/blm_jobs.html

- **Recreation Resource Management** is a private company that operates campgrounds and other recreational facilities in National Forests and State Parks
  Go to http://www.camprrm.com/

- **United States Department of Agriculture:** For a listing of volunteer job opportunities and an application,
  Go to http://www.fs.usda.gov/volunteer

- **Recreation Resource Management:** For a listing of job opening and an application,
  Go to http://www.camphost.org/

Seasonal Job Opportunities for RVer's

"Somebody asked me the other day, "What do you do?" "I amuse myself by growing old," I replied. "It's a full-time job."-- Paul Leautaud (Journal litteraire)

Many people traveling the country in their home on wheels support themselves with their monthly income and some retirement assets. Others establish home businesses to supplement their income. At the end of this chapter, you will find more information on job opportunities for boomers, retirees, and the Greatest Generation

In Death Valley, down by the Racetrack, an open expanse of flat desert, rocks from the surrounding mountainsides, slide across the desert floor leaving trails in the dry surface. For an RVer with a photography business it is an ideal place to take unusual photographs. Joe and Rose started their photography business during their RV travels and now sell their photography on-line to supplement their income.

How to Get a Job as a Campground Host

Several magazines and publications list available jobs for people who love to travel or wish to stay in one place for an extended period. Hiring for many summer positions, such as campground hosts, begins in February and March. There is a job application that asks the usual questions – name, address, telephone, experience, and references. It asks what position you desire – camp host, interpretive services, store or marina work, or maintenance. It requests information on CPR and First Aid qualifications and training and may run or request a criminal, credit and reference check.

As these position usually do not have residences, you will need to supply information on the type of RV you will live in – is it a fifth wheel, travel trailer, or a motor home? Does it require utilities or is it self-contained? Some positions provide a vehicle, exclusively for your work duties, but not for personal purposes. If you use your own vehicle, you will need insurance coverage that meets that state's Department of Motor Vehicles requirements.

A classified advertisement in the Medford Mail Tribune (2011), Medford, Oregon newspaper read: "J. County Parks is seeking to fill three vacant Park Host positions at J. County Park. Light duty work in exchange for full service campsite. RV's or trailers must be visibly pleasing and no older than 1990 models. Background check required.

Volunteer Campground Host Positions

In exchange for 10–20 hours per week of work, collecting fees, assisting campers with questions or problems, retirees can find seasonal campground work through the State and county parks, National Park Service, National Forest Service, or the Bureau of Land Management. In some states, it is possible to obtain a campground lease for the low fee of $1. As the campground duties will vary depending on your location, is important to read the lease and know what your responsibilities are before committing yourself to being a campground host. Your duties can include visitor contacts and orientation, traffic control, light maintenance, and responsibility for the fees collection from campers at an entrance station, and interpretive services. The National Park Service sees, *"The goal of all interpretive services is to increase each visitor's enjoyment and understanding of the parks, and to allow visitors to care about the parks on their own terms."*

In exchange for volunteering as a campground host, you can receive a free campsite, usually in a highly visible location, often near the park or campground entrance, so campers can easily find it. Utilities (electric, water, sewer hook-up) and reimbursement for expenses related to campsite maintenance might also be included. For northern locations, the season usually runs from March through November; in the south, the season can be yearlong.

Richard, age 68 years, is the campground host at a county campground in Oregon. Recently retired on Social Security and a pension, he maintains a home with his wife in a nearby community. However, his love of the land and camping led him to lease a 66-acre campground from the county from April–November. Patrolling the grounds on his ATV, a portable oxygen tank hanging on the side and a plastic oxygen tube dangling from his nose, he makes contact with hikers, campers, and anyone interested in camping or renting one of the several cabins on the property. Living in his mobile home parked at the campsite, he spends his summer at the campground, returning to town for supplies and family visits. He works with the county and also with the Bureau of Land Reclamation if major repairs at the campground are necessary.

Paid Campground Host Positions

Private companies or government entities such as a county, state, or federal agency, operate most paid campground host positions. In exchange for free on-site RV camping (usually located in a central well-marked area) and utilities, paid hosts also receive a small wage for their work. The workweek can be up to 40 hours per week and include more responsibilities than a volunteer position. Duties can include light maintenance, restroom and shelter cleaning, trash pick-up, grounds maintenance and upkeep, cleaning up campfire rings, minor repairs, fee collection, and regulation enforcement. A Park Ranger or Sheriff Deputy is available for back up if there is a dangerous or threatening incident that requires assistance from law enforcement. Collection of data, managing reservations, and maintaining account information and records for the Forest Service can also be required.

More job websites are listed at the end of this section under *Employment and Volunteer Opportunities for Older Workers.*

At Home on the Water

(houseboats, floating homes and eco-sea cottages, live-aboard power cruisers and yachts, passenger cruise ships, luxury residential ocean liners, world-traveling freighters)

"Twenty years from now you will be more disappointed by the things you didn't do than by the ones you did do. So throw off the bowlines, sail away from the safe harbor. Catch the trade winds in your sails. Explore. Dream. Discover."

-- Mark Twain

The active boomer seeking a new and adventurous way to live and travel during his/her retirement years may opt to live in a home on the water. You may enjoy becoming part of a houseboat, floating home, eco-sea cottage or live-aboard yacht community on a river, bay, lake, or harbor. You may be tempted to book back-to-back cruises on a passenger cruise ship or luxury residential ocean liner for an extended period. You may seek adventure by living on a world-traveling freighter, traveling from port-to-port, wherever the ship schedule takes it. When you consider living in a home on the water, you will find that some options are more realistic for you than others. Explore the possibilities.

- **Houseboats, Floating Homes, and Eco-Sea Cottages** are floating dwellings with utilities, permanently stationed, or tied to moorings on an inland lake, a river, a salt-water port or a secluded bay.

- **Live-Aboard Yachts and Power Cruisers** are power propelled or sailing boats designed for long-distance travel.

- **Passenger Cruise Ships** are passenger ships or "floating hotels" used for pleasure voyages. Passengers can usually use canes, walkers, and wheelchairs on these ships, although there can be some limitation with access to parts of the ship or ports-of-call. These cruise ships offer short trips and longer trans-ocean voyages. You can often book passages back-to back for longer trips, taking advantage of many discounts offered by the cruise lines.

- **Residential Luxury Ocean Liners** are the more expensive and opulent passenger ships that take longer, often round-the-world cruises. Although many of these residential ships are quite expensive, some offer fractional ownership plans that allow you to travel on the ship for 2 weeks or more per year. At this time, The World of ResidenSea offers cruise ship condominium living; several other cruise ship condominiums are in development.

- **Freighters** are working commercial cargo ships that take a few passengers as they travel from port-to-port. For the active and healthy retiree with a flexible schedule, it is an inexpensive way to travel the world.

Houseboats, Floating Homes, and Eco–Sea Cottages

"I feel like I'm always on holiday."
-- Houseboat owner, Lake Union, Kentucky

Although I always thought that slowly cruising across a pristine lake in a houseboat as an excellent way to spend a family vacation, I never considered what it would be like to live aboard a houseboat full-time. Yet, there are communities of people permanently living on their boats by inland lakes, calm river ways, salt-water ports, and on secluded bays.

There is a difference between a houseboat and a floating home: a **houseboat** has an engine and can travel to other locations. Permanently stationed in one location and tied to either a mooring or a wet slip, it connects to land-based services, including water, sewage, electricity, gas, telephone, and cable television. A **floating home** sits in a permanent berth, has no self-propulsion, and is connected to all utilities and land-based services. It is subject to property taxes. Houseboats and floating homes can sit on airtight pontoons or twin hull catamarans. Similar to a modest-size apartment they can be as large as a mansion or as small as a cottage. They have all the home essentials - a galley or kitchen, a head or toilet, a berth or bedroom. Larger houseboats can have offices, a dining area, family room, deck or patio, a spa, and more. They do not have attached garages, attics, or lawns. There is a hierarchal system for floating homes. At the top of the tier are the homes described above with connected services. Older models are more often closer to the water on cedar logs, Ferro cement or Styrofoam floats. The lower end floating homes are old school barges which sit on hulls, lack engines and sewage systems, depending instead on holding tanks. Referred to as aquatic RV's, they need to be towed from one location to another.

Economically priced, **Eco-sea cottages** are mini-luxury homes set on rugged catamaran hulls that can be transported short distances on flat water.

Eco-Sea Cottages:
Go to http://www.eco-seacottage.com/
Tele: 1-877-WE-R-CATS

The Floating Neighborhood

"It's like living in a college dormitory. You have your own space and whatever you need is down the hallway (or dock.)" --Houseboat owner, Sausalito, CA

The neighborhood is the dock at which the boat lies and your neighbors are the other people living on boats and floating homes around you. Neighbors look out for neighbors. Neighbors stop by in their boats; fishing is outside your door; kayaking means lowering your boat into the water; sunrises and sunsets are enjoyed on your deck, and dock parties may complement the feeling of a neighborhood.

There are implicit rules for those living on houseboats such as no construction noise before 8 a.m., no loud parties late at night, and averting your eyes from your neighbor's windows and decks to give them privacy. Still, as you are living close to your neighbors, be prepared to overhear music, personal moments, conversations, and arguments.

Is Living on a Floating Home Right for You?

Although living on a houseboat or floating home is ideal for some people, it is not for everyone. For people with motion sickness, the constant movement of a boat on the water may be enough to make you queasy. On the smaller houseboat, expect cramped living space. It is essential to be very organized and uncluttered. Belongings need to be in a secure setting so they do not move around during tidal surges or storms. You should be able to climb ladders, stairs and walk on a slightly moving and uneven surface. You should be able to conserve water or be ready to re-fill your water tank continuously. You should be aware of how the tides or currents affect the water around your boat. Maintenance is comparable to a land-based home, but different. Your boat may need painting twice as often; it is necessary to check for cracks and leaks. In the fall, it will be necessary to winterize your boat. You will clean the windows at least once a year. You will need to check the mooring lines constantly. If you plan to take the boat into open water, be sure your engine and boat maintenance is up-to-date.

SeattleCondo.com:
Go to http://www.seattlecondo.com/houseboats

Seattle Afloat:
For information about the houseboat and floating home communities around Seattle, WA. Go to http://www.seattleafloat.com/

OurSausalito.com
Presents information about living on a houseboat.
Go to http://www.oursausalito.com/houseboats-in-sausalito.html

The Gangplank on the Potomac:
A floating home community and marina located in Washington D.C.
Go to http://www.gangplank.com/

Floating Home Economics

The cost of the floating home has a wide range. Initial purchase cost can be as low as $60,000 and as high as one million dollars, depending on the size of the boat, where it is located, and the boat's condition. There is a fee for moorage rental, wet slips, dry storage in the winter, and sometimes homeowner association, cooperative, or condominium fees. If you decide to transfer your boat to another location, you may encounter transfer costs. Owners pay property taxes and berth fees.

If you decide to purchase an economical eco-sea cottage, the prices may range from $110 K to $249 K*. These homes built on catamaran hulls are primarily designed for flat-water conditions and not for rough weather or water. When equipped with an optional twin motor and helm, they can travel 4–6 knots. *prices are subject to change.*

Floating Home Insurance

You must purchase insurance to cover any claims or losses on your floating home. As anyone who has purchased insurance knows, there are many aspects to insurance coverage. You can insure your floating home for actual cash value that will pay at the time of loss or claim, less depreciation or an agreed amount value that is predetermined and includes the value of the hull, and attached equipment and hardware. Research insurance brokers and the coverage they offer. The insurance should cover perils of the sea (excluding tidal waves), fire, wind, hail, lightening, aircraft damage, riot and vehicle damage, explosion, smoke, vandalism, malicious mischief, theft, accidental discharge or overflow from plumbing, sinking, damage to watercraft or floatation devices and reimbursement for alternative housing while your floating home is being repaired.

Red Shield Insurance Company Floating Home Insurance
Go to http://www.redshield.com/floating.html / Tele: 1-800-527-7397

Floating Home Insurance
Article by Ron Moreland, March 2010 has an insurance coverage comparison chart. Go to http://www.floatinghomes.org/insarticle.htm

---

Finding a Floating Home Community

Floating home communities are located throughout the United States and overseas. In Sausalito, California, there are five marinas with beautiful views of the mountains, the waterfront and San Francisco Bay. Over 400 floating homes adorn the waterfront with flower boxes and garden benches. By Portage Bay and Lake Union near Seattle, Washington, 500 legal floating homes with moorages remain, down from their high of several thousand following World War II. On Lake Erie, the Lakefront Marina in Port Clinton, Ohio offers thirteen modern 400 square foot floating homes with large decks for $80,000 each. Residents have the use of the marina facilities that includes security, paved parking, and a pavilion with propane grills, a community room, and an in-ground heated swimming pool.

Floating Homes Association in Sausalito, CA:
Go to http://www.floatinghomes.org

Seattle Floating Homes Association:
Go to http://www.seattlefloatinghomes.org/

Lakefront Marina, Port Clinton, Ohio:
Go to http://www.lakefrontmarina.com/Amenities/FloatingHomes/
tabid/910/Default.aspx

Live-Aboard Yachts and Power Cruisers

(cruisers or power yachts and luxury, super and mega yachts)

"If you have to ask how much it costs, you can't afford it."

-- Commodore J. Pierport Morgan

The idea of living aboard a yacht anchored in a calm harbor or settled in a harbor slip appeals to many people. There are many types of yachts, some of which are appropriate for live-aboard and long distance travel; others are more appropriate for day or weekend cruising. *Wikipedia* splits yachts into 5 categories: day cruiser yachts, weekender yachts, cruising yachts, sport fishing yachts, and luxury yachts. This section focuses on live-aboard cruising and luxury-plus yachts. If you are exploring the possibility of living aboard a cruising or luxury yacht, it is important to be comfortable with all the aspects of living in a home on the water. Broad knowledge of sailing, ocean currents, GPS navigation, radar, and general boat maintenance and repairs, on land and at sea is necessary.

A **cruising or power yacht** is a recreational boat or watercraft, usually propelled by sails or a power motor. Cruising yachts are usually at least 46-feet long, designed for on-board comfort and easy handling in the water. Designed with a wide flat bottom and a deep single fin keel, they maintain stability on the water. Typically, they have a single mast with a single foresail jib or Genoa and a single main sail. Sometimes an additional sail called a spinnaker is unfurled for down-wind sailing. Many are equipped with GPS navigation systems, radar, echo sounding devices and an autopilot control. A dinghy for moving back and forth across the water and for emergencies at sea is a necessity. Some dinghies are lowered by hand into the ocean; others are pulled behind the boat, and some have a motorized system for raising and lowering the dinghy.

Luxury yachts can be 82-feet or longer and designed with fiberglass hulls. Super or mega yachts can reach over 200-feet in length. They may have an automated and computer-controlled navigation system, an electric-powered winch for raising and lowering sails (instead of raising and lowering sails by hand), and a sophisticated power generation system, helipads, and more. A crew is often necessary to operate a yacht of this size.

You can live aboard a cruising yacht anchored in a calm harbor, settled into a harbor slip at a dock, or while sailing or cruising at sea. Performing necessary maintenance and repairs such as fixing leaks and varnishing wood is easier when the boat is not underway in open water. When it is more land-based, it is easier to move about the boat and go to a store for tools, parts and supplies. It is easy to clean laundry, shop for groceries, and even work a land-based job. As some harbors do not allow long- term live-aboard, be sure to check with the harbormaster about the harbor policies.

Cruising boats offer many amenities: electric lighting, hot water, a head (toilet), a hot water shower room, a galley (kitchen), a sitting area that can also serve as a sleeping area, berths (bedrooms) at the bow and the stern of the boat. Some yachts may include televisions, air conditioning, electric refrigeration (not an ice-based system), propane cooking, a BBQ, and Internet and cell phone reception. You may find some sport fishing set-ups on these boats as well. Super or mega yacht amenities can include helicopter pads, swimming pools, gymnasium, granite kitchen countertops, Jacuzzi tubs, and more.

There is a wide variance in the cost of owning a power cruiser or luxury yacht. Although you may have no yearly taxes to pay, you will pay for dock fees, boat insurance, maintenance, and lodging (if you don't have a second home) when repairs are needed that necessitate you temporarily living off the boat.

If you are seriously considering purchasing a power cruiser or a yacht, many boat owners recommend starting out with a private charter with an experienced crew to sample yachting. Chartering a yacht as a bare-boat (you are the crew) or with a captain (you pay for the expertise of the captain and crew and may have a chance to learn about sailing a yacht or cruiser) has a fixed cost and a minimal time commitment. Talking with local marinas, yacht brokers, yacht owners, and joining a private yacht club can provide useful information.

If this experience is positive and you remain interested in purchasing your own yacht, there are many yacht brokers available to help you gather information on potential sales. It is important to look at the age of the vessel, its condition, the make of the yacht, the length, and amenities. Is the engine noise loud when the boat is cruising? Does it feel stable and comfortable? How much time do you plan to be on board the yacht? Could you live on the yacht for a few weeks, a month, or a year? What type of weather should you expect? Will it necessitate you changing your home base? How often? Do you plan on hiring a crew or sailing by yourself or with a minimal help? Look carefully at the operating costs. What are the dock fees? How much will fuel cost? What is the cost of the crew's salary? What are the costs for food and water? What are the costs for boat insurance? How much should you expect to pay for general but necessary maintenance and repairs? What should you save in reserves for unexpected costs?

Overall, the estimated cost of owning and maintaining a yacht is approximately 10% of the initial purchase ce of a new boat. If you purchase a used yacht, expect to pay 10% of the replacement value. Some yacht owners warn that maintaining a super yacht can be very expensive.

An On-line Yachting Magazine with Yacht Forums:
Go to http://www.yachtforums.com/forums/

Yacht Clubs of the World:
Go to http://www.yachtclub.com/

Yacht Club of America:
Go to http://www.ycaol.com/

Yachting Magazine.com:
Go to http://www.yachtingmagazine.com/

If you decide to live aboard a yacht or power cruiser, you will meet many people who also love the ocean and the lifestyle of living aboard a boat. Each time you sail or cruise, you will experience new adventures, sweeping panoramas and scenery, and the freedom of the seas. You may find living on a boat relaxing and comfortable and a time for reflection. You may enjoy the shift from yard work in a land-based home to boat work involving repairs and maintenance such as, polishing, painting, and varnishing the wood. Many super and mega boats designed for business are equipped for conference calling, email, and Internet access even while at sea.

For some, living aboard a boat may seem confining and cramped. On a smaller boat, the distance from the bow to stern is 40+ feet. On a super or mega yacht, there is more room to walk, but it is still limited. You may miss puttering in a yard with flowers, grass, and trees. You may not enjoy the steady demand for boat maintenance. Living part of the time in a harbor slip with neighbors in close proximity may not appeal to you. You may feel that you are too far away and unavailable for family and friends. On a larger yacht, a crew may be necessary. The cost for purchasing and maintaining a yacht can be very expensive. Living on the water or at sea may not be for everyone. Some people experience bouts of seasickness much of the time they are traveling across the ocean. You will need to be prepared for inclement weather. Still, if you are interested in pursuing life aboard a yacht, there are many informative websites to get you started.

Living on the Sea

(passenger cruise ship lines, residential luxury ships, world-traveling freighters)

For people who are active, independent with their activities of daily life, and comfortable with continuous travel, living on a cruise ship or freighter can be an option. While cost may be a primary consideration, think through the other aspects of living a life at sea. If you live on a cruise ship or freighter that is sailing the world, constantly moving from port-to-port you may feel a sense of adventure. The ship becomes your home as you spend your days with other passengers and crew. You may become engaged in on-board activities and develop friendships with other passengers. You may feel content and relaxed and enjoy the good food, camaraderie, and travel. Or you may find that living on a ship or freighter feels more transitory and not really like home. You are living with strangers instead of friends and family; friendships made on a cruise ship can be short-lived. You may feel isolated from your family and friends. Crew, although attentive, are working a job and it is unlikely that long-lasting friendships will develop. The accommodations can seem small and confining if you are not in one of the elegant suites. You may miss the familiarity of items such as family pictures from your home. Engine noise can run 24-hours a day eliminating quiet times. The atmosphere on board can include loud parties and noise from the bars, restaurants, and clubs. There is not a curfew for that allows for quiet time. Still, the memories during your adventure at sea will stay with you through the years.

Passenger Cruise Ship Lines

"My soul is full of longing for the secret of the sea, and the heart of the great ocean sends a thrilling pulse through me."

-- *Henry Wadsworth Longfellow*

There are many commercial cruise ships lines - Carnival, Cunard, Royal Caribbean, Holland America, Windstar, and Princess - to name a few.

To arrange a lengthy voyage, it is necessary to find a ship that travels the world. In 2010, Cunard offered 101-day world cruises aboard the Queen Mary 2 from New York, across the Atlantic Ocean to ports in England, and Portugal. It cruised the Strait of Gibraltar and the Mediterranean Sea, transited the Suez Canal, crossed the Red Sea and the Arabian Sea, stopping in Dubai, United Arab Emirates. Before crossing the Pacific Ocean on its return to New York, it sailed the Indian Ocean with ports-of-call in Indonesia, Hong Kong, China and Japan. The cost without any discounts, staying in a standard ocean view room was about $300 per day per person or $8500/month.

Early booking can save 10% and often, additional discounts and upgrades are available. In addition, full-world cruises offer on-board credits up to $2000 per stateroom for use at the spa, drinks in the bars and lounges, or dining in the specialty restaurants. Fares are based on double occupancy, cruise only and exclude air, air taxes, and transfers, government fees and taxes, fuel supplement, optional travel protection, and incidental charges.

Passengers with disabilities are welcome aboard the ship. Although people using walkers, wheelchairs or with vision impairment can find it difficult to access certain areas and disembark at some ports-of-call, the ships try to accommodate these passengers. They may recommend a hired companion to help on the ship. Notify the cruise ship at the time of booking if you require a service dog. These animals may not be able to disembark at certain ports and countries.

For passengers with ongoing medical conditions, the ship can request a confidential medical certification from their physician. Medical facilities on board are primarily to treat illnesses and accidents, not ongoing pre-existing medical conditions. You can also request special dietary meals at the time of booking.

Frank, age 90, and his 80+ year old wife decided to take a short cruise to Mexico. A friend joined them to provide extra support and assistance. Although Frank used a walker and a power scooter, he negotiated the hallways and dining room, and easily moved about in their handicapped accessible stateroom. When Frank became ill with an intestinal bug, the ship's physician prescribed medication and requested that he stay in the cabin until he was well. The physician and his nurse closely monitored Frank's medical condition. However, Frank's condition deteriorated and at a port-of-call, the ship personnel transported him to a land-based hospital for continued medical care. After receiving treatment, Frank and his wife were able to fly back to the United States with most of their expenses covered by their trip insurance.

Living Full-time on a Passenger Cruise Ship

In 1995, Robert and Beatrice Muller, a couple in their 70's and 80's, embarked on a romantic world cruise aboard Cunard's Queen Elizabeth 2. For four years, they traveled the world until Mr. Muller succumbed to ill health in 1999 and passed away aboard the QE2. Shortly after his passing, Mrs. Muller sold her primary home and belongings and signed on to the QE 2 for a yearlong cruise as a permanent resident.

Aboard the QE 2, Mrs. Muller lived in a small cabin with a closet-sized private bathroom along with her personal belongings, family photographs, a small stereo, and a color television. Gourmet meals were included in the price of the cabin. She had access to all the on-board amenities and activities. In addition, she continued to travel the world instead of settling into a land-based private home, moving in with her family or to a retirement community, assisted living facility or nursing home.

While some aspects of this story circulated on the Internet are folklore, *Snopes.com*, a website that sniffs out facts from fiction, reports that Mrs. Muller did not buy a yearly or monthly pass, but instead booked her cruises one at a time. Adding up her accrued frequent traveler discounts, her cost was comparable to living in an assisted living facility or a retirement or nursing home charging $5000/month. (Costs are probably higher now, than reported in 2004.) Her accommodations were not luxurious, but cramped quarters in a small and windowless room. Hallways and cabins were accessible with a cane, wheelchair or walker. With the price of the cruise, Mrs. Muller received full-time house cleaner and laundry services, three gourmet meals daily in the numerous dining rooms, access to medical care and physicians in the ship's medical center, a health spa, beauty salon, and computer center and a long list of social activities including lectures, live entertainment, cultural activities, dancing, and bridge.

Cruise Hopping

Cruise hopping involves setting up a series of cruises back-to-back. Costs are estimated at $100 per day per person. You may want to discuss the necessary scheduling with an experienced travel cruise specialist.

Discount Cruising

As cruise ships are always seeking repeat and first-time passengers, many offer discounts and promotions that lower the cost of a cruise. The term, "Cheap Cruise," indicates a fare that can be purchased below book rate, the price published in the cruise line catalogs. Reduced group rates are also available. Some cruise lines offer discounts for people 55+. On the other hand, your travel agent may offer to reduce their level of commission. When comparing fares, be sure you are looking at all costs – taxes, port charges, and fees – not just the cost of the cruise. For more information on discount cruises, type *"discount cruises"* into any Internet search engine.

Residential Luxury Ships at Sea

In 2002, Residensea launched a residential luxury cruise ship, *The World*, a 644-foot luxury ocean liner that continues to journey across the ocean. Created by Knut U. Kloster Jr. and designed by Petter Yran and Bjorn Storbraaten, it as an environmentally-friendly ship that boasts the use of marine diesel instead of heavy bunker fuel and a green waste-water cleaning system. On-board, *The World* offers luxurious rooms, stylish amenities and services, elegant dining, top entertainment, high-tech medical facilities, and world travel. Expect all the bells and whistles – cigar lounge, boutiques, salons, fitness centers, yoga classes, jogging trails, multiple pools, tennis, racquetball and basketball courts, entertainment, travel to other ports, and more.

The 12-decked *World* offers 165 private on-board residences ranging from a 337- square foot studio to an 8375 square foot 6-bedroom penthouse suite. In between, you can choose from 674-1011 square foot 1 to 2-bedroom apartments and 1758 square foot 3-bedroom apartments. Each apartment is fully furnished and equipped with a kitchenette or full-size kitchen, sitting areas, and private verandas. Privately owned by the residents of *The World*, the 130 families from 19 countries plan the itinerary for the year. An average length of stay on the ship is 4-months.

In 2011, with 150–200 residents and a crew and hospitality personnel of 250, *The World* traveled to the Antarctic, through the Chilean fjords, up the South American coast, through the Panama Canal, into the Caribbean to the east coast city of New York. From there it is cruising across the Atlantic Ocean to Western and Northern Europe, into the Mediterranean, across to Turkey, Africa, the Seychelles, and ending in Capetown, South Africa. It visits 53 countries and averages 2.5 days in the ports-of-call. Sightseeing and on-shore excursions are available.

The resident/owners on *The World* are able to enjoy on board luxuries and experience fine dining in a selection of restaurants with a selection of international wines. For entertainment, select from cultural performances, music and dancing, movie theaters, and a library. For those looking for physical activity, head to the on-board bowling alley, golf simulator, a fitness center, sports courts for tennis, racquetball, and basketball, and swimming in a choice of pools. Or shop in a 250,000 square foot complex with an art gallery, grocery shopping in a 150,000 square foot store complete with bakery, delicatessen, and fresh produce. Spoil yourself in a full service spa facility with massage, facials, waxing and hair treatments. For residents preferring meals in their apartment, they can cook for themselves or use the Call-a-Chef ™ program and request a chef to cook a meal in their residence. Housekeeping and laundry services are also available. A chapel is open for worship. If medical needs arise, a 120,000 square foot hospital is located on the ship, complete with x-ray and emergency services capability and staffed 24-hours a day with medical personnel. Some cruise ships allow residents to bring very small pets. It is always best to inquire about the pet policy when you are considering living on a residential cruise ship.

The World, a Residential Condominium Ship:
Go to http://www.aboardtheworld.com/

Ownership Programs

As the economy recovers from the recent recession, some residential ships are establishing programs operated, managed, and maintained by an independent ship management company where you can buy a cabin now and rent it until you retire, eliminating the purchase payment and monthly resident's care fee until you actually move into your home at sea. Be aware that some ships postpone their launch dates and others will not launch at all. If you decide to pursue living on a residential ship be sure that it is in a solid financial position.

You can purchase full ownership in a residential cruise ship that circumnavigates the world. You could buy a basic cabin, a suite, a stateroom, a villa, or a resort residence and then rent it. The person you rent to must pass a security clearance, necessary to protect all residents and guests. Or you could purchase fractional ownership which gives the owner a share of the ownership for a fraction of the year. Essentially, you share the investment with others who have a similar desire to have an additional residence and plan to use it as part of their retirement or as a vacation home. Most residential cruise ships suggest that you speak with an attorney and a certified accountant before purchasing a share. The cost of living on-board a land-based condominium resort residential ocean liner will depend upon what services, utilities, and meals you actually use. It may be possible to short-term rent for a week or more. Many potential residential cruise ships failed to launch or are planning to launch in the future.

World-traveling Freighters

"If you have the time to relax and a cruising spirit, a friendly freighter waits for you."

-- *Motto of Freighter World Cruises*

If the idea of living on the water is appealing to you consider spending part of the year on a cargo ship or freighter, *"any sort of ship or vessel that carries cargo, goods, and materials from one port to another."*(Wikipedia) Booking passage on a multi-purpose passenger/cargo vessel is an informal way to see the world. It is a slower way to travel the world; one day of travel on a ship is equivalent to one hour of air travel. Although you may not travel in luxury, it is affordable, accommodations are clean and simple, amenities are few, companionship is with the other passengers and the crew and officers and the itinerary is flexible. In addition, this way of travel is comparable to the cost of living in a retirement community or assisted living facility.

Compared to a typical cruise ship, freighters are less crowded, have fewer passengers, and are more casual, informal, and a cheaper alternative. Passengers must be extremely flexible as these working ships often have unexpected changes in their schedules or extended waits between sailings. They may have no set itinerary. Boarding dates can change. Ports of call can cancel or be added en-route. On ships designed for passengers and cargo service, port times can extend 1- 3 days, longer than the time allowed for fully containerized ships. There is more time to visit exotic destinations and spend time on shore exploring other countries. Crews on freighters tend to be much smaller than on the larger cruise ships. In the event of an emergency on the ship, all able-bodied persons assist.

Routes and Destinations

Destinations are dependent on the ship line and the cargo it carries. There are new regulations for international ocean freight to prevent the spread of plant pests and disease to other parts of the world. Ships must fumigate or heat treat any wood products such as pallets, crates, dunnage or padding, drums, and wood cases. Some ships depart from various cities in Europe and travel to Southeast Asia, China, Korea, Japan, and then across the Pacific to the United States Gulf and Eastern coasts before returning to Europe. Additional ports-of-call and destinations include India, Indonesia, Thailand, Vietnam, and Taiwan, the Caribbean, South Pacific, Far East, Australia, New Zealand, and passage through the Panama Canal to South America.

Rickmer's Pearl String Around-the World service operates 9 passenger/cargo ships with international crews, each carrying up to 7 passengers for a 126-day cruise. These are multi-purpose heavy lift vessels which speed across the ocean at 19.5 knots and carry over 29,000 tons of cargo. There is no way to know in advance what cargo is on board or what cargo will be picked up en-route.

Passenger Requirements

Traveling on a freighter is only for passengers in good health who are also independent walkers. As a passenger, be prepared for steep gangplanks and stairways between the decks. These cargo vessels are working ships and do not permit assistive devices such as canes, walkers, and wheelchairs. Depending on the ship line, passengers can be as young as 13-years and as old as 79-years. For older passengers, a medical certificate stating you are in good physical health is required from your physician 90-days prior to sailing. Passports and visas are required.

Baggage and Vehicles

Each passenger can bring up to 200-pounds of hand-carried baggage. Check with the shipping line regarding their specific baggage rules. Vehicles such as passenger cars or motorcycles ship as freight. Check with the shipping line about their policy on personal vehicles.

The Physical Layout

These are working cargo ships with 4-6 decks and steep angled gangways and stairways. If there is an elevator, it may not be usable during rough seas. Stacks of containers ranging from 2-40 feet across can be stacked as high as 10-stories on the ship. In addition to the working and storage areas of the ship, there may be a small outdoor pool, an officer's and crew's mess room, a recreation area with a bar, games, VCR and DVD players, and a small library area.

Accommodations

Lodging on a freighter is not as luxurious as what you might find aboard a passenger cruise ship. Expect an air-conditioned single room, a double room, or a small suite, all with private bath and outside windows. The room sizes range from a 322-square foot suite to a 194-square foot double room to a 161-square foot single room. Room sizes will vary dependent on the ship. Most rooms are designed with an outside window; the higher the room on the ship, the more likely you will have a view unobstructed by containers. A weekly change of linens is usually included.

Medical Facilities

Freighters are not equipped with comprehensive medical facilities. If there are less than 12 passengers onboard, a physician is not required. For medical emergencies, the ship will travel to the nearest port of call and drop the passenger off to ensure that they receive proper medical care. The mandatory emergency medical insurance plays an important role here. Vaccinations and inoculations are required prior to travel. The shipping line will notify you of the itinerary so that you can receive the proper shots before you embark.

Amenities

Aboard a freighter, there are few amenities. With the Captain's permission, you may have access to the bridge and receive a tour of the engine room. You can enjoy the company of the crew and officers. You can access a small library, a DVD and VCR, recreation area, and a small pool. No entertainment, no television, no radio (except short wave), and no internet services are provided. Self-service laundry service is available. Overseas mail can take over two-weeks for delivery.

Booking Your Voyage

Specialized freighter agents are available to arrange travel aboard a freighter. Some people will book back-to-back voyages with stopovers; others will travel round trip on the same ship. It is standard to arrange booking 3-6 months in advance, but voyages can be reserved up to a year in advance. Bookings are not accepted less than one month before departure. Some shipping lines will offer discounts for advance bookings. Prior to departure, a signed contract stating that you understand the terms and contracts of the shipping line is required.

Booking Freighter Agents

The Cruise People, Ltd.:
For information of ultra-luxury cruises, small ships, freighters, and round-the-world or longer voyages,
Go to http://www.cruisepeople.co.uk/freighters.htm and
Go to http://thecruisepeople.wordpress.com/tag/rickmers-pearl-string/

FreighterCruises.com:
Go to https://www.freightercruises.com/

Internet Guide to Freighter Travel:
Go to http://www.geocities.com/freighterman.geo/mainmenu.html

---

Looking at Cost

When you book an extended trip, you will receive an offer of space. At this time, a $500 deposit will be required.* Shorter trips may entail a smaller deposit fee. Final payment is due six-ten weeks before the ship sails. Expect to pay-in-full if you book within eight weeks of sailing. If you book early, discounts are often available. Be sure to check the shipping line's refund policy.

Extended trips on freighters cost is approximately $135 per day/per person. This includes accommodations, and meals. One shipping line offered roundtrip fares for 124- days for a double room at $13,020 and a single room at $15,675.

Additional fees include port taxes and deviation insurance of $563 per person and $12.50 for United States Customs and Immigration fees for passengers disembarking in the United States. Total cost is close to $3750 per month, a small figure when compared to the fee Bea Muller paid to live on the Queen Elizabeth 2.* (*These cost figures are approximate and will fluctuate with the various shipping lines.)

Required Insurances

(deviation, emergency passenger medical and evacuation, and trip cancellation insurance)

There are two types of required insurance. **Deviation insurance** protects the ship from changes to their itinerary due to any passenger related circumstance that forces the ship to change its schedule. This can occur if a passenger becomes ill or needs to reach a port not on the planned route. It is part of the fare cost. As the operating cost of the ship may be over $20,000 per day, this mandatory insurance is essential to the ship. **Emergency passenger medical and evacuation insurance** is also mandatory. This insurance will cover medical costs in foreign ports and the cost of transporting a passenger to a country with good medical care.

Optional and recommended insurance is **trip cancellation or interruption insurance** that reimburses the full or a partial amount of your cost if you need to cancel your trip for any reason.

If you are seriously thinking about traveling the world on a freighter, review the information on-line and call one of the freighter-booking agents to get answers to your many questions. Certainly traveling by freighter is an adventure and any adventure works best when one is prepared with realistic expectations.

If you choose to experience a calmer and less adventurous home on the water, consider houseboats, floating homes, eco-sea cottages, live-aboard yachts, and passenger cruise ships.

Living and Working Overseas

"Travel is more than the seeing of sights; it is a change that goes on, deep and permanent, in the ideas of living."

-- *Miriam Beard*

A plethora of books exists for people interested in moving to another country. This section will discuss the basic information you need if you are contemplating a move from the United States to a foreign country Whether you decide to move overseas with the intent of being a full-time expatriate, a seasonal overseas resident, or a time-limited volunteer, it is important to be sensitive to the customs and culture where you reside. For information on living in a recreational vehicle overseas, refer to the section on *Taking to the Road in Your Recreational Vehicle.*

Becoming an Expatriate

"An expatriate (in abbreviated form, expat) is a person temporarily or permanently residing in a country and culture other than that of the person's upbringing or legal residence."

-- *Wikipedia*

There are many reasons why a person might decide to live abroad.

- you're retired and ready for a travel adventure;
- you're a baby boomer who has worked hard, saved, watched your savings decline,and is now trying to decide whether to downsize, travel, or stay put;
- you're excited about traveling overseas;
- living in another culture promises to be new and different experience;
- you anticipate a lower cost of living and a slower or faster pace of life;
- you can save money on your daily living expenses and taxes;
- you previously visited the country and contemplated "moving there someday";
- a change of climate is important and you are thinking of settling in a country with warm weather;

- you struggle to pay for healthcare and find it is more affordable or free in another country;

- labor is inexpensive in another country and you can build your dream home.

The reasons for moving to another country are endless. The *American Association of Americans Residents Overseas (AARO),* a volunteer, non-partisan service organization estimates there are over 5.08 million Americans (excluding military personnel) living abroad in 160 countries. Countries with over 100,000 American residents include Australia, Canada, China, Dominican Republic, France, Germany, Greece, Israel and the West Bank, Italy, Mexico, Philippines, Spain, and the United Kingdom. For more information, go to http://www.aaro.org/

Looking at Your Expectations

Consider your expectations and feelings about living in a country that is very different from your home country.

- Are you seeking an adventure, a chance to live new and different life abroad?

- Are you moving without a plan, expectations, or adequate finances just to experience something new and different?

- Do you plan to retire abroad permanently?

- Are you planning to maintain your United States residence and spend some time abroad?

- Are you looking for a country with an established expatriate community?

- Is a warmer or colder climate desirable?

- Are you seeking a lower cost of living?

- Is access to good healthcare a requirement?

- Is it necessary for you to be able to speak the language?

- Are you planning to bring a pet?

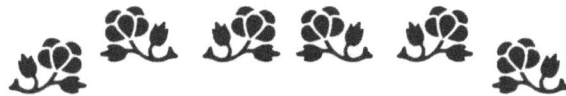

Many years ago, I drove to the coastal tourist city of Puerto Vallarta, Mexico. A mask collector, I found myself in a small store eyeing traditional Mexican masks. The owner was an expat who had lived there for over 10 years. While in the store, an elderly Mexican woman entered and requested a donation for one of the local schools. The owner of the store turned to me and said, "I don't speak Spanish. What is she saying?" I patiently explained that she was raising money for a school. As he waved her out of his store, he added, "I never wanted to learn the language and I don't like the food." I wondered to myself, "Why is he living here?"

The shop owner may have settled in Puerto Vallarta for any or none of these reasons: the beautiful surroundings and beaches, the warm climate, a lower cost of living, inexpensive labor, an array of up-scale shops, an opportunity to own his own business or the desire to live in a large expatriate community.

At Lake Chapala near Guadalajara, there is an established expatriate community with over 25,000 gringo retirees. Many Americans have lived there for years. Sit on a bench in the main plaza and you may see more expats than local Mexican residents. The area draws educated retirees looking for a slower pace of life and a lower cost of living. Many are willing to go without the modern conveniences they had access to in the states. Others are seasonal travelers, drawn to the warmer climate during the colder months.

International Living: This website includes many resources, articles on retirement in other countries, a quality of life index, a global retirement index, a subscription magazine, advice for expats, and more.
Go to http://www.internationalliving.com

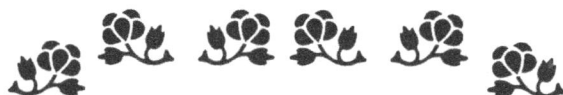

Choosing a Country to Live In

(customs and culture, political climate, language, location, transportation, climate, housing conveniences, food, finances, healthcare, family and friends, pets)

The world is your oyster. You can do or achieve anything you want in life as you have the ability, freedom, and opportunity to do so. You can decide to live in Central or South America, Europe, New Zealand, Australia, Southeast Asia, or a myriad of other countries.

It is important to research the countries you are considering, weighing what is essential for you to make a smooth transition into another culture. Consider the following:

- **Customs and Culture**: Are you content with the American way of life and hoping to recreate it in another country? Do you plan to research the customs and cultures of other countries or immerse yourself when you get there? Are you open to new customs and traditions, holidays, food, and a "local" way of life?

- **Political climate:** Is the country politically stable? Has the United States State Department released any recent travel advisories?

United States Department of State Home Page:
Go to http://www.state.gov

International Travel Section of the Bureau of Consular Affairs:
Go to http://www.travel.state.gov

- **Language:** Is it necessary for you to speak, read, and/or understand the language? If not, how will you communicate? Will you enroll in a language school? Will you "just pick up the language" as you go?

The Pimsleur Language Program:
Go to http://www.pimsleur.com/

Rosetta Stone:
Go to http://www.rosettastone.com

- **Location:** Is it difficult or easy to get to and from the United States? Is there an airport in a nearby city with reasonable air rates?

- **Transportation:** Are you planning to bring a car, bicycle, or motorcycle? Will you need a car for transportation? Would you consider buying a car in your new country? Would you need to learn how to drive a manual transmission or how to drive on the opposite side of the road? If you do not need a car or motorcycle, how do you feel about walking and using local transportation? Are bus and train services readily available?

- **Climate:** Are you moving for a change in climate? Have you considered becoming a "seasonal" retiree, spending several months at different locations throughout the year? Do you want a certain type of climate for health reasons?

- **Housing:** Are you looking for an established expat community? Are you hoping to immerse yourself in your new country? Can you afford to build a home? Do you plan to rent a home until you are sure moving to another country is the right choice? Have you researched the cost of housing and rules governing real estate in the countries you are considering?

- **Conveniences:** Are you content to live without modern conveniences if they are not available? Is it important to you to have ample amenities and services?

- **Food:** Do you love the food you now eat? Are you open to fresh culinary surprises? Do you have any religious or dietary restrictions that would be difficult to maintain in the country of your choice?

- **Finances:** Do you have sufficient income and assets to move to another country? Have you researched the rules for taxpayers living abroad?

Internal Revenue Service:
Go to http://www.irs.gov/businesses/small/international/index.html

- **Healthcare**: Are you in reasonable health? Do you have existing healthcare issues that will need medical follow-up? Are you concerned about receiving affordable healthcare services in a new country? Have you researched healthcare services in the countries you are considering a move to?

International Health Insurance

AARP International:
Go to http://www.aarp.org/intl

BUPA International:
Go to http://www.bupainternational.com

- **Family and friends:** Are you concerned about the distance from your family and friends? Is communication through the postal service, Internet and by telephone adequate for you to keep in touch?

- **Pets:** Do you have a pet that you plan to take with you to another country? Have you checked on the countries policies, restrictions, and quarantine requirements? Is it a pet-friendly country?

Getting Ready to Move Overseas

"Life might be difficult for a while, but I would tough it out because living in a foreign country is one of those things that everyone should try at least once. My understanding was that it completed a person, sanding down the rough provincial edges and transforming you into a citizen of the world."

-- David Sadaris

A move overseas is not as easy as buying a ticket, packing your suitcase, driving to the airport, and flying to your new home. It takes careful preparation as once you leave the country the distance between your new home and your home in the United States is vast. For a smooth transition, think about the following:

Home

- If you own your home, are you planning to rent or sell it?
- With the current slowed housing market, what is a reasonable time for you to place it on the market and sell it?
- Do you need to make essential home repairs to prepare it for the market or a renter?
- Can you afford to move before you rent or sell your home?
- Who will manage your rental property?
- Can you afford to pay your homes maintenance and yearly property taxes?
- Do you have plans to return to your home?
- Do you plan to purchase a home when you are living abroad?

Employment

- Do you plan to continue working?
- Can you perform your job overseas?
- Can you take a leave of absence from your current job?
- Are you interested in finding work abroad?
- Do you need to find work overseas to supplement your income?
- Will you need work documents that will permit you to work overseas?
- Do you know if it is difficult to obtain work in your new home country?

Income

- Do you have ample resources to fund the transition from your home country to living abroad?

- Have you considered how much income is necessary for you to live comfortably abroad?

- If you are maintaining your previous residence, have you estimated the monthly cost for utilities, repairs, taxes, no occupancy or rental income *(if you are renting),* or real estate management service fees?

- What is the cost of living in another country? What is the exchange rate with the U.S. dollar?

Healthcare

- Are you currently covered by healthcare insurance? If yes, can you continue to receive benefits if you live overseas? If no, what are your options for receiving healthcare benefits in your new country?

- Are you affected by any pre-existing conditions that require care from a specialist in your home country? Can you manage this condition as well overseas?

- If you take medication, can you receive this medication in your new country?

- Have you researched how to access to the healthcare system in your new country?

- How do you feel about the healthcare system in your new country? Do you feel it will meet your medical needs?

Communication

- Are you prepared to communicate with your family, friends, businesses, and others from another country? Will you miss face-to-face contact with your friends and family? How will you feel if there is an emergency and you and they are far away from one another?

- Do you plan to communicate via telephone, Internet e-mail or Skype, or snail mail?

- Will you bring your own computer (laptop) to enhance your ability to communicate?

- Will you bring a cell phone with the capacity to place international telephone calls?

- Is access to a home country newspaper important to you? Would you mind receiving your news online?

Newspapers Worldwide:
Go to http://www.onlinenewspapers.com

World Newspapers:
Go to http://www.world-newspapers.com

If you are interested in exploring living overseas, there are some excellent paperback and eBooks with detailed information about living in specific countries. In these books, the authors discuss the cost of living, health insurance, housing costs, realistic budgets, tax implications, reasons to go abroad or not to go abroad, checklists to help you determine what is important to you, and more.

Helpful Living Abroad Travel Books

The Moon Guide Living Abroad Series covers China, Italy, Guatemala, Spain, Japan, New Zealand, Panama, Costa Rica, Nicaragua, Belize, and more. Go to http://www.moon.com/books/moon-living-abroad

The Successful Expat: The Most Common Expat Mistakes and How to Avoid Them by Barbara Bruhwiler Kindle version, (Jun 28, 2012)

The Grown-ups Guide to Running Away From Home: Making a New Life Abroad by Roseann Knorr, Ten Speed Press, (03/01/2008)

How To Retire Overseas: Everything You Need to Know to Live Well (for less) Abroad by Kathleen Peddicord, Hudson Street Press, (03/29/2011)

Retirement Without Borders: How To Retire Abroad – in Mexico, France, Italy, Spain, Costa Rica, Panama, and Other Sunny Foreign Places (And the Secret to Making it Happen Without Stress) by Barry Golson, Scribner, (12/09/2008)

Employment and Volunteer Opportunities for Older Workers

"If my dreams could all come true, paradise/retirement would be - in a little bungalow- somewhere by the sea."

-- Unknown retired person

If you are not ready to pick up and move overseas, you may want to explore volunteering over an extended period. Throughout the world, there are volunteer and educational opportunities for boomers and retirees interested in other regions. By making a 6-month commitment you can get a feel for living abroad while contributing your skills to people in another country. Through a volunteer organization, you can immerse yourself in a new culture, customs, beliefs, and language firsthand. In this way, you can choose your country with clear and realistic expectations.

The Internet has made it easier for everyone to search for employment on-line. Some websites, may charge a nominal fee for their services; others are free of charge. Many offer help with resume writing, helpful articles, books, and magazines, and expert advice. These websites will help you locate flexible, temporary, full-time, part-time, and work at home jobs in your area of expertise or in a new and challenging career.

Many people over the age of 55 choose to continue working for different reasons: to supplement their income, to increase socialization, to stay actively engaged in a changing world, to find a new career path or continue on an old career path. Studies have shown that those who continue working as they age have improved health, increased mental capacity, and an improved quality of life.

Peace Corps Overseas Positions for U.S. Citizens:
Go to http://pcoverseasjobs.avuedigital.us/overseas-recruitment-process

2006 Essential Guide to the Peace Corps: Workbooks and Publications, Toolkits and Guides, Volunteering Overseas, Global Assignments, Benefits, Country Profiles, Cultural Information, (DVD-ROM, CD-ROM) by The Peace Corps. Available at Amazon.com

Become a Peace Corps Volunteer

"To promote world peace and friendship through a Peace Corps, which shall make available to interested countries and areas men and women of the United States qualified for service abroad and willing to serve, under conditions of hardship if necessary, to help the peoples of such countries and areas in meeting their needs for trained manpower."

-- Peace Corps Act, authorized by Congress on September 22, 1961

Established in 1961, The Peace Corps was a call to Americans to serve their country by promoting peace through living and working overseas in developing nations all over the world. Initially issued as a challenge by Senator John F. Kennedy to students at the University of Michigan, the program has provided over 200,000 volunteers in 139 countries. At this time, there are just under 9,000 volunteers serving in 77 countries. Although the average age is 28-years, 7 % of the volunteers are over age-50 and 7% are married.

Volunteers use their expertise in six program areas: education, youth and community development, health, business and information and communications technology, environment and agriculture. They work closely with government agencies, schools, entrepreneurs, non-profits, and community outreach programs, developing regional databases, encouraging and educating people about conservation and health.

Volunteers with the Peace Corps receive a pre-tax stipend of approximately $7425 after completing 3-months of training and 24-months of service. In addition, they receive free travel to and from their country of service, a monthly stipend living allowance for housing and living expenses, two vacation days per month, medical and dental care, and affordable healthcare insurance for up to 18-months following service.

How to Apply to Serve as a Volunteer in the Peace Corps

The Peace Corps may present an opportunity for you to live overseas if you are:

- 18-years of age or older (and retirees certainly are);

- have received an undergraduate education (although this is not required, over 93% of volunteers have a college education);

- can speak a foreign language fluently, have received two years foreign language experience or possess an affinity for learning language;

- are open to serving in a myriad of countries with different cultures and beliefs;

- are able to commit to 24-months of service.

The application process is multi-tiered and can take from 6 months to a year. It includes reference checks, medical and dental evaluations, an interview followed by a nomination, an evaluation by a Peace Corps placement officer, and lastly, an invitation to join the Peace Corps program.

Step 1 consists of completing the on-line application. To apply, go online to http://www.peacecorps.gov/learn/howvol/stepstoapply/

Applications are reviewed within two weeks or so. If you are a potential candidate, an interview is scheduled.

Step 2 consists of an interview with a Peace Corps recruiter who will discuss your work skills, personal interests, your social skills including flexibility, adaptability, cultural awareness, motivation, commitment, and more.

Step 3 consists of a nomination or recommendation that propels you to the next level of consideration. After nomination, you will complete a medical forms package that includes lab work and an exam by your physician and dentist, information about legal matters such as your marital and family status, financial obligations, and criminal history check. You can be disqualified, deferred, or have country limitations place on you at this time. If you meet the qualifications under the medical and legal guidelines, you advance to Step 4.

Step 4 consists of an invitation to join the Peace Corps. It provides detailed information about a specific country, a job description and assignment, a date of departure, and additional information. If you accept this invitation, you will receive further information about your host country and pre-service orientation information 2-3 months in advance of the start of your program.

Volunteers are employees of the Federal Government and with this status come Federal retirement, education, and employment benefits. Joining the Peace Corps and making a 2-year commitment is an excellent way to share your expertise and skills with a developing nation, an opportunity to experience living overseas while receiving a bit of income and some Federal benefits, medical and dental benefits, paid travel, housing costs and living expenses.

Federal Retirement Benefits:
Go to http://www.peacecorps.gov/index.cfm?shell=resources.returned.benefits.fedretire

Working Overseas Guide: A Guide for Staff and their Families: Look at bottom of page under Frequently Asked Questions and click on Working Overseas Guide

Go to http://www.peacecorps.gov/jobs/overseasop/countrydir/

Peace Corps Employment

If you are not interested in volunteering with the Peace Corps, there are time-limited opportunities to work as an employee of the Peace Corps. These positions are limited to a maximum of 5 years and include a housing allowance, and reasonable relocation expenses. These positions offer a competitive salary, paid holidays and sick leave, health, dental, and vision insurance, retirement benefits such as tax deferred savings plans, and more. Fluency in a language may be required. A recent listing of available positions included a country director, program and training officer, administrative officer, and an associate Peace Corps director for programming. Check out the website to view details about the hiring process and current job opportunities.

Peace Corps employment:
Go to http://www.peacecorps.gov/jobs/workingpc/fedemp/

More Job Websites for People Over 50

There are many job websites for boomers, retirees, and others over the age of 50 who are interested in working part-time or full-time in their area of expertise or in a new and challenging area of interest. They list seasonal and temporary jobs, such as work from home, on the road consulting, charitable or non-profit positions work, positions for veterans, and federal government employment. The next sections provide some ideas and websites. Also, check out seasonal job opportunities – caretaking and campground hosting - for Rver's in *Part 1: Entering the Retirement Years –Taking to the Road in Your Recreational Vehicle –Finding Employment on the Road.*

Fire Tower Lookout Positions (seasonal)

Every year, the Federal government advertises positions for individuals interested in manning fire tower lookouts throughout the western United States. A seasonal job, you live in an often secluded and dramatic natural setting with outstanding views while providing a community service. Fire season runs from May to October. There are volunteer and paid positions available. The schedule runs 5 days per week on /2 days off. Due to the skill-set necessary to staff these towers, you need to feel comfortable living in a secluded area.

The towers range from 66-foot towers with ground cabins to a 14' x 14' live-in lookout. Some are accessible by car; others are located in very remote wilderness. Position descriptions recommend you be comfortable with an emergency radio and that you have some knowledge of wild land fire behavior and fire prevention education. You should be able to observe smoke, estimate the distance, size and characteristics of the blaze, and locate it on a detailed map using references to landmarks. You should be able to observe ground lightning strikes, thunderstorms, and the massing of cloud formations. Additional responsibilities can include maintaining the lookout or cabin, and greeting and providing visitors with information about the forest.

In the Desolation Peak area of the North Cascades National Park in Washington, the fire tower is located in a remote section of the park. To get there, you must travel by boat across Ross Lake and then hike six strenuous miles to the lookout. The only water is snowmelt from the previous winter.

Being a fire tower lookout is not a position most people would think about applying for on a long-term basis. However, for the adventurous boomer, taking 3-6 months to experience nature on an intimate level may be the retirement adventure you are seeking.

For most recent **Job Postings** as a Fire Tower lookout or Fire Prevention and Detection volunteer or paid position.
Go to http://www.firelookout.org/

If working as a fire tower lookout is not the position you are looking for, consider reviewing some of the websites listed below.

- **Retirement Jobs.com** helps people over age 50 locate employment with companies interested in hiring an older work force. Go to http://www.retirementjobs.com/

- **Workforce50.com** helps baby boomers and older workers over 50 years of age find work that is compatible with their experience. This website lists jobs that are flexible, full-time, part time and work-at-home. This website lists jobs by location or type of employment, recommended books, magazines and resources and expert advice. Go to http://www.workforce50.com/

- **RetiredBrains.com** offers a website with listing of temporary jobs, work at home jobs and employment for boomers or retirees. You can post a wanted job, receive resume assistance, and more. Go to http://www.retiredbrains.com/Home/default.aspx

- **The Dinosaur Exchange** website is for dinosaurs, those retired with expertise, and dinosaur hunters or employers. You can find work as a consultant, mentor, or general employee. If you choose to work only for a charitable or benevolent organization, and you can post your resume free of charge. Go to http://www.dinosaur-exchange.com/index.php

- **Military.com** helps find employers looking for Veterans with a military background. Go to http://www.military.com/veteran-jobs

- **JobsOver50.com** is a free web-based employment service for baby boomers and retirees looking for employment. Go to http://jobsover50.com/student/

- **National Older Worker Career Center (NOWCC)** provides full-time and part-time opportunities to experienced workers, ages 55 and older, through two programs: the Senior Environmental Employment Program and the Agriculture Conservation Experienced Services (ACES) Program is focused on environmental conservation and natural resource maintenance. Go to http://www.nowcc.org/

- **Experience Works,** funded under Title V of the Older Americans Act, allows low-income persons, 55-years of age and older to find employment at eligible faith-based and community organizations. Usually, seniors receive minimum wage for an average of 20-hours a week at a variety of positions ranging from teacher's aides to emergency dispatchers, caregivers, and office assistants. For information, go to http://www.experienceworks.org

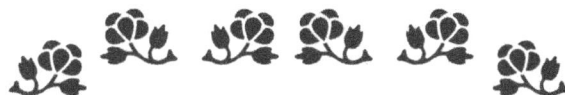

Part 2

Aging in Place
Make it Work for You

The stages of life, aging in place, levels of care, making your home safe, successes and challenges, warning signs, finding in-home help, community movements, federal, state, and local programs, home health-care and hospice services

The Stages of Life

"Question: What walks on four legs in the morning, two legs in the afternoon, and three legs in the evening?"

"Answer: Man. He crawls on all hands and knees as a baby, walks on two legs as an adult, and walks using a cane in his old age".

-- The Riddle of the Sphinx

Although the definition of "family" has changed dramatically, most baby boomers have grown up in a single-family home, living with our parents and siblings and sometimes grandparents or relatives. A continuum of care exists as we age in place, beginning with childhood and transitioning through adulthood to our retirement years. We have moved from a child's complete dependence on others to the modified independence of a teenager and young adult. However, as we get older, aging in place takes on a new and different meaning. We may start our adult years completely self-sufficient and independent. As we approach our retirement years, we may see our health decline or personal circumstances compel us to adapt a life-style of modified independence, a transition that requires us to seek more help and assistance.

Stage 1: Our childhood years are now memories. We may remember playing street football and hide n' seek with our friends, climbing trees, picnicking in the park, playing kick-ball and softball, buying penny candy from the local candy store, and attending elementary and middle school. These were carefree years, as we knew our parents would take care of us - preparing our meals, helping us with homework, taking us to after-school activities, checking our temperature when we were sick, and tucking us in our beds at nighttime. We were free to be kids, yet given some responsibility to complete simple household chores such as making our beds, cleaning the house, or helping with cooking. We did not manage bank accounts and were not required to find employment and travel daily to a job. We attended school to see friends and further our education. We depended on our parents and we enjoyed our days. Our immediate goal was to play and our abstract assumption for the future was that someday we would grow into productive and responsible teenagers.

Stage 2: We enter our teenage years and with them come increased responsibility to ourselves and our family and community. We still live under our parent's roof. "House rules" dictate how we behave at home. We feel independent, but remain dependent on our parents for our room, board, and an allowance. We have more responsibility. We enjoy sleeping late, staying up until the wee hours of the morning, and hanging out with friends. High school becomes the focal point for socialization and education. We may decide to work a part time job for extra spending money. These years are a mixture of dependence on our parents and a desire to break away to determine our own independent path. Our high school diploma or GED marks a turning point. We can decide to continue living at home or to move into our own apartment or house. We can decide to attend college or vocational training programs, apply for a job, move to some place new, travel, or we may become paralyzed by the numerous decisions confronting us. We are transitioning from semi-dependence to semi-independence.

Stage 3: We have truly turned the corner. By this time, we have graduated from college, graduate school, or vocational training and established a career path that uses skills acquired through many years of hard work. Some of us remain single, live with a partner or spouse, and have chosen a life without children; others have raised a family and watched our children grow and eventually leave home to establish themselves in the world. We are empty nesters. Our children are no longer very dependent upon us (although most parents hope that our kids will always find a reason to come home and visit.) Or our children may decide or be compelled to live in our home, working and contributing to the household or using it as a base as they consider their options. Our aged parents may require more care than before, a condition that adds to our responsibilities.

We are looking down the elusive road to retirement. Our responsibilities have shifted but not disappeared. We enter our retirement years struggling for a balance between living the retirement dream, preserving our relationship with our children and being present for our parents. There are many decisions to make about how we wish to spend our retirement years. We can stay in our current home which may be near our children and parents, move closer to our out-of-state children or parents, downsize our home for a more practical living space, move to a new setting with helpful services, or travel, volunteer, work part-time, or do something never previously considered.

Stage 4: As we approach Stage 4, we hope that we can maintain our independence for many more years. We are now in the throes of our retirement years. We may start to feel the creep of aging with a less flexible and stiffer body. We may forget more frequently and suffer memory lapses. The possibility that we will someday become dependent on our children, spouse, partner or family looms over us. We watch our friends lose their driving privileges because of health or vision issues. We see friends relocate to assisted living facilities or retirement communities or move closer to their children to receive additional support with personal care, shopping, home maintenance, and more. We have come full circle from being dependent at birth, seeking independence in our youth, finding independence in our grown-up years, and finally reverting to a modified independence or complete dependence in our later years. Of course, many people will find themselves as active at 80-years as they were at 60-years of age, seeing their golden years as a never-ending adventure.

When Christine, age 70, lost her spouse of 45 years to a sudden illness, she wondered how she would survive her retirement years. Always interested in birding, she joined a local Audubon birding club. First, she participated in local outings to bird watch in nearby forests and parks. A year later, she found herself embarking on a birding adventure, traveling down the Amazon River in Venezuela. She never imagined that someday, in her retirement years, she would find herself floating down the Amazon River on a small boat, swatting mosquitoes and sleeping in a hammock on a boat deck.

What is Aging in Place?

"Aging in place"... is not having to move from one's present residence in order to secure necessary support services in response to changing need. We are using the term "aging in place" in reference to living where [one has] lived for many years, or to living in a non-healthcare environment, and using products, services and conveniences to allow or enable [older adults] to not have to move as circumstances change. More recently "aging in place" is a term used in marketing by those in the rapidly evolving senior housing industry."

-- Sloan Work and Family, Boston College

When I first heard the phrase "Aging in Place," I asked for clarification. It was a new term to me, although not a new concept. To age in place is the ability to remain in your home despite medical, physical, and/or emotional needs, with all the in-home services necessary to create a safe and secure home environment. Your home can be a single-family home, duplex, townhouse or condominium, apartment, a family member's home, a cooperative, mobile or manufactured home, a recreational vehicle, a home on the water, a retirement or assisted living community, an adult care home or something else.

Home is where you live. A house is not a home. Feelings of belonging, comfort, and security create a home. Home decorations can convey these feelings, with each person decorating in their own style. Framed photographs of family members and places visited, artwork collected over the years, furniture passed down from one generation to the next all contribute to this atmosphere. It is a place to kick off your shoes, pour a cool drink, read the newspaper or a novel as you relax in comfort surrounded by personal bits and pieces of your life. Anyone who has walked into a friend's house knows that no two homes are the same.

Aging in Place does not discriminate by gender, race, religion, age, income, or ability level. It is available to anyone seeking to live in a place that enriches his or her life and improves the quality of that life. It transforms a "house" into a "home," ensuring a lifetime of living in an environment of your choosing.

Where Can I Age in Place?

"When you visit with your senior loved ones, let them be the host. Don't offer help. It's the best way to learn where they need help the most."

-- Hanna Steiner,
Director, Riverview Apartments Inc., Pittsburgh, PA

Each person will find a different meaning to aging in place. Some will age in place by continuing to live in the home they have resided in for many years, preserving their independence and quality of life. Others will age in place by seeking out a new living environment that maintains their quality of life. As physical, emotional, and social changes occur, they can easily access support and services. For those in excellent health seeking an active life style and open to a novel experience, aging in place may mean throwing themselves into an adventure or new and dramatic life style.

Reasons to Age in Place

Although everyone has specific reason to age in place, the most common are:

- you enjoy living where you are;
- you are comfortable in your current surroundings;
- it is affordable;
- you are close to your family and friends;
- your location is convenient to services, culture, educational programs;
- you are satisfied with your healthcare services;
- you feel safe and secure where you are;
- you like the feeling of living independently.

Staying in Your Home

"Old age isn't so bad when you consider the alternative".

-- Maurice Chevalier,
(New York Times, October 9, 1960)

As a retiring baby boomer, you may decide to continue living in your current home without the need for assistance and support from family or community. You may still retain good to excellent health, lead an active life, and be involved in your community.

However, health alone does not determine quality of life. While many exciting opportunities and places to live exist for active and retired persons, eventually most of us slow down and become more sedentary as we age. We cannot walk as far, daily chores become more difficult and take more time, maintaining a home requires more assistance and our health takes unexpected twists and turns. Yet, many people will not seek help or recognize or admit the need for it as they may equate help with the forfeiting of independence. This can create a potentially hazardous living environment and medical problems, which may have been avoidable.

Gary, age 78, had difficulty walking. Although he could transfer from his bed to his walker, he fell on a regular basis. During family visits, he was upbeat and told funny stories. He did not share information about his fear of falling, the difficulty he had getting off the toilet seat, or the problems he had preparing his meals. After one fall, Gary lay on the floor for 6-hours, unable to get to his feet or reach a telephone to call for help. A neighbor finally heard him calling out and contacted emergency services. His family remained unaware of these issues, until they received a call from a hospital emergency department informing them that Gary had fallen at home and fractured his hip. If his family was aware of his difficulties, they could have arranged for assistance in the home from a caregiver and arranged for a meals program to deliver daily meals to Gary. In addition, an emergency call bracelet, such as Lifeline, would have enabled Gary to contact 911 instead of lying on the floor for many hours. Or, they may have explored other living options with Gary, such as having a family member stay with him, having him move in with family, or maybe into an assisted living facility.

Why was Gary afraid to talk with his family about his need for help?

Was he concerned that he would lose his independence?

Was he concerned that his family would "take over" and arrange his home in ways that he might not want?

It is common for a person struggling to maintain their autonomy and independence or the illusion of it and to resist receiving help from families and from community and government programs. Yet, to age in place in your own home, it may be necessary to communicate essential information and accept some type of assistance. Alternatively, if your home situation is unsafe and you are unable to manage even with help, it may be time to consider choosing a facility or home where you can age in place while receiving help and supervision.

Levels of Care (LOC) in Your Home

"I have reached an age when, if someone tells me to wear socks, I don't have to."

-- Albert Einstein (1879-1955)

For aging in place to be successful, it is necessary to confront objectively the needed level of care. "Level of care" refers to the amount and type of assistance, supervision and medical attention needed by an individual, as determined by an assessment. Here is a summary for in-home levels of care.

Level 0: Independent Living

People living independently are able to care for themselves without assistance or support from others. They are usually in good to excellent health and lead an active life style.

Level 1: Minimal In-home Care

On a daily basis, people requiring Level I care usually need at least a few hours of help, supervision, and assistance. Assistance can include help with some of the activities of daily life – bathing, dressing, grooming, toileting, meal preparation, grocery shopping and light housekeeping. Sometimes, family and friends can coordinate provision of additional in-home supports. Alternatively, you can hire a companion, private caregiver or home healthcare aide from a licensed and bonded home care agency, a local healthy senior, or a college student. This person should be responsible, flexible, trustworthy, caring, and have some basic medical knowledge. Assisted living facilities and adult care homes can also provide Level I care.

Level 2: Moderate In-home Care

People requiring Level 2 care usually need moderate care and a significant amount of supervision and assistance with medical care, medication management, meal preparation and help with the activities of daily life (ADL's.) As care needs increase, you may choose to hire a person with some medical background such as a certified nursing assistant (CNA) or a licensed practical nurse (LPN.) If most of the care needed is non-medical, an experienced caregiver or companion can provide care.

Level 3: Maximum In-home Care

People requiring Level 3 usually need maximum care or constant help, supervision and assistance on a daily basis. They may have more complicated medical care needs and usually need a caregiver with an extensive healthcare background. Maximum care indicates that you require assistance with all or most of your activities of daily life and are unable to manage independently. Hire a caregiver with extensive experience. Consider a referral from your physician for home healthcare professionals and have them visit you in your home. They can help you evaluate your medical needs, order durable medical equipment, organize your medications, provide therapies and nursing care. Be aware that if you have extensive medical needs, you may need 24/7 or live-in care.

Age in Place Challenges

"Older: Having lived or existed for a relatively long time;
far advanced in years or life"

"Aging: The process of growing old or maturing"

-- Free Online Dictionary

Everyone ages as we get older; some age well retaining our physical, mental, and psychological abilities; others find that changes, some subtle, some obvious, require additional support and assistance from volunteers, community agencies, or providers so we can remain in our homes. These changes in our day-to-day living can sometimes interfere with our ability to remain completely independent and live alone in our homes. It is important to be aware of the following common changes and, if necessary, to arrange in-home supports to ensure success as you age in place. Common changes are:

- difficulty with memory;

- increased confusion and /or disorientation to time and place;

- difficulty with word-finding or being able to express yourself with words;

- delayed response time to questions;

- delayed reaction time when driving;

- decreased hearing and /or vision;

- difficulty with mobility;

- decreased fine motor skills;

- decreased stamina and /or strength;

- increase in health-related issues.

Warning Signs:
When to Get Help in Your Home

These warning signs are indicators of obvious or subtle changes in your behavior or mental capabilities that can affect your ability to live independently. Sometimes it is easy to rationalize or ignore these warning signs, but doing so compromises your independence by not arranging the help you need to remain in your home. If you notice these warning signs, take a closer look at how you or your loved one is managing in their home. Look for:

- **personal hygiene changes** such as a failure to bathe on a daily basis, wearing the same clothes all the time, or sleeping in their clothes;

- **a dusty and /or cluttered home** that was formerly very neat or a home no longer cleaned on a regular basis. Are piles of mail, papers, and other items stacking up all through the house?

- **a lack of food or rotting and moldy food** in the refrigerator can result from having difficulty getting to the grocery store or an inability to prepare healthy meals. This can result in unexplained weight loss and contribute to other health problems;

- **fatigue, an increased in sleeping,** a decrease in activity and constant complaints can be signs of depression;

- **passive responses** such as, "Why should I bathe/change my clothes?" "I don't go anywhere." or an "I don't care" attitude";

- **forgetfulness and memory loss** resulting in unattended food cooking on the stove, faucets left on, not taking medications as prescribed, phones left off the hook, bills left unpaid, or scheduled appointments forgotten;

- **financial mismanagement or a lack of insight regarding finances** can include products ordered that are not needed or checks written to inappropriate businesses or questionable individuals. Be alert for excessive unsolicited mailings requesting money and financial scams, as older people are vulnerable targets;

- **getting lost** in familiar settings or while driving;

- **changes in behavior** or personality or unexpected mood swings;

- **unexplained bruises or injuries** from a loss of balance or falls.

Aging in Place is more difficult for people experiencing changes in mobility, increased falls at home, and /or slowing mental process. Without family or caregiver support, this can create an unsafe home environment. Still, with community support from healthcare professionals who visit the home – such as home healthcare nurses, physical and occupational therapists, and social workers, – it is possible to develop a care plan so you can continue to live safely in your home.

Age in Place Successfully

To successfully age in place, it is often necessary to develop a supportive relationship with your family, friends, and community. With helpful people and services in place or easily accessible, the ability to continue living in your home as you age can become a reality. Most people desire the same things:

- an easily accessible and comfortable home;
- where family and friends can visit;
- an affordable home;

- the ability to perform your activities of daily life;

- the ability to obtain necessary prescription medications;

- the ability to make informed and reasonable decisions about your care and quality of life;

- the capability to maintain a clean and safe home, including any yard or garden;

- necessary in-home safety features;

- a safe and secure living environment;

- close proximity to grocery shopping, public transportation, and medical care;

- extras like theater, culture, and educational opportunities;

- participation in a community network.

RampsPlus: Key Clauses in the ADA Ramp Guidelines

- ADA Ramps should not exceed 1:12 ratio. Every inch or rise needs 12 inches of ramp.
- ADA Ramps addressing more than 6 inches should have handrails.
- ADA Ramps exceeding 30 feet must have intermediate platform.
- ADA Ramps must have side flanges of 2 inches or more to prevent accidental slipping from edge.
- ADA Ramps and Platforms must have non-skid surface and be designed to prevent water accumulation. Go to http://www.rampsplus.com/ada-ramp.html)

Handi-RAMP: How to Plan, Design and Build an Americans Disabilities Act (ADA) approved ramp.
Go to http://www.handi-ramp.com/ramp-plan.htm / Tele: 1-800-876-RAMP

A1 Wheelchair Ramp Guide: Wheelchair Ramp Resources:

Go to http://www.a1-wheelchair-ramps.com/info/ada-wheelchair-ramps-html

Your home should be easily accessible. You should be able to access easily your bedroom and bathroom, supplies in your kitchen cabinets, and food in the refrigerator. If you have to climb steps to enter your home and have difficulty walking up or down them, consider building a ramp, or, if indicated, installing an elevator. If you are having mobility issues, steps may also pose a challenge for your friends. If you have stairs inside the house that lead to bathrooms or bedrooms, consider a stair glide or lift, moving the bedroom location to a lower level or acquiring a bedside commode chair.

Stair glides can be helpful in a 2-story home where climbing stairs are necessary for you to have complete access to your home. The stair glide mounts to the stair treads. Many measurements are required so it is important to work with an experienced installer.

If your home presents daily challenges because of significant changes in your abilities, consider looking for a home on one-level, an environment that will increase your independence through greater accessibility to your activities of daily life.

Shirley and Jerry, ages 80+ years, live in a 2-level home with 14 steps leading to the front door. Although they still manage to walk up and down the steps, their disabled friends are no longer able to visit them, as they cannot climb the steps to enter or access the home. They considered installing a ramp, a stair glide or a small elevator but decided to wait until they are unable to climb the steps. If Shirley or Jerry has an accident or serious medical problems, they may have problems getting in and out of their home. By not being pro-active, this decision can affect their future ability to age in place and remain in their home. It may also affect their ability to decide where they live as an emergency could thrust them into making a hasty decision or shift the decision-making authority to their children.

Stair Lift Key Points

1. Rail mounts to stair treads, not to wall. Stairs must be in sound condition.
2. If your stairs are narrow (less than 37") than the track distance from the wall will be a key issue. This factor is also dependent on the height of the stair lift user and their leg length.
3. If you have difficulty transferring to the seat of the chair then seat height will be a key issue.
4. Seat height at bottom of stairs is an important point if you are short.
5. If you have lower back pain and a soft start and stop are important then DC powered residential stair lifts maybe more appropriate.
6. If user is tall then seat depth of the access stair lift is important.
7. Stairway must have adequate lighting at top and bottom of stairs.

8. Confirm local government requirements for electrical plug.
9. Track must be allowed to come all the way to the top landing and bottom landing for safe transfer to the seat of electric stair chair lifts.

-- **Silver Cross: Recycler and New HealthCare Equipment:**
Go to http://www.silvercross.com/stairlifts.html / Tele: 1-800-572-9310

Your home should be comfortable and inviting to family and friends. If you would like your children and grandchildren to stay with you, look for a home that enables you to live comfortably and safely with room for your family when they visit. If your home is not accessible, it may be difficult for people with disabilities or difficulty walking and climbing stairs to visit you in your home.

Your home should be affordable. If you have difficulty making your monthly rent or mortgage, you may want to consider moving to a more affordable residence, finding a family member, friend or renter to share the cost, or consider refinancing. It is best to talk with a professional accountant or real estate agent if you are considering refinancing or selling your home. You should not have to choose between paying your monthly rent or mortgage and buying your food and medications.

Be independent or semi-independent with your activities of daily life. The activities of daily living (ADL's) comprise what you do every day, i.e. your daily routine. You get up in the morning, brush your teeth, take a shower or bath, groom your hair, shave, use the bathroom for toileting, and choose your clothes and dress. Moving into the kitchen, you prepare your breakfast. After breakfast, you may decide to clean your home and work in the yard. If these activities become too difficult for you to do without assistance, consider getting a part-time homemaker or caregiver to help with housework and personal care in your home. If you are a spouse or partner caring for someone you love, a few hours each week of caregiver support can improve the quality of care for your loved one and give you respite or a break from caregiving. Be aware that many family members that provide care tend to ignore their own health and can suffer from the physical and emotional exhaustion of caregiver burnout.

It is possible to remain in your home if you bring in additional support. Sometimes a family member or a friend will volunteer to live with you, providing care and supervision. Or a caregiver can be hired from a private licensed agency or on a recommended referral from someone you know.

Sharon, age 84, is the primary caregiver for her spouse of 60-years. Every morning she helps him get out of bed, perform his ADL's, prepares breakfast, assists with toileting, and manages his medication. At noon, she prepares lunch and then again helps with toileting and prepares his bed for his afternoon nap. After preparing dinner, she dresses him for bed, again helps with the ADL's and puts him to bed. All night, she sleeps lightly, ready to get up and help him with his nightly (and hourly) toileting needs. By morning, she is exhausted and starts the same routine all over again.

Sharon did not seek caregiver assistance for several reasons. She became accustomed to her daily caregiving routine and did not realize the toll caregiving took on her physically and emotionally. As a spouse of many years, she believed it was her responsibility to provide care for her beloved spouse. She valued her privacy, especially in the nighttime and did not want someone sleeping over at night. Eventually, when the caregiving responsibilities became overwhelming, she hired a daytime caregiver. Sharon began to recognize that having a caregiver help just a few hours a week relieved her of her caregiving responsibility and enabled her to recharge her batteries for the night- time caregiving duties. It also gave her respite time or time to grocery shop, get her hair done, or take a walk with friends. Eventually, she hired a nighttime caregiver to help with the constant nightly toileting needs.

There are many ways to set up caregiving in your home. You can hire a caregiver for a split shift. That is, the caregiver comes to your home in the morning and helps get you up and out of bed, assist with your activities of daily life, prepares breakfast and then leaves. At bedtime, the caregiver returns and helps you prepare for bed. The charge for this service is usually by the hour with a minimum of 2-4 hours each time the caregiver comes to your home. If you need a 24/7 caregiver, many private agencies will have a 24/7 charge instead of an hourly rate.

For low-income, seniors, and disabled people, contact your local State Senior Service or Disability Services Office about their in-home assistance programs. If you have adequate income, it is possible to hire an individual or a privately licensed and bonded caregiving agency to provide homemaking assistance and a caregiving in your home.

Administration on Aging caregiver programs:
Go to http://www.aoa.gov/aoa_programs/hcltc/caregiver/index.aspx

Agingcare.com:
Go to http://www.aoa.gov/aoa_programs/hcltc/caregiver/index.aspx

American Association of Retired Persons (AARP):
Go to http://www.aarp.org/

CaregiverList:
Go to http://www.caregiverlist.com/RequestServices.aspx

Eldercare Locator: A public service provided by the U.S. Administration on Aging to help families locate local community services or go to http://www.eldercare.gov/eldercare.NET/Public/index.aspx or call 1-800-677-1116

Helpguide.org:
Go to http://www.helpguide.org/elder/caring_for_caregivers.htm

LIVHOME is a caregiving agency with locations in CA, GA, IL, MD, MA, TX, and VA. In addition to setting up in-home caregiving services, it provides credentialed geriatric experts in social work, nursing, and mental health to perform clinical assessments in your home. Based on the interview, the agency develops a personalized plan of care. For more information, go to http://www.livhome.com/

Medicare.gov caregiver support:
Go to http://www.medicare.gov/campaigns/caregiver/caregiver.html

---

Adult Day Care programs provide a structured setting for seniors and disabled people, providing assistance with the ADL's, social and recreational activities, basic medical care, medication management, meals, and often transportation. Some offer therapeutic services such as physical, occupational, and speech therapies. The adult day care center may provide supervision for people with Alzheimer's disease, dementia, or general confusion. They can offer respite or relief from care for family or caregivers. Many adult day care centers operate Monday - Friday with regular hours. The cost varies from facility to facility.

For **Adult Day Care Resources,**
contact the **National Adult Day Services Association**.
Go to http://www.nadsa.org / Tele: 1-866-890-7357

Be able to make good and reasonable decisions on your own behalf. Often family or friends notice changes in mental status and behavior. These changes can affect your ability to live independently, especially if you do not have adequate support from family, friends and community. If you are increasingly confused, having memory problems, disoriented and sometimes getting lost in familiar areas, you may need to increase your services in your home or consider placement in a facility that offers supervision and assistance. Consider an emergency response system such as Lifeline (this is not effective unless you can remember to push the button) or a daily well-check system, a home delivery meal program, and caregiver support during the day, evening, or 24/7.

If you are getting perplexed when taking medications, consider setting up a daily medication box. Taking medication is difficult if you cannot remember the reason you take the pill, the proper dosage, or when to take the medication. If you are homebound and unable to set up a medication box on your own, ask your primary care physician for a referral to a home healthcare agency for medication management. A registered home healthcare nurse can help you review all your medications and set up an easy-to-use medication box. In addition, if you have any medication questions, she can contact your physician on your behalf. If you are unable to obtain your prescription medication due to the cost, work with your physician on completing an application for prescription assistance with the pharmaceutical company that produces your medication.

Prescription Assistance Programs (PAP's) created by the pharmaceutical companies provide free or discounted medicine to people who are unable to afford them. As each pharmaceutical company develops its own eligibility guidelines, you must check with each company to see if you qualify for reduced cost or free prescription medications. You must not be eligible for any prescription benefits. However, if you enrolled in the Medicare Part D Prescription Drug benefit, you may still be eligible for some financial assistance programs. The financial assistance application has sections for completion by you and by your primary care physician. Attach proof of income such as a Federal Tax return (Form 1040/1040EZ) or wage and tax statements (W-2) or a letter of means of support stating which assistance programs support you (i.e. Food Stamps) to the application. Your primary care physician, a physician or nurse practitioner at the Community Health Clinics can usually help you complete these applications. Be sure that you and your physician sign the document and make a copy for your records. Some physician offices designate a person to help patients apply for pharmaceutical programs. If you qualify for a prescription assistance program, the pharmaceutical company will usually mail the medication directly to your primary care physician's office or to your home.

NeedyMeds.com is an on-line information resource of pharmaceutical programs for people who are unable to afford their medications. It lists drugs by their generic or brand names and connects you to the pharmaceutical company website where you can download an application for assistance. Eligibility guidelines are on each website. Go to http://www.needymeds.org/index.htm

---

Meal programs such as Meals on Wheels, Loaves and Fishes, or Food and Friends provide meals free of charge or for a small fee. Meal delivery to your home is available Monday–Friday during lunchtime. You can request special diet lunches, such as diabetic or low-salt diets. For information on this service, contact the nearest State Area Agency on Aging.

Other places to receive meals include senior centers managed by the community or a medical or religious organization. In addition to meals, they support a wide range of activities. Hospital cafeterias sometimes have senior discount meal programs. Contact your local hospital to inquire about this program. Charity meals are often available at the Salvation Army, St. Vincent de Paul, local houses of worship, and local Missions. Social service agencies usually have lists of local free meal programs for low-income seniors and the homeless. Some Senior Centers, churches, and community centers offer congregate meals to seniors and disabled persons. If preparing meals is increasingly difficult, consider finding someone to help you prepare meals that you can freeze for later consumption or contact your local restaurants and grocery stores and inquire about their delivery services.

Be able to maintain your home and yard. If you can hire a person to help with house cleaning and basic yard work, this can help you stay in your home. Usually there are yard services available or you can hire a private housekeeper or homemaker to help you with yard work, housekeeping services, and simple meal preparation. Some Senior Services Offices offer homemaking assistance for low-income, senior, and disabled persons that includes basic yard work to those unable to remain in their home without additional community support.

Place safety devices in your home. Supportive durable medical equipment (called DME) - such as walkers, wheelchairs, lift chairs, bedside commode chairs, hi-rise toilet seats, grab bars, slide boards, and shower stools – all contribute to a safer home environment. Consider installing ramps by the front or back door for easy access to your home.

If you are falling, losing your balance, or experiencing difficulty moving around without an assistive device (cane, walker, wheelchair, power scooter or power wheelchair) and find yourself clinging to furniture or walls when you walk, or pulling yourself up steps, you are placing yourself at-risk for serious injury. Consider having a physical therapist visit you in your home for a home safety evaluation and mobility assessment. The therapist can recommend helpful durable medical equipment and if needed, can contact your physician for additional orders. If your physician writes an order for a physical therapist from a home healthcare agency to see you in your home, Medicare, Medicaid, and most private insurances will cover the cost. You must be homebound and have skilled need for any home healthcare services. For more information on home healthcare agencies, go to *Part 4: Finding Medical Care in Your Community and at Home.*

To find a company that provides durable medical equipment in your area look in the *Yellow Pages* under *"Medical Equipment and Supplies"*. Not all communities print the Yellow Pages, but they are available online at http://www.yellowpages.com. Some pharmacies rent or sell basic durable medical equipment and offer home delivery at no charge. Or search online for "durable medical equipment" with your zip code. *i.e. durable medical equipment 97504.*

For information on **Medicare Coverage of Durable Medical Equipment and Other Devices:** Go to http://www.medicare.gov/what-medicare-covers/part-b/durable-medical-equipment.html

Many communities sponsor a free loaner medical equipment program from which you can borrow medical equipment, returning it when you no longer need it. Contact the State Agency on Aging or any community program that offers information on local resources.

Transportation Services are essential to aging in place in your home. At some point, either with or without our consent, we may decrease driving or stop altogether. Easy access to grocery shopping, medical appointments, religious services, cultural, and educational opportunities becomes essential. Most communities will offer a local taxi service and low cost transportation through the transportation district or Senior and Disabled Services Office.

- **Local Taxi Services** provide excellent transportation services at a reasonable rate. Wheelchair vans are often available and provide door-to-door service. Some taxi companies have taxi script or senior discount books available for purchase that reduce the cost of each ride.

Cindy and her spouse George, age 80+, loved to go to the downtown theater. As George used a walker and could only walk very short distances, attending performances became difficult. Usually, Cindy would drive them to the theater, drop George at the sidewalk, park the car, and walk several blocks to meet him. George would stand, alone, leaning on his walker, while he waited for Cindy to rejoin him. Following the event, they would reverse the process. When Cindy contacted a local cab service, she found they offered a senior discount program. She could buy a set of vouchers at a discounted rate to use whenever she needed transportation. The cab would pick Cindy and George up at their home, drive them to theater, and pick them up after the performance to return them home. It was economical, safer for George, less stressful for Cindy as she did not have to worry about George falling in her absence, and allowed the couple to resume their active theater life.

- **Public Bus Service** is available in many communities, often including wheelchair lifts. Although this mode of travel is not convenient for many seniors or disabled persons, it is available at a reasonable cost. Discount books with significant discounts may be available for seniors and disabled persons. Contact your local transit district office for information on senior discount programs and schedules.

- **Local Private Transportation** and assistance services are available in some communities. Usually these are private businesses designed to help seniors and the disabled with transportation, grocery shopping, and more. Check your local Chamber of Commerce for these services in your area.

- **Non-emergency ambulance** services provide transportation when a person is medically stable. They do not carry emergency equipment and do not offer paramedics. Most provide wheelchair and gurney transport and can transport a person requiring oxygen. If you require portable oxygen, inform the ambulance staff that you will require oxygen and ask if your family needs to provide your personal portable oxygen for the transport. Non-emergency ambulances commonly transfer people to medical appointments and from a hospital to home, a nursing facility, or another residence. They are more economical than using an emergency ambulance, but less economical than taxi or van service.

- **Emergency ambulances** are for emergencies only. Occasionally they transport a person to another hospital that offers care not available in your current setting. If you have an emergency medical crisis, dial 911. Emergency ambulance services operate 24/7, 365 days a year. Charges include all medical equipment used and the cost of the ambulance personnel. This service is very expensive and is for an emergency only. Medicare covers 80% of the fee if the ambulance is used to access necessary emergency care. Please note that Medicare carefully reviews these charges and can deny payment for this service, if it determines it is not a medical emergency. Many local emergency ambulances offer a yearly ambulance service program at a modest fee. Be aware that for non-emergent transports, emergency ambulances may charge a much higher rate than a non-emergency ambulance, even if you are a member of the ambulance program. Contact your local ambulance service for more information.

Emergency Call Services

LifeFone Personal Response System:
Go to http://www.lifefone.com/index.html /

Tele: 1-877-814-0130

LifeStation:
Go to http://www1.lifestation.com /
Tele: 1-866-665-5313

MobileHelp:
(no landline required)
Go to http://www.mobilehelpnow.com/

Tele: 1-800-800-1710

Philipps Lifeline Medical Alert Service:
Go to http://www.philips.lifelinesystems.com/content/home /
Tele: 1-800-797-4191

Rescue Alert:
Go to http://www.rescuealert.com /
Tele: 1-800-688-9576

Senior Alarm: Senior Medical Alarm System:
Go to http://www.senioralarm.com /
Tele: 1-866-725-8683

Emergency call services and medic alert bracelets and necklaces are useful for people who live alone and have a history of falls or other medical issues that may require a rapid emergency services response. You have probably seen or heard the commercial for a medic alert device. A senior person falls and then pushes a waterproof button on a cord around his neck or on a bracelet on his wrist and says, "Help me. I've fallen and I can't get up." This button automatically activates a 24-hour emergency response service. Wear these waterproof devices at all times, especially in the bath or shower where falls are statistically more likely.

When you apply for this service, the agency obtains a confidential medical history and personal information, including medical contacts. If you do not respond after pushing the button, trained personnel at the emergency response center will contact your emergency contact or call an ambulance, the fire department or other emergency personnel.

When Charlene helped her spouse, Nick, step into the bathroom tub-shower, she removed his Lifeline and placed it on the sink counter, 3-feet from the tub-shower. In the middle of scrubbing Nick's back, his legs gave way, and Charlene found herself holding him up to prevent a fall, and unable to reach the Lifeline button to call for help. Luckily, a family member was visiting and heard her cry for help. Together, they were able to lower Nick to the bathtub floor, and safely get him out of the tub-shower.

As these devices are designed to get wet, the Lifeline device should always remain on the person, especially since most falls occur in the bathroom area. The fee for this service is very reasonable. There is usually a set-up fee (although this fee is often waived or free with a voucher) and a small monthly charge. For those with limited income, agencies often have a sliding scale or flexible fee or a "charity" Lifeline at no charge. For information on this important service, contact the Senior and Disabled Services Office, the State Area Agency on Aging, a local hospital social work, case management, or discharge planning department, or the Eldercare Locator.

Many communities support senior hot lines or welfare-check services for the senior or disabled person who is living alone. For a small fee, an agency (or sometimes a church, synagogue, religious organization or service clubs, such as the Rotary, Elks, or Kiwanis) will call you at your home at a specific time of day. If they do not receive an answer or they determine that you are in danger or having a difficult time, they will notify your first or second emergency contact. If there is no response from your emergency contact, the Senior Hot Line staff will contact 911 emergency services. Alternatively, you can set up an automatic inactivity time that buzzes at specific time intervals. If you do not respond to the timer, it will notify your primary contact or call emergency services. Emergency personnel will respond with a physical welfare check at your home to check on your well-being.

Imagine this scenario. A woman falls in her home and is unable to get up. The telephone is on a table and out of reach. She expects no visitor or a well-check telephone call for at least a day. As she lies on the living room floor, she yells, "Help me. I've fallen and I can't get up," but no one can hear her. Instead of waiting hours or days for a visitor, she presses a button on a cord around her neck or a button on a bracelet strapped to her wrist. This emergency call system immediately connects her with either her emergency contact or 911. Help soon arrives and she receives necessary medical attention.

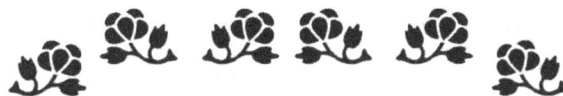

Community Movements:
Live Life Your Way

"Remember, if you ever need a helping hand, it's at the end of your arm, as you get older, remember you have another hand: The first is to help yourself, the second is to help others."

-- Audrey Hepburn

As neighborhoods and communities around the country learn about aging in place, they are developing programs to support this idea. It is not just for the Greatest Generation, but also for the boomers who are thinking about where and how they want to live when they retire.

At Riverview Towers, an independent *Housing and Urban Development* (HUD) apartment community for seniors in Pittsburgh, Pennsylvania, residents and staff replaced the term 'aging in place' with the phrase, *'Live Life Your Way'*. The residents and staff sought to find a more active and positive way to increase sensitivity within their community. With primarily low-income residents in their mid-80's and younger residents in their 60's and 70's with multiple health issues it was important for visitors to understand the vitality and dignity of each resident whether frail or active and engaged. Meetings with residents and community members were the source of an innovative vision from which to develop new programs, make changes to old programs, and introduce a nursing home diversion program that brought medical services into the residence. Even architects presented and discussed with residents plans regarding changes to the physical layout of the building.

Residents developed individualized care plans that they could choose or not choose to put in to practice. Riverview offered homemaking services, shared floating private duty nurses to lower the cost of care for residents, a day care program, practical support from four service coordinators, and assessments by nurses and social workers that emphasized safety first. These care plans helped residents set realistic goals about where they wanted to go or what they wanted to achieve in their remaining lifetime.

To celebrate the lives of the tenants of Riverview Towers and their strong sense of community, a project director, a designer, and a portrait photographer created a permanent, photography exhibit. Fifty–two black and white images of Riverview residents in three different portrait sizes hang in the lobby area, integrated into the living space of Riverview residents. They greet guests as they enter the lobby and extend through the hallways into Riverview's dining room and social hall.

A plaque by the Riverview Towers photography exhibit reads, *"This exhibit celebrates the people who live at Riverview Towers. We are inspired by their warmth and strength and the vibrant community they have created by living life their way."*

-- Riverview Towers, Pittsburgh, PA, 2007

In Bannockburn, Maryland, a program called *Neighbors Assisting Neighbors* (NAN), a grass roots effort in the small community, recently presented NAN to the Senior Services Office in Montgomery County, Maryland. Among their observations was that more residents offered their services to help others than people who requested help. The program is about neighbors helping neighbors, state agencies offering low cost caregiver support, and private caregiving agencies being available to help the disabled and older people with the basic needs of daily life.

The *Village-to-Village Movement* has gathered momentum in the past years and now has over 50 villages throughout the United States. These villages are membership –driven, grass roots organizations run by volunteers with a few paid staff. Members pay an annual due of a few hundred dollars to $1000. This fee supports the paid staff that assists residents in need of support and community services. With one call to a vetted concierge number, a resident connects with a volunteer or a screened paid provider for any services they may need. Services can include yard work, house repair, light housekeeping, legal services, financial services, computer assistance, pet care, senior check-in programs, transportation for grocery shopping or for medical appointments, and more. When paid providers are used, discounts are often available.

When a resident requests services from the concierge staff, a telephone call or email is first sent to volunteers within the community. If volunteers are unavailable, the coordinator then provides the resident with the numbers for the paid providers. If the resident requires help arranging services, the concierge will make the calls on their behalf. These community movements and programs are only one option for finding support in your community.

Community Movements

Ashby Village, Berkley, California:
Go to http://www.ashbyvillage.org

Gramatan Village, Bronxville, New York:
Go to http://www.gramatanvillage.org

Supporting Active Independent Lives: Madison, Wisconsin
Go to http://www.sailtoday.org

Village to Village Network:
Go to http://www.vtvnetwork.org/

Move Managers

If you decide to move to a new home or to age in place where you currently live, the move managers offer a variety of services. With staff from the areas of gerontology, healthcare, social work, nursing, and psychology, these mover professionals work with you and your family to make your move or reorganization or downsize seamless.

There are now over 750 companies throughout the United States, Canada, and abroad offering services to help elders pack and unpack, move household items, make decision about what to keep when moving to a smaller home. Although they do not do the actual moving, these experts work with reliable movers and provide you with emotional and physical support as you move. Look for a move manager company that is a member of the *National Association of Senior Move Managers* at http://www.nasmm.org.

Geriatric Care Managers

Geriatric care managers (GCM's) are a combination of social worker, nurse, financial and legal advisor. They can represent the absentee family – the adult children who live or work in other states and have limited time to travel to manage their parent's or relatives affairs. Look for a social worker, nurse, gerontologist, counselor, or health professional with experience, a background in health, and extensive knowledge of community resources and government programs.

Geriatric care managers usually charge an initial assessment fee. The assessment helps identify current and potential problems for which, the GCM will provide practical solutions. A GCM can help locate new housing situations, arrange personal and medical care, make referrals to helpful community agencies, set-up caregiving assistance, assess safety risks in the home, handle general legal issues such as obtaining advanced directives, guardianships, power of attorney and more. *The National Association of Professional Geriatric Care Managers* offers certification in this field. To find a GCM in your area, go to <u>http://www.caremanager.org/</u>

Private Caregiving Agencies

If you hire an individual to provide care, consider contacting a private certified caregiving agency that employs or contracts with licensed and bonded staff. These agencies perform criminal background checks and carefully screen their employees. They also provide additional training for complex cases, and, if you are not satisfied with the assigned caregiver, you can request a replacement. These agencies can provide 24/7 coverage with a 24/7 rate below the hourly rate. Unfortunately, most insurance policies do *not* pay for this service. However, some long-term care insurance policies will provide benefits. Contact *the Eldercare Locator* to locate many in-home and community services. Go to <u>http://www.eldercare.gov/Eldercare.NET/Public/Index.aspx or call 1-800-677-1116</u>

Long-term care insurance helps to fill gaps in the medical benefits you can receive in your home. Many people purchase this insurance as a safety net to ensure help in the home when they need it. Although most policies do not entirely cover the cost for in-home private caregiving assistance, these policies may pay a portion of the cost. For example, a policy may pay $95/day for care when the true cost of care exceeds this amount. Policies may have a waiting period before they provide benefits. Be sure to check out specific benefits and determine the waiting period before you purchase a policy.   Review the premiums and determine if there are any changes in the policy cost as you age. Talk with an experienced insurance broker about the differences in the policies.

For more information on long-term care insurance, contact the
National Association of Insurance Commissioners
(NAIC.) NAIC represents state health insurance regulators and has a publication called *"A Shopper's Guide to Long-Term Care Insurance."*
Go to <u>http://www.naic.org/index.htm</u>

State Area Agencies on Aging (AAA)

The State Area Agencies on Aging (AAA) can provide free assistance to people age 65 and older who meet the eligibility guidelines. They offer information and referral to social service agencies in your community, including homemaker services, transportation, home-delivered meals programs, senior centers, home healthcare services, chore and home repair services, and legal advice. They offer free or low fee assistance in the home to low-income seniors and disabled persons. To find the State AAA office nearest you, go to http://www.seniorslist.com/search/area-agency-on-aging-g.php

Disability Services Office

These state agencies provide a wide list of services for people who are over 65 years of age or disabled. If you meet the low-income financial requirements, this agency can help you obtain in-home help, meal programs, financial assistance, and medical benefits. Some offices maintain a list of trained caregivers who are available at a lower rate than those provided by a private agency. Other states have programs that pay a family member to provide the necessary caregiving. Contact your nearest Social Security Disability Services Office to obtain eligibility and income guidelines as they vary from state to state. For Social Security help and a free disability evaluation, go to http://www.socialsecurity-disability.org/

The United States Department of Veteran's Affairs

Non-service connected: *"With respect to disability or death, such disability was not incurred or aggravated, or the death did not result from a disability incurred or aggravated, in the line of duty in the active military, naval, or air service."*

Service-connection: *"With respect to disability or death, such disability was incurred or aggravated or the death resulted from a disability incurred or aggravated in the line of duty in the active military, naval, or air service."*

-- as defined by the United States Department of Veteran's Affairs

The U.S. Department of Veterans' Affairs Office (VA) provides services and benefits to both non-service and service-connected veterans. Veterans with a non-service connected may be eligible for Aid and Attendance, a program designed for aging veterans and widows. This benefit may help pay for home healthcare, assisted living, and skilled nursing care and can include a monthly pension. As the Veteran Administration is a complex system, contact your nearest veteran's facility and ask to speak to someone in the social work or benefits department. They should be able to assist you or refer you to the department that can answer your questions.

The American Legion, a non-partisan, not-for-profit service organization chartered and incorporated by Congress in 1919, offers veteran's organizational tools, free advice and guidance from service officers, and a benefits calculator to help the veteran determine and file a Veteran's benefits claim. Go to http://www.legion.org/services

The Elks Lodge sponsors a Veteran Resource Center. For an overview of their services, go to http://www.elks.org/programs/vetsprograms.cfm

The U. S. Department of Veteran's Affairs

For information on the items listed below call: 1-800-827-1000

- Burial;
- Death pension;
- Dependency indemnity compensation;
- Direct deposit directions to VA benefits regional offices;
- Disability Compensation;
- Disability Pension;
- Education;
- Home loan guaranty;
- Home modification program;
- Medical care;
- Aid and Attendance benefit;
- Vocational rehabilitation and employment

For information on **Veteran Services**,
Go to http://www1.va.gov

To find the **nearest Veteran Facility**,
Go to http://www2.va.gov/directory/guide/home.asp?isflash=1

United States Department of Veteran Affairs Caregiver Programs,
Go to http://www.caregiver.va.gov/

Home Healthcare and Hospice Services

"Never underestimate the difference YOU can make in the lives of others. Step forward, reach out and help. This week reach to someone that might need a lift."

— Pablo

If you are homebound or unable to leave your home easily, have recently had a hospitalization, accident, or live with a chronic or progressive disease that sometimes requires skilled nursing care, you may be eligible for visits from home healthcare professionals. With a physician order, these experienced nurses, therapists, and social workers can provide medical care in your home. For more information, go to *Part 4: Finding Medical Care in Your Community and at Home.* For a **Home Healthcare Directory**, go to http://www.home-healthcareagencies.com/directory/.

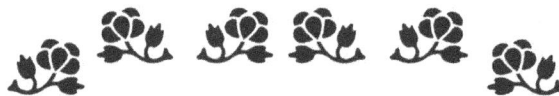

Part 3

Preserving Your Independence with a Little Bit of Help

Standard, continuing care, and theme-based retirement communities, assisted living facilities, adult care homes, and specialized memory care facilities

"To know how to grow old is the master-work of wisdom, and one of the most difficult chapters in the great art of living."

-- Henri Amiel

Many people approach the transition from independent living to assisted living with trepidation. They are reluctant to admit they need the help, unwilling to sacrifice any independence, and view such a move as a major and unwelcome turning point in their life. Some people wait for a crisis such as a hospitalization to make this change; others plan the move before they are actually dependent on receiving help. By being pro-active and recognizing the need for help in the near future, they are able to visit communities and facilities, choose their surroundings, and control the transition from an independent lifestyle to an assisted one.

In this section, you will learn about these communities and facilities that offer both independence and care and assistance. These include living in standard, continuing care or theme-based retirement communities, assisted living facilities, adult care homes and memory care facilities. For each type of community or facility, we will look at the standard features and amenities, the level of care provided, admission requirements, and more.

Living in a Retirement Community

(standard, continuing care, and theme-based retirement communities)

A retirement community is an independent, self-sufficient mini-village specifically designed to meet the needs of boomers and seniors who no longer work full-time and can volunteer their leisure time for work, hobbies, educational seminars, travel, and social activities. The type of retirement community you prefer will depend on many factors – your personal preferences, your commitment, personal finances, the location of the community, its proximity to family and friends, and the amenities and services offered by the retirement community.

Finding the retirement community that is best for you can be a lengthy process. If you know someone who is having a positive experience in one, that is an excellent way to narrow the field. If you have special interests or activities, there are university-based retirement communities that cater to people seeking lifelong learning, equestrian retirement communities for horse lovers, artist communities that encourage creativity, golf and beach oriented communities, and military retirement communities for Veteran's, government employees, and their spouses. There are also communities under development for gays and lesbians, ethnic groups, and aging musicians, to name a few. If a community is under development, be sure to check it out carefully before submitting a deposit, as some communities, despite extensive planning, do not always become a reality.

Standard Retirement Communities (SRC's)

In a Standard Retirement Community, residences are designed similarly to an apartment building or townhouse complex. Some impose an age restriction and seek people aged 55 years or older or younger disabled people who are capable of independent living. They offer some personal care assistance but are not equipped to handle chronic or serious medical problems. Although SRC's may offer their residents different levels of care, healthcare needs should be minimal and preferably temporary. If your healthcare issues require extensive medical care or daily supervision and assistance you may be required to hire a private caregiver to provide the extra care you need. These retirement communities usually charge a monthly room fee and a monthly maintenance fee which pay for home maintenance, security, grounds upkeep, linen service, at least one meal a day, activities, and other basic services. They do not require an upfront entry deposit or buy-in fee.

Continuing Care Retirement Communities (CCRC's)

"As for living our older years in a CCRC - Continuing Care Retirement Community - I can't rave enough about our quality of life, the things that are offered to us, the care we receive, the "no hassle" life we live. In fact this is really a Life Fulfilling Community!!"

-- Maje, age 87,
lives with her spouse in a Florida CCRC.

Continuing Care Retirement Communities usually take the form of large complexes or mini-villages for people aged 55 and older or those younger and disabled interested in a long-term housing commitment. Residence types include independent homes or cottages, apartment-type complexes, duplexes, villas or townhouses. The CCRC complex can range from an exclusive gated community complete with a golf course, shops, and banks to a rural facility with gardens and walking trails to a theme-based community that accommodates individuals with similar interests.

Admission requirements often include a confidential financial statement, a physical exam by a staff physician, an interview by CCRC staff, and a sizable deposit or entrance fee. This fee (also called an endowment or buy-in fee) is required in addition to a monthly service or maintenance charge. When you desire additional care due to increased personal needs and medical care, you can hire a private caregiver or move to a higher level of care within the same community. CCRC campuses include independent living, assisted living, and usually a skilled nursing facility. Sometimes, a CCRC will contract for services with a skilled nursing facility in the local community.

Many CCRC's are non-profit and sponsored by church groups or organizations such as the *Episcopal Ministries to the Aging, Inc., Presbyterian Senior Services, Jewish Homes for the Aged, and Catholic Retirement communities*, or by other non-profit corporations such as the Corporations such as *The Marriott Corporation* manage CCRC's strictly for profit. Some of these communities do not have an endowment or entrance or buy-in fee. However, their maintenance or monthly service fee can be substantially higher than those communities with an entrance fee.

Each CCRC determines its own requirements for admission. By becoming familiar with the standard requirements, you will be more aware of unusual features, deposits, fees, contracts, and requirements.

Episcopal Ministries to the Aging, Inc.:
Go to http://www.emaseniorcare.org/

Presbyterian Senior Services:
Go to http://www.pssusa.org/

Jewish Homes for the Aged:
Go to http://www.jche.org/Programs_Services.shtml

Catholic Retirement Communities:
Go to http://seniors.lovetoknow.com/Catholic_Retirement_Communities

Sunrise Senior Living:
Go to http://www.sunriseseniorliving.com

Theme-based Retirement Communities (SRC's or CCRC's)

(university-based, arts-based, golf and beach-based, equestrian-based, military/veteran-based, diversity-based, culturally–based, musician -based)

If you are looking for a community where you can continue to enjoy your passion for learning, engage in outdoor activities such as golf, beaching, horseback riding, or live with people who have similar interests and backgrounds, there are many theme-based retirement communities. Developers are calling these theme-based communities, niche or affinity housing.

A study on creative aging by the **National Endowment for the Arts and George Washington University** in 2001 found that people 65 years and older who were involved in participatory arts programs had fewer doctor's visits and less need for medication and were less prone to depression.

University-based Retirement Communities (UBRC's)

"Anyone who stops learning is old, whether this happens at twenty or eighty. Anyone who keeps on learning not only remains young, but becomes constantly more valuable regardless of physical capacity."

-- Harvey Ullman

University-based retirement communities draw both boomers and members of the Greatest Generation by presenting life-long learning in an intellectually stimulating environment. By linking with the local university, the retirement community is able to build a relationship with the university. The retirement community and university link in several ways.

- **The distance to the university** should preferably be less than a mile from the heart of the retirement campus. This makes it easy for residents to access the university programs and services.

- **Educational programs** integrate into the retirement community curriculum. While residents attend classes, mentor students, and volunteer in programs, students can participate in research studies related to people living in a continuing care environment. Student internships and paid and volunteer opportunities at the retirement community reinforce an intergenerational feel to the community. Free transportation provided to CCRC residents allows easy access to university classes and activities.

Road Scholar: Elderhostel Programs, Adventures in Lifelong Learning

Go to http://www.roadscholar.org/
Tele: 1-800-454-5768

- **A continuing care environment** that provides all the levels of care, from independent to assisted living and skilled and dementia care allows a resident easy access to all the levels of care, permitting a resident to age in place. Residents can access university healthcare centers such as a Wellness Clinic through the School of Medicine, a Dental Clinic through the Dental College, or for pets, an on-site Pet Clinic through the School on Veterinary Science.

- **Many of the university-affiliated residences are CCRC's** and offer all the levels of care in addition to educational opportunities. These residences can be expensive, ranging from studio apartments for $2,000 per month to villas for $6,000 per month. As with any CCRC's you are considering, there can be extra hidden fees. Be sure to read the fine print and review the contract with an attorney before signing it.

- **A percentage of residents should have an affiliation to the university.** Alumni, retired faculty, or staff and their families reinforce the feeling of living in an inspiring and academic environment. Although not everyone will have a relationship with the university before moving to the retirement community, the setting may draw more people seeking educational and cultural activities.

- **A formal financial relationship** should exist between the university and the retirement community. Working together by sharing some costs can help foster an educational experience for residents, students and faculty.

Residences for Life-long Learners:
For a listing of examples of collegiate-affiliated retirement communities already built,
Go to http://www.campuscontinuum.com/resources.htm

Best Guide Retirement Communities provides links to Over 55 retirement living, equestrian, military, and university affiliated retirement communities.
Go to http://www.bestguide-retirementcommunities.com/Collegelinkedretirementcommunities.html

---

Arts-based Retirement Community dedicated to fostering creativity in older residents encourage seniors to explore new ideas, activities, and artistic talents within themselves, many of whom have never explored their inner creative self. Through workshops and classes in music, art, and acting, residents can discover new abilities and ways to express themselves.

Burbank Senior Artist's Colony: This community is dedicated to independent living in a creative arts environment. Creative older residents participate in classes on poetry, writing, computer skills, and anti-aging exercises. Located in downtown Burbank, 70 % of the apartments rent from approximately $1450-$2200. Thirty percent of these units are reserved for low-income residents and rent from $500-$650*. There is an extensive waiting list. (2009) Go to http://www.seniorartistscolony.com / Tele: 818-955-9391 *(Prices are subject to change.)

NoLo Senior Arts Colony: For independent and active seniors preferring an art-focused setting. Go to http://www.apartments.com/California/North-Hollywood/NoHo-Senior-Arts-Colony/978606

Golf and Beach Retirement Communities cater to people interested in pursuing their love of golf and/or retiring in a warm climate.

Best Retirement Destinations: This website lists national retirement communities. Go to http://www.bestretirementdestinations.com/

Equestrian Retirement Communities, usually set in rural areas with access to nearby cities, accommodate the horse enthusiast with on-site equestrian centers, barns, and paddocks, trail riding and instruction, and caretakers who feed and care for the horses, clean the stalls, and maintain the facility.

PrivateCommunities.com offers a wide selection of equestrian communities around the United States: Go to http://www.privatecommunities.com/private-communities-with-equestrian-facilities.htm

Military Retirement Communities are available for retired, honorable discharge officers, and their spouses, surviving spouses over age 55 and retired civic government employees with a GS-7 or higher rating.

Military Connection.com can connect you with retirement communities for veterans. Go to http://www.militaryconnection.com/military-retirement-communities.html

Military Officers Association of America (MOAA) is a non-profit that advocates for all the military community. It publishes the Military Officers Magazine. Go to http://www.moaa.org/ , then Publications and click on the magazine website.

My Army Benefits website includes information on **The Armed Forces Retirement Hom**e offers retirement communities to enlisted military retirees and veterans. Its homes are located in Washington, D.C. and Gulfport, Mississippi. Go to http://myarmybenefits.us.army.mil/Home/Benefit_Library/Federal_Benefits_Page/Armed_Forces_Retirement_Home_.html?serv=148

Diversity-based retirement communities are springing up and breaking ground in 2012. Designed for people ages 40 to 80 plus years, they will be open to gays, lesbians, and straight persons. This high concept project is under development and describes itself as *"A home for people who live the life they want."* A new development in Palm Springs, CA, called BOOM is not yet for sale. To follow the progress of this new development, go to http://www.boompalmsprings.com/.

Cultural-based retirement communities cater to different ethnic groups. The community shares life values and beliefs, customs, language, and activities. At *Aegis Living*, Asian seniors live in an environment sensitive to Chinese culture, dining on Asian foods, receiving help from staff who speak other languages and dialects, receiving care from healthcare providers from China, practicing activities like Tai Chi. These facilities located in California, Nevada, and Washington offer assisted living and memory care with 24/7 care management. For more information go to http://www.aegisliving.com/

Aging musicians may find a not-for-profit retirement community designed for musicians age 62 and older in Franklin, Tennessee. Also under development, this community will offer independent living, assisted living, and a skilled nursing facility. Amenities include an on-site recording studio and performance venues. Scheduled to open in 2013, you can follow this retirement community development at http://www.activelifestylecommunities.com/community/the%20crescendo/the-crescendo-at-westhaven/

Choosing a Retirement Community

(certification and accreditation, commitment, location, atmosphere, residents, staff, features, services, meals, housekeeping, security, transportation and parking, social activities, interdenominational services, healthcare, and insurance)

Choosing a retirement community is a personal decision. Each person will see the atmosphere, residences, residents, staff, security systems, activities, and social programs from their own viewpoint. The retirement community that feels right for you may not feel right for another. If you have friends who are happy and satisfied with their retirement community, certainly this is a positive sign. However, it is still necessary to take some time to evaluate fully several facilities before making a decision and signing a contract. You will want to think about the following issues:

- **Certification and accreditation:** *Has the retirement community received approval from a national organization?* The *Office on Aging* (also called the *Area Agency on Aging*) now offers accreditation of retirement communities. To meet these standards, each facility must perform a self-study with its staff, board of directors, and residents. Before a national commission based in Washington D.C. grants accreditation to a facility, they require an on-site visit and evaluation by trained continuing care professionals. Although this does not constitute a recommendation or endorsement, it indicates that the facility meets certain state requirements. *(These requirements may vary from state to state.)* Look for a certificate at the retirement community that states, *"Accredited by the Continuing Care Accreditation Commission (CCAC) for the American Association for Homes and Services for the Aging."* Look for a certificate or statement from the *Equal Housing Opportunity* stating: *"Does not discriminate against any person because of race, color, sex, familial status, disability, or national origin."*

- **Commitment:** *Are you ready to live in a retirement community on a long-term basis, or are you interested only in a short-term commitment while you decide if retirement community living is the right choice?* Standard retirement communities (SRC's) permit people to change their minds and easily move to a different living situation. You are not locked into living somewhere because you placed a large down payment on admission to the community. Continuing-care retirement communities (CCRC's) can require a substantial financial investment that may or may not be refundable or pro-rated, depending upon the terms of the admissions contract. Moving from a single-family dwelling to a CCRC is a decision that requires thoughtfulness. When you consider the life changes you make by moving to a retirement community, you may quickly realize that this is not an easy decision. By moving into some retirement communities, you are making a commitment or pledge to live in the retirement community for all or most of your remaining years. If you are unsure if a retirement community is the right place for you to live, consider a short-term commitment, maybe in a Standard Retirement Community (SRC.) You may ask at the retirement community if you can rent an apartment or house for a temporary period while you decide if retirement living is right for you.

- **Location and closeness to family, friends, shopping, and medical services:** *Is the retirement community close to friends and family, or will you feel isolated from them? Can you easily access the grocery or department store or medical appointments, or are you dependent on others for transportation?* It is important to consider the location of the retirement community in relation to family, friends, church or synagogue, shopping, and medical care. If you are self-sufficient and drive a car, it is easy to get to activities and appointments. Without your own vehicle, you may need to rely on the services provided by the retirement community staff, using the community van or local taxi service. Family and friends are more likely to visit if you are located nearby. If visiting involves an hour's drive, many people may not want to take the time for a lengthy excursion. If Sunday church services or Friday night or Saturday morning services in a synagogue are important to you, check with the community regarding the nearest congregations. Many retirement communities maintain a chapel on the premises. Others provide transportation to a local house of worship. If going to town to shop or attending theater is important, the closer you locate to a city, the more opportunities are available. Many communities arrange activities outside the retirement community and transport residents to these activities.

At the Mountain Meadows Retirement Community in Ashland, Oregon, residents have access to a daily events and classes calendar that lists happenings on and off the retirement community grounds. For a small fee, residents can sign up for van transportation to activities such as shopping expeditions, walking in the downtown area, theater or lectures at the local university.

Mountain Meadows Retirement Community:
http://mtmeadows.com/

- **Atmosphere:** *Does the retirement community make you feel comfortable or do you feel out of place?* When you visit a retirement community, you should get a feel for its surroundings. Some surroundings will showcase beautiful gardens, new buildings, and a luxurious setting. Accommodations can be private, palatial and formal, requiring residents to dress more formally for meals in the dining area where they are served by waiters. Other retirement communities promote a home-like and informal environment. It is important to visit these communities with a family member or friend, spend a day walking around the grounds, sharing a meal, and talking with residents and staff. You should not feel you are being harassed or pushed into making a decision. Some communities encourage you to sample the food in the dining room, and spend at least one night sleeping at the residence.

- **Residents:** *Are the current residents the type of people you would like to socialize with on a daily basis?* Residents and atmosphere go hand in hand. Some seek the faster country club life, filled with many amenities and social activities. Others desire a slower lifestyle, preferring solitude and comfort. You may find that your politics and way you view the world are different from other residents. If you cannot relate to the people living in the retirement, it may not be the right choice for you. The extent to which you participate in activities and share mealtimes with others can depend on relationships you develop with other residents.

- **Staff:** *Is the staff at the retirement community helpful? Is staff available on a twenty-four hour basis? Are the staff healthcare professionals easily reached and responsive?* The staff in the retirement community plays an integral role in determining the atmosphere. Many communities maintain a front desk office for management and a concierge service to help residents arrange activities, transportation, and more. Staff should be accessible, considerate, patient, and flexible. You should feel comfortable asking questions and requesting services and assistance. The staff will consist of non-professionals and professionals. In addition, a registered nurse or licensed practical nurse may be on the premises during regular hours to help evaluate residents' medical needs. Non-professionals can assist with homemaking activities, unskilled medical care and medication management, meal preparation, security, and transportation. Often, a social worker or case manager is available to help residents with transportation and medical, social, or community issues.

- **Features:** *Do you like the physical characteristics of the residences?* A standard residence may be a studio, one, two, or three-bedroom apartment, a townhouse or condominium, a small cottage, or a single-family home. Many of the residences include a complete kitchen area, independent heating and air-conditioning controls, window coverings, cable television, and safety features, such as smoke detectors, safety grab bars in the tub or shower, and a twenty-four hour emergency call system. Some communities provide partially furnished units and encourage residents to bring their own furniture to give their unit a touch of home. Others provide an unfurnished unit and expect residents to furnish it with their own belongings. Check with each facility for their guidelines regarding pets, making physical changes to the residence at the resident's expense, and extra charges, such as utilities, parking fees, and major maintenance or repair work.

- **Services:** *Does the retirement community offer services you will use? Is there adequate staff at the retirement community to provide all the offered services?* The basic services in most retirement communities are similar and include meals, housekeeping services, security, transportation and parking, interdenominational services, and other on-site services. Retirement communities often operate as independent mini-villages, with a multitude of stores, businesses and social centers located on the community grounds. When you visit, note which services are available in each retirement community. On-site services can include a bank or credit union, post office, grocery store, pharmacy, a fitness center, beauty salon, or barber shop.

- **Meals:** *Are you interested in cooking your own meals or eating some or all meals in a communal dining area?* Both types of retirement communities offer meals to residents. SRCs and CCRC's can provide up to three daily meals. Dining areas are often set up cafeteria or buffet-style; in others, servers deliver the meals to residents at their tables. Some CCRC's provide one daily meal, often in a communal dining area. Others provide one to three daily meals daily, usually with a full-course dinner. Some CCRC's may expect a resident to eat a certain number of meals in the dining room each month; others do not require a minimum number of meals in the dining area. Take-out food may also be available. The dining atmosphere can vary at different retirement communities. One community may expect residents to dress up for dinner in appropriate clothes, such as jackets for men and a nice dress or pants for women. Others may adopt a more casual approach to mealtime. For residents needing assistance at mealtime, a staff member may be available to bring residents to the dining area in their wheelchairs and assist them with setting up their trays, cutting food, and hand feeding. Some communities discourage the use of assistive devices such as walkers and wheelchairs in the dining room. Check the facility's policy on dining room protocol. Ask if the facility prepares special diets and, if you are unable to eat in the dining area, whether staff can deliver meals to your residence. Check the terms of your contract for any extra fees for additional meals or assistance during mealtimes.

- **Housekeeping**: *Are you interested in receiving weekly housekeeping services?* Most retirement communities provide a weekly housekeeping and linen service. Others are equipped with washers and dryers, available in common areas for residents' use. Installing a washer and dryer in your unit is possible in some communities. Although many retirement communities include housekeeping services in the fee, others may charge an additional charge for this service.

- **Security:** *Is living in a retirement community with significant security important to you?* Security systems vary at different communities. Some maintain a 24/7 security guard or responsible staff member and a security alarm system. Security guards stationed at an assigned post or patrolling the retirement community grounds watch for and handle problems as they arise. In gated communities, the "gate" provides residents with extra security. Any person entering or leaving the grounds must pass through a locked gate, usually staffed by a security guard 24 hours a day. This helps to prevent unauthorized people from entering the retirement community.

- **Transportation and Parking Services:** *Will you depend on transportation through the retirement community or will you drive your own vehicle?* A community van may be available free or for a small fee to transport residents to medical appointments, shopping, church or synagogue, social community events such as lectures, theater, and group outings. These vans are usually wheelchair-accessible. For residents who use their own vehicles, parking in the community can include valet parking, covered and/or illuminated parking spaces. There can be an extra fee for a parking space.

- **Social Activities:** *Is maintaining an active social life with other residents important to you? Are there activities that would be of interest to you?* Many retirement communities offer an extensive selection of activities for their residents. The listed social activities that follow were compiled after reviewing many facilities and include – arts and crafts, book clubs, bridge and scrabble groups, ceramics, fitness centers, exercise classes, water exercise classes, yoga, square dancing, tennis, shuffleboard, golf, needlework, quilting, photography, library, lectures, woodworking shop, movies, music, game rooms, and garden plots.

- **Interdenominational Services:** *Is attending a house of worship important to you?* For many people attending a local church or synagogue is a vital part of their life. Attending services can help you practice your faith, maintain spirituality, and connect to a community. While some facilities maintain a chapel on their grounds, others provide free transportation or charge a small fee to transport you to a house of worship.

- **Healthcare and Insurance:** *Are you looking for medical care within the retirement community? Do you have a chronic medical condition that requires or will require medical services?* If you prefer a specific physician or hospital, consider how far the retirement community is from the doctor's office or hospital. Many communities provide transportation to medical appointments within a reasonable distance. Some charge a small fee for this service; others provide the transportation free of charge. In a continuing care retirement community, skilled nursing care is usually available at the health clinic on the premises.

Following treatment for cellulitis, Seth, 90-years old, transferred from the hospital to a skilled nursing facility on the campus of the CCRC, exactly .3 miles from his home. His wife could walk to visit him, and happily, there were no strict visiting hours. Seth received "all the best nursing care he could want", three meals served to him, (and to his wife if she was visiting), and free transportation to the infectious disease facility for his home infusions.

Although many Standard Retirement and Continuing Care Retirement Community residents enjoy good health and an independent, active lifestyle, there may be times when you need medical care and services. For this reason, most retirement communities require their residents to subscribe to health insurance. Medicare and supplemental insurance benefits help pay for hospital care, skilled nursing care, home healthcare services, durable medical equipment and supplies, and prescription medications. Some of these insurance benefits apply to residents who receive care in a CCRC healthcare center. They may also apply to care in the resident's home or in a community nursing facility after a hospitalization, accident, or injury. The amount of supportive and medical care a resident requires determines their level of care. Many SRC's provide all the levels of care *except* for skilled nursing care in a healthcare center. If you require skilled nursing care, it is usually available in the local community.

As part of the continuum of care, a CCRC can provide all the levels of care and 24/7 medical care to residents recovering from an accident, surgery, illness, or hospitalization. Some residents can receive healthcare in their home while others with a need for skilled care may need to stay in a healthcare center within the retirement community. The CCRC healthcare center should be state-licensed and Medicare-certified, especially if it provides skilled nursing care, which is considered a high level of nursing care. Medicare Part A will pay for medical care received in a skilled healthcare facility if the resident meets the standard requirements for skilled nursing care. (See *Part 4: Finding Medical Care in Your Community and At Home*)

- **If you require more than 100 days of coverage in a skilled facility**, check with the CCRC on their policies regarding your benefits in the skilled nursing facility. Determine the facility's policy or fee for care above your allotment of Medicare days.

- **Medicare does not pay for intermediate or non-skilled custodial care.** However, for a limited stay or a fee, some CCRC's will provide the necessary nursing care in the healthcare center. If you must live in the healthcare facility on a permanent basis, some facilities charge the standard monthly fee. Others add an additional fee for the medical care on top of the cost of medications, supplies, and therapies.

- **Some CCRC's will consider other care options**, such as returning the resident to her home with supportive home healthcare services. The home healthcare services can be provided by the CCRC healthcare center or a community home healthcare services agency.

- **Many healthcare centers in a retirement community require a resident to maintain a supplemental insurance policy** to offset health or related charges not covered under Medicare. Some healthcare centers are not Medicare-certified, which means they cannot accept Medicare payment for the medical care you receive at their facility. If the healthcare center does not accept payments from Medicare, you should have subscribed to a supplemental insurance policy with benefits for skilled nursing care. Be prepared to pay an extra charge for nursing care at the healthcare center or to receive medical care outside the retirement community at a Medicare-certified skilled nursing facility that accepts Medicare payments.

- **There can be additional charges** for services, supplies, medication, and care you receive in the healthcare center.

- **If you require long-term assistance** with your activities of daily life (ADL's) and medical needs, consider hiring a private caregiver or moving to a higher level of care within the retirement community.

- **If you are unable to resume safe independent living**, the management at the SRC can suggest you receive a higher level of care or that you move to an alternative living situation that can provide increased supervision, assistance and medical care. Or the SRC may require you to hire a paid caregiver to help you with your care. In a CCRC, you should be able to move to a higher level of care within the community. For example, if you are residing in independent living at a CCRC but find you need assistance with bathing, dressing and more, consider moving to the assisted living unit within the retirement community.

- **If you are admitted to a hospital**, a nurse from the retirement home may visit you during your hospital stay to evaluate your mobility and medical care needs and determine your ability to manage safely in your residence. If the nurse determines that you would benefit from a higher level of care, she can recommend post-hospital care in the CCRC healthcare center or a community skilled nursing facility. The nurse may confer with hospital staff. Prior to your discharge from the hospital, hospital discharge planners and social workers may act as a liaison between your retirement community and the hospital. Helping you transition smoothly from the hospital to home. They can help you arrange temporary supportive care in your home through a home healthcare agency or private caregiver service. Some retirement communities retain a list of available private caregivers to assist you when you return to your residence.

Best Guide Retirement Communities provides links to Over 55 retirement living, equestrian, military, and university affiliated retirement communities.

Go to http://www.bestguide-retirementcommunities.com/collegelinkedretirementcommunities.html

---

Levels of Care in a Retirement Community

Levels of Care: *What are the levels of care provided in a retirement community?* While some retirement communities offer different levels of personal care, many prefer residents to be as independent as possible. A typical resident is in good physical and mental health and requires little or no assistance with their activities of daily life. For residents who require help, some retirement communities try to anticipate health changes in their residents by offering up to five levels of care.

Level 1: Independent Living (SRC and CCRC): Independent living is the ability to live without assistance from others. This means you are active and capable of caring for yourself by performing all the activities of daily living (ADL's), such as personal care, bathing, dressing, grooming, toileting, medication management, and attending meals in the dining area. You are able to walk without an assistive device (walker, cane) and are not at-risk for falling. If you use a cane or walker, you can use it without help from another person (to ensure you do not fall.) You may drive a car, attend theater, shop, and travel without assistance.

Level 2: Supportive Services (SRC and CCRC): Supportive services or the need for help with basic personal care and/or ADL's means you are capable of independent living with a minimal amount of help and stand-by or contact guard assistance. Stand-by or contact guard means you may need someone to stand near you or have a hand on you while you walk to ensure your safety. You may need occasional help with your personal care needs. This means you require help with some of your daily activities of life - dressing, eating, toileting, grooming, and mobility - but you do not have a skilled medical need. This type of care is referred to as *custodial care* and is *not* a Medicare covered benefit.

Level 3: Assisted Living (SRC and CCRC): Although you may continue to live independently, you now require moderate assistance with your personal care and activities of daily living. You may need someone to help you with many of your ADL's in the morning and later at night. You may need someone to check on you during the day or in the evening. You may need assistance with mobility and use a cane, walker, or wheelchair. Without assistance, you can be a fall risk or at-risk for harm or injury. In some retirement communities, you may be required to hire a private caregiver.

Level 4: Alzheimer's or Memory Care Special Units (CCRC): Some retirement communities have specialized units set up to provide extra assistance and supervision to people with Alzheimer's disease or dementia-related disorders. These locked specialized units prevent confused people from wandering off and getting lost. In addition to units within a CCRC, there are also community-based memory-care facilities and some adult care homes that specialize in providing care to those with Alzheimer's disease.

Level 5: End-of-Life Care (SRC and CCRC): As people approach the end of their lives, many prefer to stay in their own homes, receiving supportive healthcare services at their bedside. Some SRC's remain open to end-of-life care within their community as long as 24/7 care and supervision is provided by family and private caregivers. Others will encourage families to seek an alternative setting for end-of-life care in the home of a family member, in a skilled nursing facility, outpatient hospice center, assisted living, or adult foster care home. Hospice staff can see patients in any of these settings.

As CCRC's provide a continuity of care, residents may be able to stay in their own home within the retirement community with hired private caregivers and family support for end-of-life care. In a CCRC, this is possible to arrange end-of-life care either in your home with family, caregivers, and support from community hospice programs. Or the retirement community may provide end-of-life care in their assisted living section or healthcare center. At this time, Medicare pays for hospice care in a skilled nursing setting, *but it does not pay for the room and board.* Room and board in a skilled nursing facility can cost more than $300 per day. Check the policies of the CCRC regarding their services and coverage for hospice care.

Receiving medical care and services on the premises where you live is convenient. However, the CCRC staff cannot provide all medical treatments. Although the healthcare clinic can provide basic medical care, you will also need to arrange and travel to off-site medical care. For instance, you will need to travel to your primary care physician and travel to receive procedures such as x-rays, laboratory work-ups and some therapies.

For homebound residents with a skilled need such as nursing care, physical, occupational, or speech therapies, your physician can complete a referral for a home healthcare agency to provide these services in your home. A visiting nurse, with an order from your physician, can sometimes complete lab draws in your home.

If you have an emergency medical condition, the healthcare center can assess your condition and may recommend that you receive a more comprehensive evaluation and treatment in a nearby hospital emergency department.

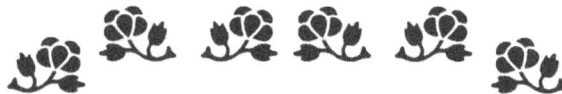

Similarities and Differences between Standard and Continuing Care Retirement Communities

Standard Features and Requirements in a Retirement Community	SRC	CCRC
Age requirement: Must be 55+ years of age or younger and disabled	Yes	Yes
Health requirement-Must be in good physical and mental health	Yes	Yes
Requires physical exam by physician	Not usually required	May be required
Requires long-term care health policy	Recommended but usually not required	May be required
Financial requirement: Must be financially secure	Yes	Yes
Monthly service fee	Yes	Yes
Requires large deposit or endowment or entrance buy-in fee	No	Usually required
Commitment to living in a retirement community	Can be short-term or long-term	Yes – More likely to be long-term due to financial investment
Offers different levels of care	Yes -includes independent living	Yes – includes independent and supportive and assisted care living, supportive, and assisted and often skilled healthcare
Residential units	More condo-like or apartments	Large complex similar to mini-village, with separate family homes, apartments, or condo-like units
Location	Rural or city	Rural or city
Services such as meals, linens, security	Yes – may include hidden fees or charges	Yes – may include hidden extra fees or extra charges; may charge fees for clubhouse, medical clinic, stores and more
Transportation, other extra charges	May offer free van or charge a fee	May offer free van or charge a fee
Activities – interdenominational services excursions, social programs	Yes	Yes – may offer more extensive programs

Admission Requirements and Guidelines

*"People tell me I look good these days. I look good because I feel good.
I know people who are older than I am who are twenty-five.
It's all about attitude. To me, age is just a number."*

-- Rita Moreno

As living in a retirement community is expensive, you should carefully consider the financial investment and commitment before you sign a contract. The following are general admission guidelines used by many retirement communities. When you begin to look at retirement communities, you will find a wide variance in the admission requirements. In many facilities you must be:

- **at least 55–62 years of age** or have a spouse at least sixty-two years of age. There is no maximum age limit provided you meet the other admission criteria. The age requirements will vary in different residences;

- **in good physical and mental health**;

- **capable of independent living**;

- **financially capable of fulfilling the residency agreement or contract** with the facility. Some facilities offer a free personal and confidential financial analysis to help you determine if you can afford to live in their community;

- **insured with a long-term care health policy** either through an insurance company of your choosing or through a health policy offered by the retirement community. *(Requirements may vary but long-term care or supplemental insurance policies provide essential medical coverage and benefits.)*

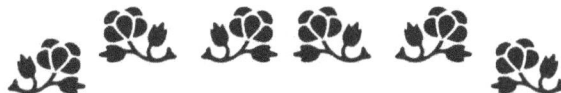

Applying for Admission to a Continuing Care Retirement Community

There are three types of CCRC communities: LifeCare, modified, and pay-as-you-go. In a LifeCare community, you pay a large entrance (also called endowment or buy-in) fee plus a set monthly fee that covers your meal plan, utilities, housekeeping, maintenance, transportation services, and activities. The monthly fee should not increase if you require additional healthcare services. In a modified community, you pay a lower entrance fee and an initial monthly fee that covers a certain amount of higher-level healthcare plus the above-mentioned amenities. In a pay-as-you-go community, you pay a still lower entrance fee and a monthly maintenance fee. However, if you require assisted living or skilled nursing care in the healthcare facility, the additional charges are substantial. Be aware that the monthly maintenance fee may increase with inflation each year. Entrance fees can be refundable minus a percentage of the fee or can be completely non-refundable. While the application process and the deposit requirements will differ in each retirement community, the following guidelines will help you understand the basics of the application process:

1) **Choose the type of living accommodation** you are interested in residing.

2) **Submit an application form** with a generally non-refundable application-processing fee.

3) **Read and sign the residence and care agreement or contract**. Some facilities request you sign and return the agreement within ten to fifteen days. At this time, half of the entrance fee may be due and payable. Place a deposit on the residence of your choice.

4) The **second half of the entrance fee** less the deposit may be due on or prior to occupancy.

5) **An additional application fee or refundable deposit** may be required. If the application is withdrawn, this additional deposit is usually refundable. (*Application fees will vary in individual retirement communities.*)

6) **Submit copies of insurance cards** (front and back) to the admissions office.

7) **Request an interview** with the admissions liaison at the retirement community to answer any questions and to tour the community. Some communities offer a free night lodging with meals so you can get a first-hand feel of the community life.

8) **A physical exam** by a retirement community physician may be required prior to acceptance. The applicant may receive this exam free of charge or may be financially

responsible for its cost. Check with your individual health insurance policy to determine if the exam is a covered benefit.

9) **A confidential financial statement** may be required. Some facilities offer a free or low-cost analysis of your financial situation to help you determine if their facility is a viable choice.

10) **The retirement community determines the occupancy date**.

11) **The first monthly maintenance or service charge** may be due on the occupancy date.

(The guidelines listed above will vary according to the policies and requirements of each retirement community.)

To consider realistically living in any retirement community, you must be financially secure. In a CCRC, the monthly service fees can range from $2,000 to over $10,000 per month, depending on the size and location of the residence and the activities and services provided by the retirement community. Some retirement communities may raise the monthly fee after you move in. You may also be responsible for property taxes and other "hidden" fees. In addition to the monthly service fee, there can be additional charges for assistance with personal care, transportation to shopping and medical appointments, meals, parking, and cable television. Rates vary depending upon the resident's needs: The greater the need for assistance, the higher the monthly fee. For example, if you are independent and require no assistance, the monthly rate will be lower than if you require some help with personal care.

Living in an SRC is usually less costly than living in a CCRC, as they tend to be smaller communities with fewer services and activities on the premises. If a married couple decide to move into the retirement community together, sharing a residence, one person pays the full cost for living in the retirement community while the spouse usually pays a reduced fee.

Types of Refund Contracts

There are several types of refund contracts offered to the potential resident. They provide an opportunity to change your mind, leave the community, and still receive a prorated or portion of the entrance fee. The terms of retirement community refund contracts vary widely. Standard declining-refund contracts allow 24-50 months for a decision. For example, if you moved into a Continuing Care Retirement Community under a thirty-six-month declining-refund contract,* you could leave the center, move somewhere else during that thirty-six-month period, and receive a refund portion of your entrance fee. If you stayed for twelve months, you would receive a pro-rated amount for the twenty-four remaining months. However, if you decided to move after thirty-six months, you could lose your entire entrance fee. In the event of your death or the withdrawal of your application, the entrance fee might be refundable.

Some retirement communities will pay the refund only when a new resident occupies the residence. This means another person, not necessarily related to you, moves into the apartment unit you have vacated by choice, illness, or death

*(Please note: These contracts will vary at individual retirement communities.)

On the following pages, you will find helpful questions to ask when you visit the retirement community.

Questions to Ask about the Retirement Community

Location and Grounds

- How convenient is the facility to the nearest town or city?
- Is bus /public transportation easily accessible?
- What is the size/acreage of the retirement community?
- Are the grounds well maintained?
- Are walkways easily accessible for canes, walkers, wheelchairs, and electric scooters?

Residences

- How many occupied units or residences does the community maintain?
- Is there a waiting list for units within the retirement community?
- How long is the waiting list for residences?
- Can you move into a temporary unit while waiting for your unit to become available?
- Is there a fee for changing units?
- Can you easily change from one floor plan to another?

- Are units furnished or unfurnished?

- Does the community pay for the initial design changes to your residence?

- Can you make changes to your unit such as painting walls, installing new carpet? Are there any restrictions on interior design such as carpet quality, color, or design, or wall color or type of paint, or use of wallpaper or design?

- Who provides and pays for maintenance and upgrades? Who determines when an upgrade or repair is appropriate?

Residents

- What is the average length of stay among residents?

- What is the average age of residents when they move in?

- Are most of the residents: female_____ male_____
married/with partner_____ single _____ divorced ___ widowed___

- Are most residents local or have they moved there from other areas?

- What is the average health status of residents?

- What is the average level of education for residents?

Guests, Children and Pets

- Are there guest accommodations?

- Can guests join the resident at mealtime? Is there a cap to the number of times this is possible? Are there any age restrictions such as no children under the age of 18?

- Is there a charge for guest accommodations or for meals provided during the guest's stay? If yes, what is the charge?

- What is the policy regarding pets living/visiting in the residences or buildings?

- What is the policy regarding children staying/visiting in the residences and/or eating in the dining room?

Staffing

- Is staff available twenty-four hours a day and seven days a week?

- What is the staff to resident ratio?

- Is staff professional, friendly and helpful?
- Is staff easily accessible to residents?
- If you need staff to address a problem, how long is the average wait time?

Services

- Which services are included in the monthly fee?
- Which services are subject to extra charges?
- Who determines which supportive services a resident needs?
- If you require a special diet, can the retirement community meet your dietary needs?
- Is meal delivery to the residence available for residents with temporary health problems?

Health

- Is nursing care available on the retirement community grounds?
- Is a supplemental long-term healthcare insurance policy required?
- Does the retirement community work closely with local home healthcare agencies?
- Is there a policy on hiring temporary live-in help or caregiving? Does the community retain a list of licensed caregivers?
- Can a resident receive skilled nursing care in the healthcare center?
- Can a resident receive intermediate nursing care or custodial care in the healthcare center? Are there additional fees for this service?
- Is there a maximum length of time a resident can receive care in the healthcare center? Is yes, what is it? _____
- If significant long-term nursing care is required, is a resident allowed to live on a permanent basis at the health care center? If not, what options are available to the resident?
- If a resident is hospitalized and requires increased assistance and/or skilled nursing care at discharge from the hospital, can they return to their residence? If not, will they receive care in the skilled nursing healthcare center? Will Medicare or other insurance cover this care? Will the resident be required to hire private caregivers to provide care?

- Is an evaluation required to determine the residents' ability to return to their residence after a hospitalization? *Retirement communities often require a medical evaluation at the hospital before allowing a resident to return to their residence. The evaluation may include talking with the hospital nursing staff, a medical social worker or case manager, the primary care physician, the family, and the patient. The evaluation may focus on the mental and physical capabilities of the resident, including nursing care needs, such as incontinence care, injections, dressing changes and mobility. This includes the ability to transfer or get in and out of bed or into a wheelchair.*

Cost

- Is a financial report of the retirement community available for your review?

- Can the retirement community increase the monthly fee?

- What are the conditions for increasing the fees?

- How often does the retirement community increase the monthly fee?

- As a resident, how much notice will you receive regarding fee changes?

- Are resident's responsible for paying property taxes?

- Are there any hidden costs? *Additional expenses may include utilities, telephone services, medication, medical care outside the retirement community, garage or carport rental, additional meals or delivery of meals, excursions, and some transportation services.*

Legal Issues

- *Should I consult with an attorney before I sign a residence contract?* When you sign a residence and care agreement, you are signing a complex legal document. Review this contract with an attorney before signing it.

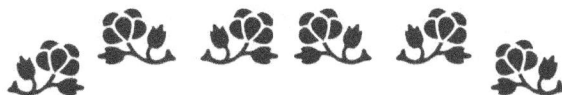

Living in a Home or Facility
with Supervision and Assistance

*(assisted living facilities, adult care
homes, and specialized memory care units)*

"There are only four kinds of people in this world. Those who have been caregivers, those who are caregivers, those who will be caregivers, and those who will need caregivers."

– Rosalynn Carter, Former First Lady

In the continuum of care, living in an assisted living facility, an adult care home, or a specialized memory care facility falls between independent living and skilled nursing care. With over 40,000 assisted living facilities in the United States, they encompass a variety of living options. It is a bridge for those in need of daily help and supervision with personal care, meal preparation, and their activities of daily life – bathing, dressing, grooming, and toileting, medication management and basic nursing care.

For people experiencing a decline in personal health, difficulty with managing basic care needs, or deteriorating mental function, assisted living offers an alternative to living in an unsafe home environment.

If you are considering moving to an assisted living environment, you should understand the types of assisted living settings, admissions procedures, the levels of care, licensing, cost, insurance benefits, and available features and services. In addition, it is important to consider many of the factors you reviewed for retirement communities: location, environment, resident characteristics, and staffing. This information can help you make a realistic and informed decision, as well as determine if assisted living is the best choice for you and for what you need.

Types of Assisted Living Care Facilities

The term, "assisted living" is used to describe a facility or home that provides assistance and supervision with daily personal care and non-skilled or custodial medical care. The facilities offering this care range from larger assisted living complexes to home-like adult care homes. Specialty-care facilities focus on those with disabilities, dementia or Alzheimer's disease, or the mentally challenged. These facilities differ in their size, staffing, atmosphere, room set-up, levels of care, and more.

Assisted Living Facilities: *(Also known as residential care.)* These moderately-sized residences provide studios and apartments for residents over 65-years old, and those younger than 65 with disabilities. You can live independently in your own residence, receiving only the services that you need. Residents usually require help with at least three activities of daily living – personal care, bathing, dressing, grooming, toileting, mobility, medication management, and basic nursing care. The facilities are staffed 24/7 and provide three meals daily, usually in a communal dining area. Some facilities will deliver meals to your room, if needed. While many assisted living facilities include independent residences, assisted living sections are provided as part of the continuum of care found in a continuing care retirement complex. Assisted living facilities may also be found attached to a skilled nursing care facility.

Adult care homes: *(also known as board and care homes, adult foster care homes, domiciliary homes, personal care homes, community residences, and rest homes.)* An adult care home is a private home that accepts no more than six residents needing daily support and assistance. As these homes provide different levels of care, you should choose one with the specific needs of the resident in mind. Residents requiring minimal help may need a Level 1 home: those requiring moderate assistance should consider a Level 2 home; those needing significant help with most or all of their ADL's should consider a Level 3 home. These homes provide basic nursing care and sometimes offer end-of-life or hospice care. Some offer private rooms with a private bath. Often you will share a bedroom and bathroom with other residents. It may also specialize in providing care for people with dementia and mental health issues who require supervision where they live.

Some owners/caregivers in the adult care homes have a nursing background and are comfortable with basic nursing care; others may not be comfortable giving diabetic insulin injections, providing catheter care, or changing dressings. Be sure to check for any medical care restrictions with the adult care homeowner.

Specialty-Care Assisted Living: *(also called memory care)* is found in an assisted living facility, an adult care home, or in a skilled nursing facility with a specialized unit. Sometimes a facility will specialize in caring for people with Alzheimer's disease, providing a locked and secure environment to prevent residents from wandering away from the facility.

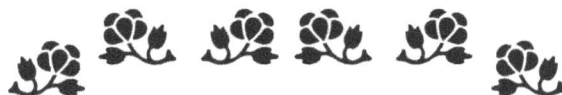

When to Consider Living
in an Assisted Living Facility

If you are living at home and beginning to have difficulty with the following, it may be time to consider an alternative to living in your home. There are several common warning signs that indicate a living situation is becoming unsafe. They include:

- **increased need for supervision and assistance** with the activities of daily living such as bathing, grooming dressing, feeding, personal hygiene and toileting;

- **difficulty with mobility**, such as walking, transferring from bed to chair, climbing stairs;

- **frequent falls** resulting in fractures, contusions, bruising, or abrasions. Frequent falls place you at high risk for a serious injury or accident;

- **prolonged illness, injury, or recent or repeated hospitalizations**, resulting in the need for additional medical care and supervision that family and community agencies are unable to provide;

- **inability to manage medication**, resulting in an accidental overdose or skipping necessary medication If medication management is necessary, look for an assisted living facility with a staff registered nurse or an adult care home which has an owner or caregiver with nursing training or healthcare experience;

- **increased mental confusion or disorientation,** resulting in a need for additional supervision. Basic cognitive skills such as critical thinking, remembering, reasoning, the inability to recognize danger or summon assistance, express needs or make decisions regarding basic healthcare are all indicators;

- **significant depression, anxiety, or fears,** which interfere with your ability to manage independently;

- **poor eating habits** that cause a significant weight loss or gain due to an inadequate diet. Sometimes a person with dementia may not be able to feed themselves without direction and cues or assistance from another person;

- **increased social withdrawal or isolation from friends and family** caused by decreased attendance at social activities and fewer visits from friends and family;

These are indicators that it is time to consider moving to a safer home environment where you can receive the help you need. If you are determined to stay in your current home, it may be time to increase your in-home services.

Many assisted living and adult care residences offer a continuum of care that makes it possible for you to age in place. That is, even as your medical care increases, you can remain in your own apartment or room. Some assisted living facilities and adult care homes offer end-of-life care with support from family, private caregivers, and home healthcare or hospice services.

If you currently live in an assisted living facility or adult care home, you may find a home that once met your needs no longer does. This could result from changes in the residence and its staff or residents or from our own changing health needs. When this happens, consider a move to a residence that can meet your daily care needs. Factors that can affect your care include:

- inadequate staffing;
- limited assistance and supervision, especially at night-time;
- less personal attention;
- increased medical care needs;
- an unsafe living environment.

Pam lived in an assisted living facility for one year. During that time, the staff and other long-term residents knew her well. She had her own studio apartment and a small kitchenette. In the morning, staff helped her get dressed and ready for the day; in the evening staff helped her get ready for bed. During an unexpected family visit, Pam's family found her in her room confused and disoriented to her surroundings. She had knocked over her nightstand and was trying to pick it up. She had a bleeding cut on her arm that required a bandage. Due to reduced staffing, no staff was aware of her predicament. Despite living in an assisted living facility, her family felt that she did not have adequate supervision, making it an unsafe environment. Her family decided to move her to a different assisted living environment that provided increased supervision.

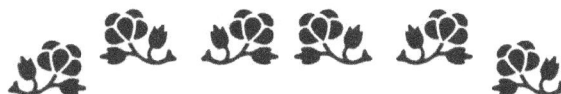

How to Choose an Assisted Living Facility

The amount of physical care and supervision needed by a resident, the type of accommodation and the resident's financial situation can determine which assisted living facility you choose to live in. Look at:

- **admission guidelines**;
- the **resident's required level of care and assistance**;
- **licensing and regulations**;
- **the location**;
- the **type of buildings and accommodations**: private room versus semi-private room;
- **standard residence features**;
- **basic services, including social activities**;
- the **resident's characteristics**;
- the **staff** including their relationship with residents;
- the **cost of living in the residence and insurance benefits** – private pay versus Medicaid. If you have a long-term care policy, check the benefits for care in an assisted living facility. *(Please note: Only some states offer Medicaid benefits for living in assisted living facilities and adult care homes Check with the local State Area on Aging to determine if your state provides this benefit.*

Admission Guidelines for an Assisted Living Facility

Each assisted living facility will determine its own admission guidelines for new residents. By evaluating each resident, the staff can gain a better understanding of the resident's personal care and medical needs. After you visit several assisted living facilities and decide on the facility that meets your personal requirements, contact the facilities admissions office. An admissions coordinator will give you an application to complete which includes information about your personal, financial and medical history. By completing the *Getting to Know You Worksheet* at the end of the Introduction section, you will have the information you need to complete application forms.

Because some facilities maintain a waiting list, it is important to ask about availability when you first visit the facility. Even if you have not decided on the best facility for you, it is helpful to place your name on the waiting list. This should not obligate you, but ensure that the facility will notify you when an opening becomes available.

If the room or apartment you choose is unavailable, some facilities will temporarily place you in a different room until your first choice becomes available. If units have turnover infrequently, this may give you priority. However, if the temporary room is significantly larger than the room you will be moving into, it may cost more.

The monthly fee is determined in part by room size, and in part by the level of required care. As your care needs increase, which is often the case for people living in an assisted living facility, the monthly cost can also increase. Because of limited staffing, some facilities will not accept residents with a high level of care needs. Alternatively, they may recommend temporary placement in a higher level of care, such as a skilled nursing facility in order for you to receive skilled medical care. When the level of care you need returns to its original or baseline level, you can usually return to the assisted living facility.

When you have been in the hospital, many assisted living facilities will send a social worker, admission coordinator, or registered or licensed practical nurse to the hospital to review your medical record and talk with hospital staff about your medical care needs. They can determine from this information if it is appropriate for you to return to the assisted living facility. If they determine that your healthcare needs are greater than what they can provide, the facility may recommend you receive a higher level of care until you are able to resume your normal activities and usual level of care. Most facilities will work with you and hold the room until you can return.

Following a hospitalization or illness, the assisted living facility can help you arrange for visits by home healthcare professionals. These professionals, registered nurses, therapists, and social workers, can visit you in your apartment if you have a skilled need – physical, occupational, or speech therapies and nursing care. You must be homebound or unable to leave your home without considerable effort and only for a short duration.

Most people living in an assisted living facility are referred to as private-pay residents. As stated earlier, **Medicare does *not* pay for this unskilled or custodial care**. In some states, **Medicaid** will pay for assisted living costs for low-income individuals. In addition, some **long-term care insurance policies** may provide partial payment toward care in an assisted living facility. **Veterans programs** can also pay for service-connected veterans to live in a facility when other options are limited.

Levels of Care in an Assisted Living Facility

"Life is what you make it, always has been, always will be."

– Grandma Moses

If you choose to move to an assisted living/residential facility, you may be partially independent or able to care for yourself without placing yourself at-risk for personal harm. Prior to admission, the admissions staff will evaluate the level of care needed. They will look at your basic personal and medical care needs, cognition, mobility, and your ability to perform your activities of daily life. The assisted living facility provides 24-hour personal care services, but you will need to function when alone in your apartment, which may be the case for significant portions of the day and night. The levels of care available in most assisted living facilities are:

- Independent - needs little or no care;
- Level 1: minimal care;
- Level 2: moderate care;
- Level 3: maximum care - This can include end-of-life care.

Independent Living

Independent living means that you are capable of caring for yourself without help from others. You can choose to live in an assisted living environment *before* you require considerable assistance with your care, utilizing facility amenities such as housekeeping services, prepared meals, social activities, and more. To live independently, you should:

- be alert and oriented to time of day, place (Where are you?), and person (What is your name?);
- move independently, safely walk with a cane or walker, or self-propel a wheelchair or power scooter;
- be able to easily and safely transfer from a wheelchair to a chair, bed, or toilet;
- require no to minimal assistance with activities of daily living such as eating, dressing, bathing, and personal care;
- not require a special diet at mealtime *(Some facilities prepare special meals, such*

as diabetic or low-cholesterol foods for residents at no charge or for a small extra fee);

- be able to take your medication properly., i.e. the correct dose at the correct time.

If you require additional care, an evaluation by assisted living staff can help determine the proper level of care needed.

Level 1: Minimal Care

To receive Level 1 care, you may:

- be alert and oriented, with minimal confusion or disorientation You should be aware of your surroundings, and able to understand information and make decisions on your own behalf;
- need occasional assistance with mobility or transfers. i.e., you may need assistance walking to the bathroom or to the dining area for meals;
- need some assistance with the activities of daily living such as bathing, dressing, grooming, or toileting;
- need an occasional reminder or assistance with personal hygiene;
- have occasional loss of control or incontinence of your bladder or bowel;
- need occasional reminders or assistance to properly take medication;
- need a special diet.

Level 2: Moderate Care

To receive Level 2 care, you may:

- be alert and oriented, with some episodes of confusion and disorientation;
- need daily supervision;
- need regular assistance with mobility or transfers;
- need moderate assistance with the activities of daily living have frequent loss of control of bladder or bowel;

- need daily reminders and some assistance with personal hygiene;
- need moderate medical and basic nursing care;
- need daily medication management;
- need daily assistance at mealtime.

Level 3: Maximum Care

To receive Level 3 care, you may:

- be moderately confused and disoriented;
- be alert and oriented but in need of constant supervision and assistance because of your physical needs;
- need constant supervision;
- need frequent intervention by staff so you do not harm yourself or others;
- have increased need for assistance with mobility;
- need total assistance with routine bathing, dressing, grooming, toileting and personal care;
- need frequent medical intervention and basic nursing care. Visits from home healthcare or hospice nurses may be necessary;
- need constant supervision and assistance at mealtime; i.e. help with setting up a plate and feeding at mealtimes;
- need constant supervision and monitoring of medication. i.e., help with taking daily medications.

Determining the Cost of
Living in an Assisted Living Facility

When you live in an assisted living facility, several factors will determine the cost. These include:

- type of residential unit;
- levels of care offered;
- method of payment.

An evaluation by facility staff determines the *level of care* or the amount of supervision and assistance an individual needs. The higher the level of care you require, the higher the monthly rate you will pay.

For example, a person who receives Level I care and resides in a studio apartment pays less than a Level I person who resides in a one-bedroom apartment. A person who lives in the same type of residential unit, but receives Level II care pays more than a person receiving Level I care.

The *method of payment* refers to the way you pay the monthly fee for assisted living to the facility. You may pay privately with personal funds from your monthly Social Security or pension checks, with funds from savings or investments, or through long-term care insurance. Alternatively, if you have a limited income, you may be eligible for financial support through the state Medicaid program policy. On average, assisted living facilities cost less than nursing homes, with fees ranging from $1000 to more than $6,000 a month. Some facilities charge additional fees for supplies and other services. If the monthly charge seems much higher than other facilities in the area, it is important to question the charges and determine why the rate is so much higher.

Assisted Living Federation of America (ALFA) provides information on assisted living services and programs.
Go to http://www.alfa.org/alfa/Consumer_Corner.asp

Medline:
Go to http://www.nlm.nih.gov/medlineplus/assistedliving.html

Assisted Living Source: Go to http://www.assistedlivingsource.com/

National Center for Assisted Living:
Go to http://www.ahcancal.org/ncal/Pages/default.aspx

Assisted Living Facilities.org:
Go to http://www.assistedlivingfacilities.org/

Insurance Benefits
in an Assisted Living Facility

Most insurance policies do *not* pay for custodial or unskilled care in an assisted living facility. *Custodial care, also known as unskilled care,* is general care and assistance with the activities of daily living, as well as supervision to prevent personal harm. Provided by an unskilled person, this care is not medically necessary or essential to the treatment and diagnosis of an illness or injury.

- **Medicare** does not pay for custodial or non-skilled care in an assisted living facility.

- **Medicaid,** in some states, provides financial benefits to assist low-income individuals living in an assisted living facility. To determine your eligibility for the Senior Assisted Housing Waiver, contact the *State Area Agency on Aging* or your *local Senior and Disabled Services Office.*

- **Private-insurance policies** generally do not offer financial benefits for assisted living care.

- **Some Long-term Care policies** may provide financial assistance for hiring a private caregiver. This amount may or may not cover the entire cost of hiring a caregiver. Review your policy to determine your long-term policy benefits. Confirm your understanding with your policy company.

- **The Department of Veterans Affairs** offers benefits that help veterans pay for room and board and personal care in an assisted living facility. Contact your nearest *U.S. Department of Veterans Affairs Office* to determine if these benefits are available in your area.

U.S. Department of Veteran's Affairs: This website contains veteran's benefit, pension, compensation, and GI Bill information. It allows you to download important forms and has a facility locator. For VA benefits, go to http://www.va.gov or call 1-800-827-1000.

Licensing and Regulations

In the continuum of care, assisted living facilities constitute one of several living options between retirement communities and nursing home care. This alternative to nursing home care is receiving praise from many but also raising concerns regarding the lack of standardized state or federal regulations governing them.

Although more than one million people now live in more than forty thousand assisted living facilities nationwide, no uniform state or federal accreditation or licensing program exists. Some states require specific training for assisted living staff, which includes certification to care for residents. Other states do not require any training and may have assisted living facilities with poorly trained staff to provide this care. Some states maintain regulations for building code or fire safety requirements. Others states have no regulations regarding building or fire codes. Some facilities comply with the *Americans with Disabilities Act* (ADA), are members of the *American Healthcare Association* (AHCA) or a state healthcare association. Others do not comply with ADA regulations and are not members of a state healthcare association. Two organizations that provide accreditation to assisted living facilities are the *Joint Commission on Accreditation of Healthcare Organizations (JCAHO)* and the *Commission on Accreditation of Rehabilitation Facilities (CARF.)* If a facility has accreditation from these organizations, it is held to above average standards.

The *Assisted Living Federation of America* (ALFA) offers a free brochure and checklist you can use to help evaluate assisted living facilities. Ombudsmen, or people who investigate complaints regarding facilities, may offer additional insight.

Assisted Living Federation of America (ALFA): This website represents the largest national organization involved in influencing public policy in this area. In addition, it offers *Source for Senior Living,* a helpful information and referral resource. Go to http://www.alfa.org/alfa

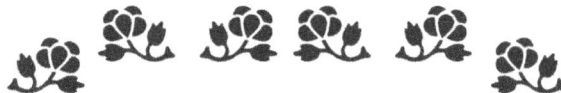

Resident Characteristics
in an Assisted Living Facility

If you choose to live in an assisted living facility, you can move there directly from your home, the home of a family member or friend, a skilled nursing facility, a retirement community. While some residents live independently, they may choose an assisted living facility where they can receive meals and easily access social activities, care and assistance. When you observe the residents, you may see a wide range of abilities. Some residents will be active and mentally and physically capable; others will require daily care and supervision for physical and mental health issues.

Many residents use walkers, canes, crutches, and occasionally a wheelchair or power scooter. Residents who need durable medical equipment and supplies can obtain any necessary items while living in the facility. Sometimes a bedside commode, a shower stool, or a raised toilet seat makes the difference between maintaining independence or necessitating a higher level of care.

Staffing and Staff Qualities in an Assisted Living Facility

A fair amount of interaction between the staff and the residents should exist. Expect the staff to maintain a care plan that contains your daily care needs, personal information, emergency contact information, names and telephone numbers of your physicians, a brief medical history, a list of medications, and other important data. The care plan should accompany you to hospital visits and medical appointments. Expect the staff to know residents by their names. Expect them to be aware of your medical issues and needs. Furthermore, the staff should be available to help you with the activities of daily living - - bathing, grooming, dressing, toileting, eating. If you have recently been in the hospital, they should be able to increase this assistance, at least for a short time.

Most families tend to visit at specific times and so may only know the staff on one or two shifts. Staff members usually work three different shifts and it is important to for you and your family to familiarize yourselves with staff members on each shift. Administrators, management, social workers, and therapists usually work during the day shift*, 7 a.m.- 4 p.m. Registered nurses and licensed practical nurses tend to work the day shift and part of the afternoon shift, 3p.m.–11p.m. During the night shift, 11p.m.–7a.m. staff is often limited to one registered or licensed practical nurse with additional support from a certified nursing assistant (CNA) or certified home healthcare aide (HHA.) It is important to check that the evening staffing is sufficient for the number of residents. *(Shifts can vary at each facility.)

Check the resident-to-staff ratio: How many staff members are available to help residents at mealtimes? How many staff members are available during the day or at night? Is there a high staff turnover? Is there a training program for staff in place

Considering the Location of an Assisted Living Facility

When you look at assisted living facilities, consider the distance to local hospitals, medical clinics, family and friends, shopping, houses of worship, and entertainment. If you function independently or receive minimal care, you may want these services and activities located close by.

Many assisted living facilities situate themselves in areas convenient to hospitals and medical care, anticipating the residents' needs for medical services from a physician, clinic, hospital or hospital emergency department. Because many residents in these facilities rely on daily help and assistance, the proximity to a medical facility guarantees prompt medical treatment when it is necessary.

A location close to family makes it more likely that you will receive family visits. Family members are encouraged to visit regularly, as too often, insufficient facility staffing can affect the staffs' ability to provide necessary supervision of residents. Frequent visits by family members allow them to evaluate your current care needs and whether changes need to be made.

Residents in assisted living facilities may require more support from family and friends than those who live in a retirement community. The facility may request assistance from family to help with transportation to a medical appointment at a physician's office or to a pharmacy to refill prescription medications.

Types of Buildings and Accommodations

Assisted living facilities come in many shapes and sizes. They can resemble hotels, large private homes, high-rise apartment buildings, or one-level apartment-like structure. Small facilities can house five to eighteen residents; larger facilities can provide care for up to several hundred. When looking at these various settings, consider the ages, health level and interests of residents, the staff members' professionalism, the resident to staff ratio, the physical environment, and the level of care and assistance provided by each facility.

Some assisted living facilities affiliate with both standard and continuing care retirement communities. When a resident is no longer capable of safely living independently and requires more assistance and/or supervision, they can easily move from independent living to a higher level of care where additional help is available. In an assisted living apartment, they can receive a higher level of care and closer monitoring from staff.

In many facilities, the residents live in a private studio or one or two-bedroom apartment. These apartments should be equipped with safety features, including bathroom grab bars and an intercom system. A common shared area may have books, television, games, and comfortable chairs and sofas for residents. Residents should be able to access the dining area easily. In other words, there should be enough space for residents to maneuver with walkers, wheelchairs, power wheelchairs, or power scooters.

Standard Residence Features

A standard residence is usually a studio or one-bedroom apartment, either semi-private or private. All or most utilities are included in the monthly fee. Determine which utilities are included in the monthly rental charge. Telephone and cable services are usually *not* included. Many residences feature the following:

- use of convenient laundry rooms;
- individual heating and air-conditioning controls in each room;
- 24-hour emergency call system;
- safety systems in each apartment unit;
- small kitchen area;
- option to add own furniture to apartment;
- satellite television with local and cable stations;
- smoke detectors;
- sound proof construction;
- wall-to-wall carpeting;
- bathroom with safety grab bars in the tub or shower.

Basic Services and Activities

Many of the services in an assisted living facility are similar to those offered in a retirement community. Basic services can include the following:

- **three meals daily in a communal dining area.** In times of illness, many assisted living facilities agree to deliver meals to the room for a temporary period of time;

- **transportation services.** Many facilities have their own wheelchair van, which can be used for transportation to medical appointments and other excursions;

- **apartment and ground maintenance;**

- **basic medical care services** as described in levels of care;

- **assistance with the activities of daily living** (ADL's);

- **housekeeping and linen service.** This service may be provided once or twice a week, inclusive in the monthly fee;

- **use of social and recreational areas.** Many facilities maintain an activities director on staff who schedules monthly activities. Religious services may take place at the facility, or the facility may provide transportation to local houses of worship.

Assisted living facilities offer a variety of daily activities appropriate for different levels of care. The most common activities include:

- arts and crafts;
- cards and bridge groups;
- bingo and other games;
- chapel/religious services;
- Bible study;
- discussion/book groups;
- garden in a provided garden area;
- reading/access to books in a facility library;
- needlework;
- movies;
- entertainment and music;
- low-impact aerobics, yoga and exercise classes;
- pet therapy;
- recreational activities and outings;
- water exercise classes.

Questions to Ask at an Assisted Living Facility

Visit several facilities *before* making a decision. Spend a day at the facility, dining and participating in activities. Take advantage of sleeping overnight in a guest unit. After talking with residents and staff members, sit down with other family members to discuss their impressions. Everyone will notice different details about the facility, but trust your instincts even if you are unable to pinpoint why you feel the way you do. When you walk into an assisted living facility, look at the general appearance of the residence.

Outside Area

- Do the grounds appear well maintained?
- Is there an outside patio or sitting area, garden plot, or paved walkways for residents?
- Is the residence taller than one story?
- Are there ramps along the curb for easy wheelchair access?
- Are outside handrails located near steps and along sidewalks?

Inside Area

- Does the front door area have a security guard?

- Is the lobby area empty or are residents sitting around? Are they interacting with one another?

- Does the facility permit smoking or designate a smoking area?

- Is the atmosphere formal or informal? Are people dressed up or dressed casually?

- Is there a dress code?

- What are the visiting hours?

- Are the hallways wide enough to accommodate a walker, wheelchair, or power scooter or power wheelchair?

- Are the hallways equipped with convenient handrails?

- Are elevators conveniently located and easily accessed?

- What is the distance from your room to the dining area?

- Are apartment units available furnished or unfurnished? If the unit is furnished, what furniture and accessories are included?

- Are single units and /or double occupancy units available to share with another person?

- Can residents provide their own furnishings and/or decorate their rooms? Are there guidelines or policies that dictate or constrain interior design or furnishings, improvements, repairs, or upgrades? Is there adequate storage space?

- Do apartment units include a kitchen area? Is it a full or a partial-kitchen?

- Do apartment units contain handicap features such as emergency call buttons and grab bars in the bathroom?

- Is there an easy-to-access shower, tub, or a tub-shower?

- Is there an extra charge for telephone, and/or cable services?

- Does the facility allow small pets? Is there a pet exercise area?

Residents

- What is the average age of residents?

- Do residents spend most time isolated in their rooms or in a shared common area?

- Are residents active or inactive? Do they interact with one another? Is there a sense of community among the residents?

- Are residents dressed in street clothes, formal attire, or sitting in their nightgowns and pajamas?

- What is the participation rate of residents in the various activities?

- Are family members or friends encouraged to visit?

Staff

- Does staff convey a professional attitude? Do they provide satisfactory answers to your questions?

- Does staff receive training to care for residents? Do they have licenses or certifications in place?

- What is the staff to resident ratio? Is it the same during the evening shift? Is the staffing on the weekends the similar to staffing during the week?

- Are you comfortable communicating with staff members?

- Are you comfortable with their interactions with residents?

- How does staff determine the care needs of each resident? Does the staff develop and maintain a personalized care plan for each resident? How frequently do they review and update the plan? Do they update the plan with input from the resident's physician?

- Does the facility maintain a house physician on staff?

- How often does the physician visit the facility?

- Can your primary care physician visit or continue to provide your medical care and treatment?

- Does the facility maintain an activities director? What activities are available to residents?

- Is a social worker or care manager available to talk with patients and their families regarding any issues or concerns?

Personal and Healthcare Services

- Can residents self-administer their own medication?

- Is medication management available to residents who have difficulty taking their correct medication at the proper time of day?

- Are staff trained and certified to help a resident with administering injections i.e. insulin injections?

- If a resident experiences a change in health, is staff available to provide additional assistance? Is staff available to escort a resident to the emergency department for medical care? What is the process? Is the process delayed or complicated if a medical crisis occurs during a weekend or holiday? Is family notified if a resident requires acute medical care?

- Do staff members maintain health and medication records for each resident? Do they send these records with residents when they seek emergency medical care?

- Is staff trained, available, and certified to help with the activities of daily living such as:

  - bathing;
  - grooming;
  - shopping;
  - personal hygiene;
  - housekeeping;
  - help eating at meal

  - time;
  - laundry;
  - walking;
  - transfers.

- Can a resident privately hire a person to provide additional care in their apartment unit?

- Do staff members encourage family involvement?

- Are home healthcare agencies available to provide basic nursing care?

- Does staff help coordinate services with a home healthcare agency?

- Can a resident receive hospice services and end-of-life care at the facility?

Cost

- What services are included in the monthly fee?

- What services are *not* included in the monthly fee?

- If a resident's care requirements change, does this affect the monthly fee?

- If a resident changes units or decides to leave the facility, what is the refund policy?

- Does the facility accept Medicaid payments? *(This is an important question. Some facilities do not accept Medicaid. Others may accept Medicaid's low reimbursement rate.)*

- What is the policy regarding residents if their funds run out? *(This is an important question. Some facilities may discharge or evict a resident who is unable to pay for care. Others may try to work closely with the resident to prepare them for reduced funds. They may help you apply for Medicaid and financial assistance through the State Senior and Disabled Services Office.)*

- Will the facility help a resident apply for Medicaid? *(Many facilities will anticipate the financial aspects of care and help a resident apply for Medicaid.)*

- Does the facility accept long-term health insurance? *(Some long-term insurance policies provide limited coverage for assisted living.)*

Transportation

- Does the facility own a wheelchair van?

- Does the facility provide transportation to medical appointments?

- Is there a fee for transportation services?

- Are there excursions to other activities, such as plays, concerts, or movies? Do they involve additional charges such as for tickets, transportation, refreshments?

- Is the facility located close to shopping for food, gifts, etc.?

Licensing and Certification

- Does the facility have a current state license and/or certification?

- Does a non-profit or a corporation manage the facility?

- What is the facilities reputation within the community?

If you are considering living in an assisted living facility, also be sure to look into the smaller and more home-like setting found in an adult care home.

When to Consider Living in an Adult Care Home

(board and care homes, adult foster care homes, family care homes, domiciliary homes, personal care homes, community residences or rest homes)

Adult care homes fill a large gap in the types of facilities offering care to semi-dependent and vulnerable seniors and disabled persons. An adult care home is a private home in which the owner of the residence, an employee, and/or a caregiver provides basic personal care and assistance with the activities of daily living (ADL's) at a reasonable cost. ADL's include grooming, bathing, dressing, personal hygiene, mobility, toileting, meal preparation and feeding, and supervision. Caregivers can provide some medication management, but there is a preference for residents to be able to give themselves their own medication with supervision. Basic nursing care covers all levels of care; end-of-life care may be available in homes licensed for Level 3 care. As there are guidelines regarding how many bed-ridden residents a home can care for at a time, it is best to check with each individual home regarding their ability to provide care for a resident who is bed-ridden requiring end-of-life or hospice care. The resident to staff ratio is seldom less than one staff to six or less residents.

It is important to note that adult care homes often have an owner who does not live in the residence or provide direct care to the residents living in the home. These owners are responsible for supervising their employees and the hired caregivers. They also act as a liaison between you, your physician, and your family, community agencies, hospitals, skilled nursing facilities, medical supply and equipment companies, transportation services, Senior and Disabled Services and home healthcare and hospice agencies.

The amount of reviews or visits by state officials to ensure that all adult care homes are licensed, hire experienced or certified caregivers, and that there is no exploitation or abuse of residents, varies in each state. Some states perform limited evaluations of these homes, meaning some operate without a license and not held to a high standard of care. That said, there are many well-run adult care homes that provide excellent personal care to the people living in their residence.

If you are considering living in an adult care home, it is important for you to assess your physical and mental condition and current care needs accurately. Visit the residence to observe the physical and social atmosphere, meet the current residents, evaluate the caregiver's performance, and review the level of care and the available services offered. Discuss the cost for residing and receiving care in the adult care home. It is also important to review the adult care home's state license and the rights and responsibilities of residents, families, and care providers.

Advantages to Living in an Adult Care Home

There are some advantages to living in an adult care home compared to an assisted living facility.

- **Residents:** In contrast to assisted living facilities, adult care homes limit the number of residents housed at one time usually no more than six residents at a time. By living in a house instead of a large facility, a resident should receive more individualized care and attention. There is less of an institutional feel in the residence.

- **Staffing:** The ratio of staff/caregivers to residents in an adult care home, usually less than 6:1, compares favorably to that of an assisted living facility. This allows for more personal care and a quick response to residents in need of assistance. Staff can be accessed 24/7.

- **Medical Care:** As the ratio of staff to residents is high, the caregivers at an adult care home become familiar with the daily medical needs of the residents. They can determine when there is a significant change in the resident's condition. Most adult care homes will provide or arrange transportation for residents and will accompany them to medical appointments. They can act as a liaison with your family and your physician. If needed, they can arrange for home healthcare professionals to come to the home to provide skilled nursing care, physical, occupation, and speech therapies.

- **Meals** at an adult care home usually taste better than larger facility food. This is because they are usually home-cooked meals, rather than food prepared for a large number of residents. Also, special diets can sometimes be prepared.

- **Social Activities:** With a smaller number of residents, it is possible for the caregiver at an adult care home to take outings with residents that are more active.

- **Safety:** As the caregiver to resident ratio in an adult care home is high, there is increased supervision. If a resident falls or is injured, a rapid response time is likely.

- **Cost:** Adult care homes often cost less to private pay than assisted living facilities. In some states, Medicaid will pay for care.

Disadvantages to Living in an Adult Care Home: Warning Signs

When you seriously begin looking into adult care homes, you will hear about their negative aspects. It is important to remember that residents living in these homes are one of the most vulnerable populations for abuse. Inadequate state licensing and regulations at this time cannot guarantee quality care in all facilities. Be alert for the following red flags or warning signs, which may indicate a substandard facility.

- **Overcrowding:** You note that there are too many residents in the home, certainly more than six.

- **Limited caregivers:** The ratio of caregivers to residents prohibits the home from providing adequate 24/7 care to all the residents.

- **Physical restraints or overmedication:** The adult care home uses physical restraints (behavioral) or medication (chemical) to keep residents calm and controlled. *By law, residents cannot be controlled with behavioral or chemical restraints.*

- **Activities of daily living:** You observe that residents are not out of bed, dressed, or assisted with their personal hygiene.

- **Activity or social programs:** You see no evidence of programs planned during the day or evening. Residents watch television or remain isolated in their rooms.

- **Safety:** The adult care home does not maintain a fire-emergency plan or drills. Cluttered hallways and rooms hamper an emergency exit. The home is not equipped with grab bars, rails, or safety features in the bathrooms or hallways, increasing the likelihood of an accident or fall.

- **Cleanliness:** The adult care home does not follow basic sanitation policies. Commode chairs are not cleaned and emptied frequently, and incontinence diapers are not properly disposed of in a covered container. Caregivers do not take precautions for infectious diseases, such as hand washing and needle disposal. You detect a pervasive odor.

- **Licensing:** There are special conditions stated on the license that directly relate to the risk of harm or potential harm to residents. For instance, it may state that the provider is not compliant with operation rules.

- **Abuse:** This can include physical abuse or neglect, verbal abuse, and financial abuse. *Physical abuse* is bodily harm inflicted on a resident by another person. With *verbal abuse,* words spoken to a resident may cause emotional harm. Yelling at a resident is not appropriate. Both types of abuse demonstrate a serious lack of control by the caregiver or an incompatibility with other residents at the home. *Financial abuse or mismanagement of funds* is a frequent occurrence. The owner of the adult care home often assists the resident with money management. Many residents endorse their monthly Supplemental Security Income (SSI), Social Security, or pension checks to pay for their care. The resident receives a portion of the check to pay for personal needs. Unfortunately, in this situation, residents are vulnerable. Adult care owners may take advantage of residents by asking them to sign over property and other assets. It is important to ask other residents how they handle their financial affairs. If the owner is responsible for their money management, ask how well they feel it is handled. Consider having a reliable family member, a close friend, or hire a certified geriatric care manager to receive financial power of attorney so they can handle your financial affairs. Talk with your local bank about a power of attorney for finances. If many assets are involved, talk with an Elder Care Attorney. *(Please note: Abuse can take place in any care setting.)*

National Academy of Elder Law Attorneys, Inc.:
For information and help finding an elder lawyer in your area,
Go to http://www.naela.org/public/

National Committee for the Prevention of Elder Abuse (NCPEA):
Go to http://www.preventelderabuse.org/elderabuse/

How to Choose an Adult Care Home

When you begin to look for an adult care home, you should consider the following factors:

- admission requirements;
- the level of care;
- whether it is a state licensed home;
- the location;
- the home's physical layout;
- private versus semi-private accommodations;
- the basic services;
- the social atmosphere and activities;
- the characteristics of the residents;
- staffing, including number of staff around the clock, training, and personality;
- the cost for room, board, and care.

Admission Guidelines for an Adult Care Home

As adult care homes are private residences, each home may adhere to its own set of admission requirements. Usually the owner of the home is the primary contact person. If the adult care home has an opening, the owner of the residence will evaluate a potential resident to determine their level of personal and medical care. As each home has a designated level of care, the adult care home will not accept a person who requires more care than they can provide. For example, a Level 1 home should not take Level 3 residents that have significant healthcare requirements.

Most adult care homes will offer tours or encourage visits from prospective residents. If you decide to become a resident, they may ask you to first complete paperwork that includes personal information, emergency contacts, medical history, and source of payment. Some may require a contract for the resident or their family to sign. For residents working with the State Medicaid program, a state caseworker will need to be involved with arranging care in the adult care home. For private pay residents, you can contact the home directly. A referral from a healthcare professional, friend, or former resident is a good way to screen the long list of providers. For service-connected veterans, you will need to work with a community social worker from the Veteran's Administration to arrange placement in an adult care home.

Levels of Care in an Adult Care Home

The owner and/or caregiver at the adult care home determines the level of care, that is the amount of physical care and supervision by reviewing the activities of daily living and medical care needs of each resident. Each licensed home provides care at a specific level. Alternatively, if a state agency is involved and assisting with placement or payments to the adult care home, a state caseworker may review your care needs and determine the level of care you require. The higher the level of care, the greater the cost will be to live in an adult care home. The owner/caregiver and the state agency review the following care needs:

> ➤ mobility and transfer assistance;
> ➤ nutrition and special diets;
> ➤ bathroom and toileting activities;
> ➤ dressing and grooming;

> ➤ personal hygiene and bathing;
> ➤ medication management;
> ➤ basic nursing care;
> ➤ Alzheimer's, dementia, or memory care;
> ➤ end-of-life care.

An adult care home provider with a Level 1 classification or license can accept residents who require assistance with up to four activities of daily living, routine oral medication management, and no skilled medical or nursing care, such as supervision due to confusion and wandering. If you are semi-independent with your activities of daily living and have no skilled medical needs, you would require a home that provides Level I care.

An adult care home provider with a Level 2 classification or license can accept residents who require assistance with *all* the activities of daily living. The provider and qualified staff may perform basic nursing tasks. If you require significant or moderate assistance with your activities of daily life and have minimal to moderate medical needs, you would require a home that provides Level 2 care.

An adult care home provider with a Level 3 classification or license can accept residents who are dependent on the caregiver with *all* the activities of daily living. However, the home cannot accept more than one total-care or bedridden resident at a time. Skilled nursing tasks can be assigned to the provider and qualified staff only with approval from the resident's physician, a registered nurse, and, if involved, the local State Area Agency on Aging. If you are dependent or unable to help with your care and have some skilled medical needs or need total care or end-of-life care, you would require a home that provides Level 3 care.

A Level 3 provider, and sometimes a Level 2 provider, can offer **end-of-life care.** As not all homes provide this specialty care, be sure to discuss this need with the caregiver before you choose a home. Some adult care homes work closely with hospice nurses and other healthcare professionals.

As guidelines for these levels of care vary from state to state, it is important to check with the nearest *State Area Agency on Aging* or *Senior and Disabled Services Office.*

Determining the Cost of Living in an Adult Care Home

Similar to determining cost in an assisted living facility, several factors influence the cost of living in an adult care home:

- the **resident's required level of care** and assistance;
- the **type of accommodations**: private room versus semi-private room;
- the **resident's financial situation** – private pay versus Medicaid or Veteran benefit. *(Please note: Only some states offer Medicaid benefits for living in an adult care home.)*

Depending on the state where you live, the state Medicaid program may pay for care in an adult care home. Check with the local *State Area on Aging* to determine if your state provides this benefit.

Ways to Pay for Your Care in an Adult Care Home

The cost for living in an adult care home varies depending upon the location, your level of care, and the type of accommodation. Payment for an adult care home can be private pay, through the state *Medicaid* program, or the *Department of Veteran Affairs Office.* Few long-term-care and private insurance policies pay for care in an adult care home.

- **Private Pay:** The range of monthly fees for your room, board, and personal care ranges from $1,500 to over $5,000 per month. If you are considering an adult care home in the high range, you may want to compare it to other alternatives, such as hiring a private caregiver in your own home, hiring a caregiver to help you in an assisted living facility, or moving to an intermediate care facility.

- **Medicare** does *not* pay for care in an adult care home.

- **Medicaid:** In some states, the Medicaid program helps supplement low-income seniors and disabled persons who need placement in an adult care home. Although the state pays most of the cost, the resident is expected to contribute a portion of their income, usually from Social Security or Social Security Disability Income (SSDI.) Caseworkers in the *Office of Aging* and *the Senior* and *Disability Services Office* will work with you to locate an adult care home that meets your needs. Although the state rates for care are lower than the amount homes charges for private pay, many homes contract with the state to accept the state rates. For heavy-care residents, the state may allow a higher allowance or rate of reimbursement to the adult care home. To determine if your state provides this service, contact the nearest *State Area Agency on Aging.*

- **Veteran Affairs:** If you are a service-connected veteran, the *Department of U.S. Veteran Affairs Office* (VA) can sometimes help pay for care in an adult care home or in a VA sponsored domiciliary care program. Contact the nearest VA office and ask for the admissions office or, if you need assistance to understand your options, contact the Veteran's Community Social Work Department. They can help walk you through the admission eligibility requirements, answer any questions and/or direct you to the appropriate department.

United States Department of Veteran Affairs Guide to Long-term Care. Go to http://www.va.gov/geriatrics/guide/longtermcare/Adult_Family_Homes.asp

---

- **Social Security Administration:** In forty states and Washington D.C., **Supplemental Security Income** (SSI), a federal cash assistance benefit for the aged, blind, or disabled low-income individuals may be used to make up the difference between the monthly room, board, and care fees and the resident's monthly income. The state may supplement the SSI payment with a **State Supplemental Payment** (SSP.) This payment amount differs from state to state. Residents in an adult care home may also keep a small portion of SSI or SSP payments each month for personal needs. The remainder of the check goes toward room, board, and care. Check with your local *Social Security Office* about this program.

To check **Social Security benefits and programs**, go to www.ssa.gov

For electronic and printed versions of **The Social Security Handbook,** go to http://www.ssa.gov/OP_Home/handbook/

Licensing and Regulations

State licensing of an adult care home is required in many states and strongly recommended. However, it does not guarantee high quality care or safety in the home. Inspections may be infrequent and enforcement of licensing requirements may be lax.

Why is licensing so important? Those homes without a license have no regulated standards for providing physical care or a safe environment for their residents. They may not receive state funding from the Medicaid program to assist residents in paying the cost of care in the home. There may not have a state or watchdog agency checking on their facilities.

Homes that are licensed demonstrate some responsibility in pursuing the state standards and upholding the state regulations and policies for providing care to older adults. They must meet structural and safety standards. In the event of fire, they must be able to evacuate residents in three minutes. The caregiver or provider must complete a training program, pass criminal-records check and be financially solvent and physically and mentally able to provide care to all residents.

The adult care home should have a current state license posted where residents and families can easily read it. The home should also provide a current summary of complaints, special conditions on the license, and a copy of the inspection report. *If the adult care home is reluctant or refuses to let your family view this information, you should consider a different facility.* A list of licensed facilities is available at the local *Senior and Disabled Services Office* or *State Area Agency on Aging.*

Resident Characteristics in an Adult Care Home

The people who live at the adult care home are usually people in need of some physical assistance and care. Each state determines the number of residents, typically no more than 6 residents at a time. If a home provides care to residents with very high levels of care, the number of residents should be lower. Depending on the level of care, residents may be able to participate to varying degrees in social activities and conversation. Be sure to meet the residents, as you will be living with them.

If you are alert and oriented, you may not want to choose a home with residents who are loud and confused. A confused resident may yell at night. If you have minor health issues, you may not want to share a room with someone with significant health problems that requires constant attention. If you are continent and have control over your urine and bowel, you may not want to share a bathroom with a resident who is incontinent and has accidents. This is especially important when you consider sharing a room or bathroom. Be sure your needs and personality are compatible with those of your roommate. Many adult care homes provide care to difficult residents with behavioral and emotional issues. Be sure to meet the residents living in the adult care home before making a decision to live in the home. As the residents living in the adult care home will change, ask the owner about her policy when placing new residents with people already living in the home. Will she continue to find compatible residents to share a room? Will the current resident have any input about a new roommate?

Staffing and Staff Qualities in an Adult Care Home

At some adult care homes, the owner lives at the residence and is one of the primary caregivers; at others, the owner lives at another residence and supervises paid caregivers in the adult care home. A caregiver should be available to residents 24/7. If a resident needs assistance, the waiting time should be short. Safety guidelines should be adhered to, minimizing the risk of falls to residents. The owner and caregivers should be approachable, accessible to residents and their family, and knowledgeable about each resident's daily and medical care. Staff should maintain a care plan for each resident, detailing their daily care, medications, physician's names and telephone numbers, emergency contact and insurance information, Good quality staffing should allow for accompanying residents to medical appointments and unexpected emergency services. The owner should consent to visits ordered by any resident's primary care physician for home healthcare nurses, therapists, and social workers.

Some adult care home caregivers will visit their residents in the hospital and work closely with the discharge planners, case managers, and social workers to ensure a continuity of care as the resident transitions from hospital to back to the adult care home. They may encourage visits from visiting home healthcare professionals.

Considering the Location
of the Adult Care Home

Adult care homes are located in many types of settings - urban/city, residential suburban communities, and rural areas. Many homes are located in well-maintained neighborhoods and others in run-down areas. In rural areas, the home may have acreage, views, and even farm animals.

When considering location, it is important to find a home that is convenient for your family and friends to visit. It should also be close to a community with shopping, activities, and a house of worship for observing religious practices, if that is important to you. Medical care in a local hospital and at a primary care physician's office should be easily accessible.

Atmosphere and Accommodations
in an Adult Care Home

The physical atmosphere of the adult care home is important. If the home is not inviting, you will not be content to stay and live there. The adult care home should be pleasing to the eye; the yard and physical structure well maintained. The home's carpet and furniture should be clean and in good condition. The home should be bright and cheerful. It should be easily accessible for walkers, standard wheelchairs, and power scooters or wheelchairs. There should be a comfortable sitting area with a communal television or activities. Residents should be able to choose where they sit from a variety of comfortable chairs.

It is important for residents to receive daily personal care and assistance with their activities of daily life. If residents are lounging about in their pajamas or bathrobes, it may signify that the home is not providing adequate staffing and care. Exceptional adult care homes will go the extra mile toward making their residents feel they are part of a family.

Robin, a retired licensed practical nurse decided to open an adult care home after reducing her working hours at a local hospital. She carefully screened new residents to be sure they were compatible with her existing residents. During one of her initial interviews with Jack, a potential male resident, she discovered he was a former air force veteran and loved airplanes. Less than a week after Jack moved to the adult care home, Robin took him on an outing to the local airport to view the display of airplanes on the airport grounds and to watch the airplanes landing and taking off. This simple gesture made Jack feel he was living in a family home where people cared about his interests.

Accommodations can range from a private room with or without bath to a shared room with a shared bath. Private bedrooms may be available to couples who choose to share a room. Private rooms, especially with private bath, are usually more expensive than semi-private rooms. Most adult care homes have a common sitting area or living room. You can bring some personal belongings, such as a television, a radio, and sometimes furniture to the home to create a comfortable and familiar atmosphere. Some adult care homes provide a telephone in each room, as well as cable service. Other facilities may include a patio, yard, gardens, and acreage.

The rooms in an adult care home are either private, with or without private bath or semi-private, with or without bath. When sharing a semi-private room, be sure you share the room with someone who has similar mental status and medical care needs. For example, an alert person should not share a room with a very confused and noisy person. A person with minimal medical care needs should not share a room with a person with extensive medical needs. Furniture from home is often welcome although some adult care homes will offer a furnished room. Many homes will accommodate personal items from home as long as they are not too bulky. Do not bring sentimental, expensive or fragile items to the home as items can be lost or misplaced.

The bathroom should be odor-free, clean, and close to the bedroom. The size and number of bathrooms should easily accommodate the needs of all residents in the adult care home. The bathroom entrance should be wide enough and accessible for a wheelchair or walker. High-riser toilet seats or commodes with arms that go over the toilet seat, safety grab bars, and shower stools in the bath or shower are necessary safety features. If a resident is unable to use a bathroom easily, the home should provide and place a portable bedside commode chair next to the bed.

Hallways and rooms should be clutter-free, making it easy for residents using walkers or wheelchairs to maneuver around the residence. This reduces the chance of an accidental fall and ensures easy access to exits in the event of an emergency. Installed grab bars and other assistive devices should be easy to grab in bathrooms and hallways. Bars placed in the hallways also provide an additional safety feature for residents who need support for balance.

It is important to check the adult care home's policy on smoking. Some homes allow smoking in designated areas only. Each bedroom, hallway, kitchen, and common area should be equipped with working smoke detectors. Check for an emergency call system and scheduled fire drills, as they are necessary safety features as well. A copy of the evacuation plan and a record of fire drills should be available for review.

Many adult care homes will allow small, well-trained pets. Check with the adult care home about their policy on bringing your pet.

Basic Services and Activities in an Adult Care Home

The fundamental services offered in a typical adult care home include:

- meals;
- personal care;
- basic medical care;
- 24/7 supervision;
- social atmosphere and activities.

Meals: Residents meet in a communal dining area for meals. They should be tasty and nutritious and should meet the needs of special diets, such as low-salt and diabetic diets as well as cultural or religious regimens. Often, the owner or caregiver prepares the meals and eats with the residents. The caregiver should offer snacks to residents several times daily. If you experience difficulty feeding yourself, the caregiver should be available to assist you at mealtime. Alternatively, they may encourage family members to help at mealtimes.

Personal care includes any assistance and supervision with the activities of daily living provided by the owner or caregiver.

Basic medical care is dependent upon the level of care offered by the adult care home, the qualifications of the care provider to provide medical care, and the type of medical care needed. If you need temporary medical care resulting from an accident, injury, or hospitalization, your primary care physician can request follow-up care at the adult care home by a visiting home healthcare nurse or therapist to meet these short-term needs. Home healthcare staff can also provide basic medical skills training to the caregiver at the adult care home. For example, if you are discharged from a hospital to an adult care home and require daily wound care with dressing changes, the home healthcare nurse can train your caregiver to change your dressings properly. The caregivers should work closely with the residents, their family, and your primary care physician. They should help you arrange medical appointments and transportation, as needed. All residents receive supervision as a necessary safety measure to help prevent injury and reduce the risk of falls to residents.

Social activities are determined by the activity level of the residents. For alert and engaged residents, daily activities and outings to the theater and concerts, craft projects, music therapy, pet therapy, supervised and planned projects, and exercise programs, can help residents maintain cognitive and physical abilities. Most adult care homes do not have activities director. The social atmosphere is important because it indicates the amount of stimulation and resident interaction offered by the home. If all the residents are in their rooms, it can increase the feeling of social isolation. In order to remain as alert and active as possible, it is important to continue to have contact with the other residents, your family, and the caregivers.

For resident's who are confused and disoriented or have Alzheimer's disease, social activities can include an exercise program designed to increase strength and endurance, maintain motor skills, improve balance and reduce fall risk. The caregiver can confer with the resident's physician about a suitable physical activity.

Where to Look for Information about Adult Care Homes

There are many state and community agencies that can help your family find a clean, safe, and reputable adult care home with a solid record for providing good care and management. There are now private agencies that help families locate assisted living facilities and adult care homes. They usually charge a fee to the home, not the person or family looking for placement. Many state agencies provide free lists of licensed homes, indicating the level of care they provide, whether they are owner-occupied, or the owner manages the home and hires caregivers to provide care, but lives in another residence. The lists indicate whether the licensed homes are wheelchair accessible, prefer male or female residents, or accept fees from the state. The state fees accepted are usually less than the amount adult care homes normally charges residents. To obtain updated information about the adult care homes in your area contact any of the following:

- The Administration on Aging (AOA);

- Senior and Disabled Services;

- Adult Care Home Associations;

- Hospital Social Work/Case Management/Discharge Planning Departments;

- United States Department of Veteran Affairs;

- Home Healthcare Agencies;

- Private Placement Services;

- Friends with first–hand knowledge.

The Administration on Aging (AOA): The mission of the AOA is to *"develop a comprehensive, coordinated and cost-effective system of home and community-based services that helps elderly individuals maintain their health and independence in their homes and communities."* The AOA maintains a website with links to federal, state, and local resources, and community-based programs for seniors, people with disabilities, caregivers, and professionals. These links include information on benefit programs, prescription drug programs, health care, housing, and more.

The *Eldercare Locator* is an excellent free public service sponsored by the U.S. Administration on Aging that links you to local, state, and federal services for older adults and their families. Topics range from information about legal services, long-term and nursing home care, financial programs, housing options, elder abuse prevention, Alzheimer's disease, and more.

The Administration for Community Living (ACL) has resources and helpful information for older adults. Go to http://www.acl.gov/Get_Help/ Help_Older_Adults/Index.aspx

Eldercare Locator: To find a listing of **Area Agencies on Aging**, go to http://www.eldercare.gov/Eldercare.NET/Public/Index.aspx or call 1-800-677-1116.

Senior and Disabled Services: The *Senior and Disabled Services* division of the *State Area Agency on Aging (AOA)* is responsible for developing and managing programs and services for seniors and people with disabilities. As each AOA is run by individual states, each program differs. Many will maintain a list of adult care homes and can inspect these homes and issue operative licenses. They may run a criminal-record check on the owner of an adult care home. If the state runs a caregiver training program, they may also run criminal record checks on individuals before issuing them certification as a state caregiver. The state can set a reasonable level of care for the home and a limit on the number of residents living in the residence at any one time. There may be limitations on the number of difficult or "heavy-care" residents that an adult care home can accept. "Heavy-care" residents may exceed the usual Level 3 care guidelines due to complex medical problems.

Be aware that although an adult care home may be listed by the state, you should still visit, meet the caregivers and owner, talk with residents, and eat a meal at the home. Bring a friend or family member with you when you visit as each person sees a home from a different perspective. Talk with a state caseworker who has been in the home. Ask about its reputation. How many years has the adult care home been in operation? Although the caseworker may not be able to state his opinion of the home, he should be able to support your decision as a good choice or suggest a different home. Additional services include ombudsmen programs, caseworker support, and hands-on community services. *Ombudsman programs* advocate and protect the health and safety of residents in long-term care facilities (assisted living, adult care homes and nursing facilities.) These trained volunteers will listen to concerns and complaints from residents and their families and seek resolution to improve the quality of life for the residents.

This agency also investigates reports of abuse. It can guide you to licensed homes and steer you away from homes with poor reputations or no licenses. Contact the *State Area Agency on Aging* to find the office nearest you.

To locate your State and/or Area Agency on Aging with services for seniors and people with disabilities, go to http://www.aoa.gov/aoaroot/aoa programs/oaa/How_To_Find/Agencies/Find_Agencies.aspx?sc=OR

Adult Care Home Associations: These associations can provide your family with information about choosing an adult care home, the licensure requirements, ombudsmen programs, and residents' rights. They can guide you through the difficult and time-consuming process of locating a safe, clean, and reputable adult care home. Their staff members help families review the long list of potential adult care homes. As these individuals are familiar with the adult care homes in their area, they can match the potential resident's needs, taking into account the medical and care needs, the personality of the resident (i.e. compatibility with other residents already in the home), the preferred location, and finances. Sometimes the agency will charge a small fee to the adult care home or the family for this service. Contact your local *State Area Agency on Aging* for contact information.

Hospital Social Work/Case Management /Discharge Planning Departments: These professionals work closely with the AOA and other community agencies, assisting with hospital discharge arrangements. Although they may not necessarily have visited all the adult care homes, they are continually assessing residents who enter the hospital for medical reasons. They can contact the resident's family, the senior services caseworker, or other involved agencies to coordinate the hospital discharge. Or, if there are concerns about the care a patient receives from the adult care home, they are mandated to report any signs of abuse. The state mandates that these professionals report suspected abuse to the appropriate agency. In addition, these experts liaise between you and your physician for prescriptions, for necessary medical equipment as well as for referral orders to a home healthcare agency for follow-up care at the adult care home.

Home Healthcare Agencies: These agencies are an excellent resource to assess adult care homes because the nurses, therapists, and social workers visit residents in the homes on a regular basis. They are alert to care problems, poor hygiene, caregiver ability, medication management, and other healthcare needs. In addition, they act as a liaison between the resident and the physician, helping to ensure a continuity of medical care. To receive this service you must get a referral from your physician, be homebound, and need skilled care. Contact a local home healthcare agency and ask to speak with a nurse case manager or social worker. (S*ee Part 4: Finding Medical Care in Your Community and at Home*)

Private Services: For families who live in another state or a great distance from their loved ones, a private geriatric care manager can help arrange care in an adult care home or other assisted living facility. They are familiar with resources in your area and trained in case management, gerontology, social work, and health and human services. A Geriatric Care Manager (GCM) can provide a complete assessment as well as assistance with placement, in-home services, financial and legal issues, crisis intervention, hospital stay management, referrals to specialists, and much more. The family or client would pay a fee to the GCM for this service.

The National Association of Professional Geriatric Care Managers can help you find a geriatric care manager in your area. Go to http://www. caremanager.org/displaycommon.cfm?an=1andsubarticlenbr=306

Friends with first-hand knowledge: Word-of-mouth is perhaps the best way to find an adult care home. Ask a friend with a family member residing in an adult care home if he is satisfied with the care in the home. Personal experience goes a long way when choosing a home for a loved one.

Visiting an Adult Care Home

Visit several facilities before making a decision. Bring a friend to share your impressions. You will find that each of you notices different details . Spend some time at the adult care home so you can eat a meal, participate in any activities, and talk with residents and staff. Discuss with your friend or family what you each liked and disliked at the home. Trust your instincts even if you are unable to pinpoint why you feel the way you do.

You can visit an adult care home anytime you wish during regular working hours, usually between 8 a.m. and 5 p.m. Most homes should be able to accommodate you. If you are interested in speaking with the owner, call in advance to set up an appointment. Use the questions on the following pages to keep track of your observations and the responses to your questions.

Questions to Ask at an Adult Care Home

When you walk into an adult care home, take a careful look at the general appearance of the home.

Outside Area

- Does the owner maintain the yard and grounds?

- Is there a patio or comfortable place to sit outdoors?

- Is the residence taller than one story? If yes, how do residents navigate between the floors?

- If more than one story, is there a fire escape on the outside of the building?
- Are there ramps along the curb for easy walker, wheelchair or scooter access?
- Are people out walking in the neighborhood?

Inside Area

- Is the atmosphere formal or informal? i.e. How are the residents dressed? What is the decor?
- Does the home enforce standard visiting hours? What are the visiting hours?
- Does the home appear clean?
- Do you detect an odor in the home?
- Does the home use air-conditioning?
- Can residents easily look outside through the windows? i.e. are the windows large, low, and clean?
- Does the home seem cheerful, filled with light or dark and gloomy?
- Is the living room area empty or are residents sitting around?
- Are the hallways wide enough to accommodate a walker, wheelchair, or power scooter?
- Are handrails placed conveniently along the hallways?
- If needed, can you easily access an elevator or ramp?
- Does the home allow smoking inside or does it designate a smoking area?
- Does the home provide easy access to a telephone?
- Are exits from the home clearly marked and easily accessible?
- Does the home regularly schedule and practice fire drills?
- Can you easily access a mailbox and postage stamps?

Watch for

- ➢ bad odor;
- ➢ safety hazards;
- ➢ residents who are not dressed or are badly groomed;
- ➢ residents who remain in their rooms all day;

➤ residents restrained or tied in chairs. *The law strictly limits the use of restraints, especially for convenience of caregiver.*

Rooms

- Are private rooms available?

- How many residents are permitted to live in a room?

- Will you share a room with another resident?

- Will you share a room with a compatible roommate? *This is an important question.*

- Can residents provide their own furnishings? Are there any guidelines that must be followed?

- Do rooms contain handicap features, such as emergency call buttons and grab bars in the bathroom?

- Does each bed include a privacy curtain?

- Does each room include a window or view?

- Is the residence pet-friendly? Can residents keep a small well-trained pet?

Personal and Medical Care

- What is the level of care provided in the home?
  Level 1__ Level 2 __ Level 3 __End-of-Life care__ Memory care___

- Does the home welcome and encourage visits from a home healthcare agency?

- If a resident experiences a change in health, is staff available to provide additional assistance?

- Is staff available to help with the activities of daily living (ADL's) such as bathing, transfers, grooming, shopping, personal hygiene, housekeeping, laundry, feeding at mealtimes, and walking?

- How are resident's prescriptions filled?
  local pharmacy_____ mail- order pharmacy____ physician's office____
  by family____ Veteran's facility ____ medication assistance program____

Some states require a pharmacist to prepare all medications in individual doses and place them in a bubble pack. All self-medication is stored in a locked box or area.

- Is medication management available to residents who have difficulty taking their correct medication at the proper time of day?

- Can residents self-administer their own medication?

- Can a resident hire a private-duty nurse to provide additional care?

- Does staff encourage family involvement?

- Can family supply medical supplies, such as incontinence diapers?

- What is the protocol followed by the adult care home for medical emergencies? Will a caregiver accompany a resident to the hospital and stay with them until family arrives?

- Does the staff maintain a care plan and health and medication records for each resident?

- Does the staff maintain an emergency information form to bring to the hospital emergency department that lists the resident's physician, medical history and conditions, medications, and emergency contact?

- Will a resident's advanced directive, living will, or POLST form accompany them to the hospital?

- What is the role of the adult care home for hospitalized residents?

Caregivers

- Is staff professional and able to answer your questions?

- How does the staff determine each resident's care needs?

- What is the resident-to-staff ratio?

- How many caregivers are on duty during each shift? How long is each shift?

- Does caregiver maintain a personalized care plan for each resident?

- Does staff cooperate with community agencies, such as home healthcare agencies, medical supply companies, and senior services?

- Do you and your family feel comfortable interacting with staff?

- Can your primary care physician visit or continue to provide medical treatment to you while you are residing at the home?

- Does the home maintain a private place for exams conducted by your physician?

Staff should be.

- ➢ helpful;
- ➢ pleasant and courteous;
- ➢ affectionate;
- ➢ honest;

- ➢ cheerful;
- ➢ respectful;
- ➢ interested;
- ➢ compassionate.

Watch for:

- ➢ disgruntled staff;
- ➢ yelling at residents;
- ➢ excessive complaining by staff;
- ➢ impatient staff;
- ➢ excessive time to respond to resident call light;
- ➢ bad attitude.

Activities

- Does the home staff have an activities director or activity program?
- Does the home post a schedule of activities?
- Does the home observe religious services in the home or provide transport to a local church, synagogue, or house of worship?
- Does the home maintain a library?
- Is there a beautician or barber who visits regularly?

Watch for

➢ no scheduled activities;

➢ excessive television watching;

➢ residents not bathed or dressed;

➢ no stimulation or support;

➢ neglect or abuse by staff.

Transportation

• Does the home own a wheelchair van?

• Does the home provide or arrange transportation to medical appointments, to shopping, religious worship?

• Does the home charge a small fee for transportation services? Is the home located close to shopping?

Cost

• What services are included in the monthly fee?

• What services are not included in the monthly fee?

• Are there hidden fees? If yes, what are they?

• If the care needs of a patient changes, does this affect the monthly fee?

• If a resident's level of care changes or she decides to leave the home, what is the refund policy?

• Does the home accept Medicaid payments? *(This is an important question. Some homes do not accept Medicaid. Others accept the low Medicaid reimbursement rate.)*

• What is the policy regarding residents if their funds run out? (*This is an important question. Some homes may discharge or evict a resident who is unable to pay for care. Others may try to work closely with your family to prepare them for reduced funds. They may help your family apply for Medicaid and financial assistance through your local state agency.)*

• Will the adult care home help a resident apply for Medicaid?

Specialized Memory Care Facilities for Alzheimer's disease and Dementia Care

- *One in eight older Americans has Alzheimer's disease.*

- *Alzheimer's disease is the sixth leading cause of death in the United States.*

- *Over 15 million Americans provide unpaid care for a person with Alzheimer's disease or other dementias.*

- *Payments for care are estimated to be 200 billion in 2012.*

   --2012 Alzheimer's disease Facts and Figures, Alzheimer's Association

Recent studies issued by the *Alzheimer's Association* and the *U.S. National Institute of Aging* in April 2011 open the door for a dramatic increase in the number of people diagnosed with Alzheimer's disease. There is a distinction between the two types of dementia: vascular dementia (related to a stroke or new medication) and Alzheimer's dementia, a progressive and irreversible neurological disease of the brain. While the two are often grouped together, vascular dementia is more common for people over 70 and Alzheimer's disease can strike people as young as 45 years old. Both share many symptoms and require similar care. As Alzheimer's disease is progressive, individuals with this diagnosis do not usually experience all the symptoms at once. Some people can function with helpful cues, daily reminders such as calendars and simple posted schedules. Medical expertise and medications may also be instrumental in aiding individuals with Alzheimer's disease. As we age, we all experience 'senior moments' when we are forgetful. You may find yourself asking, "Now, what was I looking for in the kitchen?" Or, "Where did I put my keys?" This is normal 'forgetfulness' for most people. However, when memory loss becomes progressive and begins to interfere with the daily activities of life and places you at risk for harm, it may be time to consider care in a facility specializing in memory loss.

Assisted living facilities, standard and continuing care retirement communities, some adult care homes, intermediate care facilities, and specialized memory care centers can provide a safe and secure environment to people experiencing severe memory loss. Some facilities will have secure units with alarms and locked doors to prevent wandering. You may benefit from a memory care facility if you:

- have been diagnosed with dementia or Alzheimer's disease;

- experience confusion and disorientation to time, place, and person;

- are at-risk for wandering and getting lost;

- require daily cues and reminders;

- require constant supervision;

- need a structured setting;

- need a secure setting;

- need assistance with the activities of daily life;

- require assistance at mealtimes;

- require medication management.

The New Stages of Alzheimer's disease

"My father started growing very quiet as Alzheimer's started claiming more of him. The early stages of Alzheimer's are the hardest because that person is aware that they're losing awareness. And I think that that's why my father started growing more and more quiet".

-- Patty Davis, (speaking about her father, President Ronald Reagan)

There are new guidelines for recognizing the stages of Alzheimer's disease recently released by the *U. S. National Institute on Aging/Alzheimer's Association Diagnostic Guidelines for Alzheimer's disease*. Although these new guidelines will not change the way physicians diagnose Alzheimer's disease, it will increase awareness of disease progression and treatment in the earlier stages. The three stages are:

- **Mild cognitive impairment** (MCI) or "pre-clinical": no symptoms,but physical brain changes may be noted;

- **Moderate Alzheimer's disease**: early phase with memory problems and changes in mental abilities determined by diagnostic tests,such as the presence of amyloid proteins or nerve damage in the brain;

- **Severe Alzheimer's dementia**: memory loss, visual, spatial and judgment problems.

Recognizing Common Signs of Dementia and Alzheimer's Disease

"Humans have this enormous capacity to learn, and the arts are so intrinsic within us that even with dementia we still retain that ability for imagination and creativity."

- Contribution by Executive director, Gay Hann, National Center of Creative Aging, U.S. News and World Report

Here are some of the symptoms commonly found in people with a dementia or Alzheimer's disease.

- **Memory loss** can make it difficult for a person to remember very recent events (short-term memory loss) such as their morning activities, medication schedules, appointments, turning off the stove after cooking. As memory loss increases, the person loses the ability to remember names of familiar people such as family members, the location of familiar items, and how to provide basic self-care.

- **Language and communication difficulties** can make it hard to express feelings, desires, and needs in speaking or writing. Familiar words may be hard to find and frustration over "word-finding" can occur.

- **Changes in behavior** can occur, triggered by frustration over "not being understood" and by the inability to perform simple familiar tasks. Due to the unpredictable nature of Alzheimer's disease, increasingly agitated and aggressive behavior can amplify the risk for harm to both the person and the caregiver. It is important to seek medical advice if this problem is escalating. Increased agitation and aggressive behavior can occur in a person with Alzheimer's disease. Try to reassure and remain calm. However, if the behavior escalates and places anyone in danger, seek immediate medical help.

- **Disorientation and confusion to time and place** are common. Simple calendars, large clocks, posted schedules, and maintaining a daily routine can help re-orient the individual. To help a person with Alzheimer's disease locate a specific room, you might color-code doors (for example, yellow for the bathroom and blue for a room) or post photographs on an individual room door.

- **Wandering** is common and too often, a once familiar place no longer resembles what was once well known. It is easy to get lost a few doors from home.

- **Personality change and mood swings** are common. A once docile person may display temper and aggressive behavior or become frustrated to the point of crying. They may direct distrust or hostile behavior toward a loved spouse. A once cooperative person may display a streak of increased stubbornness.

- **Loss of inhibitions** that can result in inappropriate behaviors.

- **Depression** may result from frustration at not being able to manage without help and the inability to express thoughts. They may withdraw from familiar social activities or work.

- **Poor abstract thinking** makes it difficult to perform tasks like banking and other conceptual activities. This can present challenges in planning and problem solving. Consider assigning a family member to help with financial matters and health care decisions.

- **Decreased or poor judgment** can place an individual at-risk of harm to themselves or to others. It may make them more susceptible to "elder sharks" or people who prey on the elderly, getting them to make monetary donations or purchases that are not legitimate.

Recently widowed at age 84 and diagnosed with beginning Alzheimer's disease, Lydia found she needed help to maintain her home and yard. She hired a handyman to help her with simple chores. After each chore was completed, the handyman would drink a cup of coffee with her and share his personal and financial concerns. Each time, the handyman left with a check for his services and an additional check for his "concerns". As she became more forgetful, her family began helping Lydia with managing her finances. As they reconciled her checkbook, they discovered payments to her handyman for over $60,000, well above the cost of his repair services.

- **Hallucinations** or seeing images that are not there seem very real to the person experiencing them. It is important not to confront a person with the hallucination as this can cause agitation. Reassure them and then distract them from the hallucinations. Sometimes hallucinations result from medical procedures or a change in medication. Seek medical attention if they persist.

- **Performing familiar tasks** such as dressing, grooming, bathing, toileting may become difficult. To perform them, the person may need cues and reminders, or someone to direct every step from brushing teeth to buttoning a shirt.

- **Perceptual changes** may occur. A person may exhibit difficulty with visual images and spatial relationships.

- **Insomnia** can occur. Try limiting naps and orienting with clocks, white boards with schedules, and calendars. Use a night light at nighttime and bright lights during the daytime if the home is dark. Sometimes a person can experience *Sundowner's Syndrome*, becoming more confused as the sun sets and nighttime falls. Other symptoms of Sundowner's may include restlessness, crying, anger, depression stubbornness, agitation, fearfulness, and pacing. In more extreme cases, a person may exhibit paranoia, wandering, violent behavior, and hallucinations.

  The caregiver should remain calm, speak in a soft voice, reassure the person and address any expressed needs. Re-orient the person to the time and place. Do not argue with them. It may be helpful to limit sweets and caffeine in the afternoon and evening, increase physical activity during the day, limit napping, establish a routine, set- up a quiet place in the home, structure the daily activities, and use distraction. Although the cause of Sundowner's Syndrome remains unknown, it is believed that a person suffering from it is overwhelmed by the sensory stimulation of the day. Consult with the physician to rule out a medical or medication problem.

- **For those who drive**, when you lose your way on a once familiar route, this is a clear sign that driving now presents a hazard to you and to others on the road. Be aware that listening to excuses such as blaming others for accidents or near misses, confusing changes in the road conditions, or your inability to see in the darkness, are also warning signs. Rescind driving privileges for the protection of all. Your primary care physician can help you file a form that recommends the cancellation of a driver's license with the *Department of Motor Vehicles*. **Think about turning over the car keys** if you notice the following:

➢ you feel increasingly nervous and anxious when driving;

➢ your reaction time seems slower;

➢ you concentrate, but with increasing difficulty;

➢ you get lost while driving to familiar places;

➢ you encounter a few close calls or accidents;

➢ your family and friends express concern for your safety and the safety of others.

I recently spoke with the 70-year old wife of a man diagnosed with Alzheimer's disease. As the wife had degenerative eye disease and was unable to see well enough to drive, she used cues and directions to help her spouse "drive" the car. Without her cues, he did not know where to go, when to stop, how to use the brake or accelerator, or how to obey the traffic signals. We discussed the danger of having her spouse driving, not just to the two of them, but also to other drivers on the road. I explained that the physician could contact the Department of Motor Vehicles and have her spouse's license rescinded or she could take away the car keys and not allow him to continue driving in an unsafe manner. Being able to drive enabled both of them to maintain their fragile independence. However, the wife was able to recognize the danger to themselves and others and voluntarily stopped driving with her spouse.

If you notice any of the above symptoms or changes, consider scheduling an appointment with your primary care physician for a complete physical and a review of your medications.

Levels of Care for Special-care Memory Units

Here are three levels of care offered in a special-care memory unit. Each level provides 24/7 supervision and personal assistance. The more time and care the resident requires, the higher the level of care and the higher the cost of the service.

Level 1: Special-care unit, minimum care

You may:

• experience occasional, short-term memory loss and forgetfulness. For example, you may have difficulty remembering where you live. You may turn on the oven and forget to turn it off. Or you may not remember when or if you took your medication;

- have difficulty understanding information and making decisions on your own behalf;

- have difficulty remembering normally familiar people or places;

- be at-risk for wandering away from your home and getting lost;

- be capable of walking independently, or with a cane, walker, or wheelchair;

- need minimal assistance with the activities of daily living;

- experience occasional loss of control or incontinence with bladder and/or bowel;

- have difficulty safely using standard household appliances.

Level 2: Special-care Unit, moderate care

You may:

- experience a moderate amount of short-term memory problems;

- experience difficulty following instructions, written or verbal;

- experience increased forgetfulness;

- notice increased episodes of wandering;

- experience increased difficulty recognizing familiar people and places;

- need moderate assistance with the activities of daily living on a daily basis;

- experience moderate loss of control or incontinence of bladder or bowel;

- be at-risk for harm to yourself or to others;

- create hazardous situations when using standard household appliances.

Level 3: Special-care Unit, maximum care

You may:

- experience poor short-term memory and some long-term memory problems. For example, you may not remember what you ate for breakfast less than an hour before, or you may not recognize or remember the names of close family members;

- experience difficulty with communication and with organizing thoughts in a coherent way;

- need maximum or total care for your activities of daily living;

- create unsafe situations without constant twenty-four hour supervision;

- be at-risk for wandering greater distances and getting lost;

- not understand information and be incapable of making a competent decision on your own behalf;

- not recognize familiar people or places;

- have total loss of control or incontinence of bladder and/or bowel.

Caregiving Issues

By reviewing the levels of care for Alzheimer's disease, it is easy to see why caring for a person with this disease is a 24/7 occupation.

At a rest area in Northern California, I noticed two disabled seniors, both using canes, helping guide and coax an elderly woman to the bathroom. It took much persuading, repetition, and cueing to keep the woman on task. After completing this task, they were unable to persuade her to get back in the car. The woman sat at a picnic table and adamantly refused to stand or walk. Due to their own disabilities, the disabled couple was unable to move her. My husband and I offered our assistance to the senior couple who immediately thanked us and explained that their sister had Alzheimer's disease. Initially the woman glared at us and was very suspicious and hostile. She verbally accused us of lying to get her to move. By remaining patient, using distraction, talking in a calming voice, and repeating the goal to get her into the car so she could continue her trip, she finally cooperated and allowed us to take her arm and walk her back to the car.

When a person is diagnosed with a medical issue and requires medical care, a social worker, case manager, or medical professional directs them to a nursing or rehabilitation facility. When a person needs help with their activities of daily living, options may include living with others, hiring in-home healthcare services, moving to an assisted living facility, or an adult care home. When a person is afflicted with Alzheimer's disease, they are usually directed to hire a 24/7 caregiver to provide supervision and help with the adl's or to consider living in a facility that specializes in dementia care. These special units provide ideal support for people who suffer from confusion, forgetfulness, and disorientation often associated with Alzheimer's disease. Many people with this disease do not have significant physical problems; however, mental confusion can contribute to problems with incontinence, poor personal hygiene, poor eating habits, difficulty performing the activities of daily living, and inappropriate or unsafe behavior.

Care for persons with Alzheimer's disease and dementia can be found in several settings with special-care units designed to prevent wandering from the home or facility. Nursing facilities may offer locked Alzheimer's units. Some assisted living facilities will try to accommodate persons with memory and behavioral issues. Be aware that this setting may not provide as much supervision as other facilities or homes. Some adult care homes specialize in caring for people with Alzheimer's disease and dementia and set up a designated area in which the person can be closely monitored. Other independent memory care facilities specialize in caring for people requiring a safe and secure environment. Look for a setting that includes activities such as painting, making crafts, exercise and dancing programs, music, pet therapies, and other programs.

Be aware that current Medicare programs do not provide benefits to cover Alzheimer's disease and dementia care in many of these facilities. It is *not* considered a skilled need. Some state Medicaid programs may provide benefits for Alzheimer's care. Some long-term care insurance policies may provide benefits for care.

Aging Parents and Elder Care has a helpful website with a checklist to help you determine the best facility for your loved one.
Go to http://www.aging-parents-and-elder-care.com/Pages/Checklists/Alzheimers_Chklst.html

The Music and Memory website shares research and videos about the therapeutic benefits between music and memory.
Go to http://musicandmemory.org

For family members who assume the 24/7 caregiver role in the home, the constant need for supervision and assistance can exhaust them. Family caregivers can benefit from respite or a break from the daily task of caregiving by hiring part-time help from a licensed and bonded in-home caregiving agency, hiring or receiving additional support from other family members or friends, or occasionally arranging for the person with Alzheimer's disease to be placed short-term in a residential memory care facility. It is important to avoid *caregiver burnout* , a condition whereby the caregiver becomes overwhelmed and begins to exhibit emotional and physical problems related to their caregiving activities.

Paul's spouse of 50 years received a diagnosis from her physician of Alzheimer's disease. For several years, he was able to provide caregiving to her with minimal assistance from family, friends, or outside agencies. However, as the disease progressed, he found he was unable to leave his wife alone. This made it difficult for him to go grocery shopping, run errands, or take care of household responsibilities. In addition, every day he helped his wife dress, brush her teeth, go to the toilet, and assisted with feeding at mealtimes. Paul did not feel he could take time to visit his own physician and let his own health deteriorate. Only after having chest pain did Paul make an appointment with his physician. The physician arranged for Paul to speak with a social worker about respite care and services available to assist him in his home.

The Alzheimer's Association provides resource information and available services for caregivers and persons with Alzheimer's disease. Go to http://www.alz.org/index.asp

The Alzheimer's Project of the National Caregiving Foundation offers an excellent and free **Caregiver Support Kit**. To order, call 1-800-930-1357. On-line, go to http://www.caregivingfoundation.org/

U. S. News with content developed with the Cleveland Clinic offers this excellent website for people diagnosed with Alzheimer's disease and their caregivers. Go to http://health.usnews.com/health-conditions/brain-health/alzheimers-disease/managing#13

Questions to Ask a Memory Care Facility

Memory care can be provided in a variety of settings. Look for a facility or home that feels more like a home setting than an institutional one. Remember, you are looking for a facility that offers quality care by trained and professional staff. Look for an environment that encourages residents to participate in activities, stimulates the mind, and shows a positive and caring attitude toward residents. Ask these questions.

Physical layout

- Is the facility on one level or more?
- If the facility is more than one level, are there elevators?
- Are hallways wide enough for a wheelchair or walker?
- Are hallways and rooms marked with color codes to help residents find their way?
- Are hallways well lit?
- Do residents live in an apartment or shared room?
- If they share a room, do the residents have some privacy?
- Are bathrooms private or shared?
- Is the furniture clean and comfortable?
- Are the floors and carpet clean?
- Is there an inside common area?
- Is there a secure outside garden or common area?
- Are exit doors locked or armed with an alarm system to help prevent wandering?
- Are there ramps along the curb for easy wheelchair access?
- Are outside handrails located near steps and along sidewalks?
- Does the building seem well maintained?
- Is the facility conveniently located for family and friends to visit?

Atmosphere

- Does the physical layout appear inviting to residents and their families?
- When you walk into the facility or home, does it feel comfortable?
- Are residents sitting around, watching television, or engaged in activities? Residents should be engaged in activities and not parked in front of the television.
- Are residents in their rooms? Are many resident doors shut or open?
- Does staff interact with the residents?

Activities

- Is there a professional activity director on the premises? If not, who is responsible for arranging the activity program?

- How often are activities for residents scheduled?

- Are activities available for residents with different stages of Alzheimer's disease?

- What activities are available for residents? Art? Music? Pet therapy? A more personalized project that uses a resident's former skills?

- Is participation actively encouraged by facility staff?

- Is the television on all day? Are residents lined up in front of the television? This is a red flag. Look for a facility that engages the residents in activities.

- Does staff place easy-to-read calendars and schedules where residents can read them?

Residents

- What is the average age of the residents?

- What is the level of care required by residents? Is there a mix of mild to severe dementia patients?

- Do residents interact with one another?

- Do residents interact with staff?

- Does staff help residents with their activities of daily life?

- Do residents appear clean? Are they dressed in street clothes and properly groomed?

- Do they receive assistance at mealtime if they need it?

- Do residents appear isolated or depressed?

- If a resident exhibits behavioral problems, how does the facility handle this?

- If a resident exhibits combative or aggressive behavior, what is the facility policy?

- What is the facility policy if a resident needs a higher level of care?

Staff

- What type of licensure does the facility require of its staff?
- Is there an RN or LPN on duty 24/7?
- What training does caregiving staff receive?
- What is the staff to resident ratio during the day, evening, and on weekends?
- What is the staff turnover?
- Is staff professional in their attire, manner, and attitude?
- Do they interact in a positive way with residents?
- Does staff appear aloof, tired, or stressed?

Cost

- If a resident's care needs increase, will the cost for care increase as well?
- If a resident is no longer able to private pay for care, will the facility help their family apply for Medicaid? Does the facility accept Medicaid?
- If not, what is the facility policy for residents who are unable to pay for their care?
- Will the facility work with the family and help them locate other appropriate placement?
- Does the facility accept long-term healthcare insurance?
- Are there any hidden or extra fees?

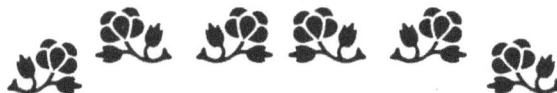

Part 4

Finding Medical Care in Your Community and at Home

Urgent care centers, community health clinics, primary care physician offices, veteran outpatient clinics, hospitals, rehabilitation programs, intermediate and skilled nursing facilities, home healthcare, hospice and end-of-life care, and home infusion services

Accessing Medical Care

A "patient-centered medical home (PCMH) is a model of care where patients have a direct relationship with a provider who coordinates a cooperative team of health-care professionals, takes collective responsibility for the care provided to the patient and arranges for appropriate care with other qualified providers as needed."

--The Healthcare Information and Management Systems Society (HIMSS) and the National Committee for Quality Assurance (NCQA)

As baby boomers, retirees, and the Greatest Generation look at creative, traditional, and non-traditional housing options, we must also consider the role of medical care and health issues in determining appropriate housing and lifestyle decisions. Many people suffer from chronic health issues, pre-existing conditions, or unexpected medical problems. This makes access to your primary care physician, an urgent care center or community clinic, the nearby hospital, and other medical services essential to maintaining a healthy and active life.

Everyone receiving medical care should seek a medical home where he or she can develop a relationship with a medical care provider. A medical home can improve your primary medical care, increase your satisfaction with care, and allow better access to your physician or medical care provider.

Retaining medical insurance benefits as you near retirement can be a complicated and often costly process. Many people will choose to work until age 65 to maintain medical coverage through an employer, when Medicare benefits kick in. For people self-employed or working without healthcare benefits, paying for medical coverage can create a financial burden. Deductibles may be high, premiums for limited coverage may be costly. For those on a limited income and not yet Medicare eligible, collecting Social Security, Social Security Disability, employment or veteran pensions, buying a medical insurance policy can be a costly affair. For this reason, many baby boomers delay retirement and work beyond the time they would normally retire.

As we see the Affordable Care Act implemented, seniors and the disabled face dramatic changes in Medicare health insurance. Premiums, co-payments, and deductibles for Americans with private health insurance continue to rise. For Americans without health insurance, it is difficult to find a primary care physician or receive medical services, even with a diagnosed serious medical condition. Costly hospital and physician bills that usurp much of their daily living budget confront increasing numbers of Americans. According to the *American Hospital Association* and the CNN Money article, *6 Reasons Health Care Costs*

Keep Going Up, by Parija Kavilanz, (July 12, 2012), factors driving up healthcare costs include:

- rising costs of goods and services used for patient care;
- rising demand for care and compliance with regulatory requirements;
- increasing numbers of Medicare and Medicaid patients (60%) which do not fully reimburse the cost of hospital care;
- increasing numbers of patients unable to pay for care who receive charity care;
- increase in the cost of physician care;
- increase in the patient share of the medical bill as seen in higher deductibles, co-payments, co-insurance, and out-of-pocket costs;
- increase in higher-cost new technologies;
- increase in the use and cost of lab testing;
- increase in the cost of prescription drugs.

HealthCare.gov summarizes the *Affordable Healthcare Act,* signed into law by President Obama on March 23, 2010. In addition, it has many helpful links to Medicare–related resources. Go to http://www.healthcare.gov/index.html

The *Affordable Healthcare Act* signed into law by President Obama in 2010 will change many aspects of future healthcare. As this is an extensive document that describes a plan that will be implemented over a number of years, it may be helpful to review it on-line in its entirety. Barring additional legislative changes to it, the new law encompasses many aspects of current healthcare services for families, children, seniors, and tightens the Medicare system to prevent fraud and abuse. To summarize a few of the aspects that relate to boomers, retirees, and seniors:

- **Prescription drugs**: The Medicare Part D "donut hole" coverage gap is slowly closing. The "donut hole" is a gap in prescription medication coverage that presented a financial burden on seniors. The "donut hole" gap will close in 2020, and you will receive full prescription coverage.

- **In 2012, free preventive care,** annual physicals, colorectal screenings, and mammograms will begin.

- **By 2014, support to Community Healthcare Clinics** will increase.

- The **Elder Justice Act** will focus on combating elder abuse and neglect, and improving nursing home quality.

- Through **state Medicaid programs**, there will be **improvements in home and community-based services.**

- **A new program to preserve and offset the cost of employer-based retiree health plans** will help those who retire before age 65 to receive affordable healthcare.

- **Through a transitional high-risk pool, affordable health insurance** will be available to people who could not purchase insurance due to a pre-existing condition.

Where to Receive Primary Healthcare

(urgent care centers, community health clinics, primary care physician offices, veteran outpatient clinics, hospitals)

At this time, there are several places where a person can receive healthcare. For people without a primary care physician, urgent care centers and hospital emergency departments provide the fastest path to evaluation and treatment. For people with a primary care physician or a provider at a Community Healthcare Center (CHC), calling the CHC for an appointment should be the first step. If a timely appointment is not available and you feel uncertain whether your condition constitutes an emergency or life-threatening situation, go to an urgent care center (more for non-emergency conditions) or the nearest hospital emergency department. Despite its name, an urgent care center is more appropriate for non-emergent conditions than a hospital emergency department. Using a hospital emergency department for a non-emergent or minor injury or illness is very expensive and should be reserved for life-threatening or serious conditions.

Urgent Care Centers

(also called intermediate care clinic, express care center,
walk-in clinics)

Started in the 1970's, 10,000 Urgent Care Centers now exist throughout the United States, many started by emergency department physicians. Urgent Care Centers provide limited and non-urgent treatment with board certified family practice and internal medicine physicians, doctors of osteopathic medicine (DO's), nurse practitioners, and physician's assistants, to anyone who walks in the door with a non-life threatening emergency. This includes cuts, bruises, sprains, minor injuries, colds, coughs, ear infections, mild asthma, rashes, and more. Many urgent care clinics offer Women's Health clinics with services such as routine health screenings, physical exams, immunizations, and free blood pressure testing. If the Urgent Care physician decides your problem is critical, you may be referred to a specialist or to the nearest local hospital emergency department for an evaluation and treatment.

These centers fill the medical care gap for people who do not have a primary care physician, are traveling and without access to their healthcare provider, newly moved to an area and without a primary care physician, or without heath care insurance. If you do not have healthcare insurance, urgent care centers may request payment at time of service. For those on low-income, the out-of-pocket expenses may not be affordable. At the time of service, be sure to ask about the estimated charges for your visit. Ask if you can speak with someone in the billing department regarding payment plans.

Unfortunately, most urgent care centers do not accept Medicare; some will accept state Medicaid benefits. Most will accept private insurance reimbursement, private pay, and payment from a health savings account or by credit card. There is usually a higher fee for new patients, as it requires more time for assessment and treatment. Procedures, x-rays, lab draws and tests, immunizations, in-office medications, breathing treatments, and other medical treatments usually result in an additional fee.

Many Urgent Care Centers are open 7-days a week, 365-days a year. You can walk-in without an appointment. After completing a registration form that includes personal information, insurance and payment information, medical history, and a release of information, you will see a family practice or internal medicine physician or a nurse practitioner. This qualified healthcare professional can treat your problem, refer you to a specialist or emergency department, write prescriptions, and provide follow-up care.

For a list of **Certified Urgent Care Centers,** go to http://www.ucaoa.org/ recognition_certification_certifiedsites.php

Community Health Clinics (CHC)

(general medical care, dental and vision care, x-ray and lab services, prescription assistance)

"Sliding scale fees *are variable costs for products, services, or taxes based on one's ability to pay. Such fees are thereby reduced for those who have lower incomes or less money to spare after their personal expenses, regardless of income."*

--Wikipedia

Community Health Clinics offer primary and preventive care to the uninsured and underinsured, persons with low-income, at-risk persons, and those experiencing difficulty establishing a medical home with a primary care physician (PCP), physician's assistant (PA), or nurse practitioner (NA.)

Many communities support non-profit neighborhood healthcare clinics to provide basic medical care and *"promote the health of low-income, working uninsured and other vulnerable adults and children."* (Community Healthcare Center, Jackson County, Oregon.) These clinics provide medical care to:

- those that are uninsured;
- low-income working poor who have no employer sponsored healthcare benefits;
- those with income above the qualifying level for the state Medicaid program;
- those that are insured, but with low-income;
- those that are underinsured;
- those having difficulty establishing a medical home with a primary care physician;

- at-risk persons with barriers to healthcare access. These barriers can include social or geographic isolation, religious, cultural or language obstacles, and /or unique needs that require individual case management services.

These clinics usually accept state Medicaid payments and use a sliding-scale based on income for the indigent who cannot afford to make substantial payments. The CHC assigns each patient to a clinic primary care physician or nurse practitioner. Many services are available including:

- 24/7 on-call services;
- chronic illness management;
- chronic pain management;
- incontinence treatment;
- gynecological services;
- general physicals;
- depression diagnosis and treatment;

- drug and alcohol referrals;
- family medical care;
- lab and diagnostic services;
- hearing evaluations;
- minor surgical procedures;
- medication assistance;
- well–woman examinations;
- behavioral and mental health counseling;
- dental care;
- vision examinations.

Dental services can include oral surgery, prevention and general dental care, and emergency care digital x-rays and dental hygiene education. Vision services may include eye exams and prescriptions for glasses.

Many clinics partner with local pharmacies participating in the *Federal 340B Drug Pricing program,* a plan that limits the cost of drugs to Federal purchasers and to certain grantees of Federal agencies. It allows the purchase of prescription drugs at 51% below retail cost for those with low-income and the uninsured. In addition, for patients without prescription drug insurance, health professionals can help you apply to pharmaceutical prescription assistance programs. As the cost of many necessary prescriptions can be very pricey, inexpensive generics such as those found at, Target, Wal-Mart, Walgreens, CVS , Giant Eagle, and Kroger and other local pharmacies, charge $4 per certain generic prescriptions. Check for a pharmacy in your area offering this service.

The Coalition of Community Health Clinics website can help you find a Community Health Clinic in your area. In addition, it provides information and a timeline for implementation of the new Affordable Care Act. Go to http://www.coalitionclinics.org/

Needymeds.org is an excellent website that includes an easy way to find free, low-cost, and sliding-scale clinics. Go to http://www.needymeds.org/free_clinics.taf

In addition, Needymeds.org lists patient assistance programs for essential medications. Go to http://www.needymeds.org/indices/pap.htm

---

Primary Care Physician Offices

Many people prefer to contact their own physician for basic medical care and questions. When a medical situation arises, it is easy to pick up the telephone, call your physician, and request an appointment. As a regular patient, you may have established a comfortable relationship with your doctor and his staff. As it is not always possible for a physician to see you on the day you call, it is important to convey to office staff the urgency for medical care. The person answering the telephone at the office does not always have the medical knowledge to understand a medical condition. If you feel you have an urgent health problem and scheduling an appointment is proving difficult, ask to speak to the physician's nurse or assistant. If you are experiencing serious symptoms such as chest pain, difficulty breathing, excessive bleeding, to name a few, call 911 or go immediately to the nearest hospital emergency department.

When planning a trip to the physician's office, be sure to bring your picture ID, medical insurance card, a list of your medications, and any other pertinent medical history. If you recently received test results or x-ray reports, bring them with you so your physician can review them. Alternatively, notify your physician's office in advance of your appointment so they can retrieve your additional records.

Many physician offices will ask for a co-payment at the time of the office visit. Others may offer to bill you for the service. If you carry private insurance or Medicare, most offices will bill the insurance company for any outstanding balance. At this time, some physician offices do not accept Medicaid due to the low payments and may accept only a few new Medicaid patients each month. Place your name on a Medicaid patient waiting list at the primary care physician's office for future openings.

To obtain a referral to see a specialist, you may need to visit your primary care physician for an evaluation.

Cindy fell on her hand three months ago. Expecting her bruised hand to recover in a reasonable time, she did not make an appointment to see her physician. When her hand continued to exhibit reduced range of motion and increased pain issues, she requested a referral to see a hand therapist. Her primary care physician set up an appointment for an evaluation, and then, completed and faxed the referral paperwork to a hand clinic. When the hand specialist received the fax, his office called Cindy to set up an appointment.

Veteran Outpatient Clinics

Serving over 5.5 million veterans, veteran outpatient clinic are available to veterans at Veteran Hospitals and facilities. If you qualify as a retiree from military service, a service-connected veteran with injuries or conditions related to your service, or a Purple Heart recipient, you are eligible for services.

If you qualify as a non-service-connected veteran or are considered less than 50% service-connected, the Veteran Administration (VA) will base your eligibility for services on financial need, with a cost of living adjustment. If you receive medical care not related to your service-related condition, you may be responsible for co-payments for this care. To apply for admission for outpatient clinic services, go to your nearest Veteran's facility admissions office. Ask the admissions office how to apply for admission, what papers you should bring with you, how long it will take to get an appointment with a VA physician or nurse practitioner. Eligible veterans are assigned to a team with a physician or nurse practitioner who then directs the medical care. Due to the large volume of veterans receiving outpatient care, you may experience an initial delay before they assign you to a team and a physician.

These clinics provide primary care, pharmacy services, behavioral and mental health services, drug and alcohol services, specialty care services such as ophthalmology, dermatology, podiatry, respiratory and pulmonary, dental care, and laboratory and radiology diagnostic testing. If you require durable medical equipment such as home oxygen, the VA clinic can help you receive the necessary medical equipment in your home. Be aware that ordering and delivering the medical equipment to your home can take time.

If you are being discharged from a hospital with essential prescription medications, you may request that the prescriptions be faxed to the outpatient VA clinic where you receive your medical care. Often, there is a delay getting prescriptions filled through the VA, especially on weekends. Sometimes the physician will write a separate prescription for a few days of medications to get the veteran sufficient medications until he can fill his prescription through the VA.

To locate a **VA Community-based Healthcare Center,** go to http://www2. va.gov/directory/guide/division_flsh.asp?dnum=1

Contact the **U.S. Department of Veteran Affairs.** Go to http://www.va.gov/

Receiving Medical Care in the Hospital

The purpose of the Patient Self-determination Act passed by Congress in 1991 is to "inform patients of their rights regarding decisions toward their own medical care, and ensure that these rights are communicated by the healthcare provider. Specifically, the rights ensured are those of the patient to dictate their future care (by means such as living will or power of attorney), should they become incapacitated."

-- Wikipedia

At some point in many people's lives, there is a need to seek medical care in a hospital. Hospitals provide emergency care, necessary or elective surgeries, procedures and tests, and diagnostic workups and treatments.

Outside the hospital, most people live independently in their own home, making their own decisions about where they live, what they eat, what to wear, and how to spend their day. In the hospital, it is easy to become dependent on nursing staff and other hospital personnel. Your room may be private or shared. You may be required to eat a special diet of pureed food instead of a hamburger. A call button brings the nurse to help you use the bathroom. Your hospital attire consists of a skimpy hospital gown with an open back, providing little privacy. (You can ask for two gowns, one to cover the front and one to cover the back.)

The abrupt change in your ability to manage independently—to walk, eat, brush your hair or teeth, tie your shoes, button your shirt, use the bathroom— presents a challenge. If you consider yourself a private person and are uncomfortable with people viewing your personal daily care, then simple, but often-necessary hospital practices, such as using a bedpan or sitting on a commode chair in your room, can seem like an invasion of privacy. Receiving a bath by a certified nursing assistant or registered nurse, who is also a stranger, may be a new and uneasy experience. It is important for you to share your feelings and concerns with the nurses who provide your care. This increases their awareness of your personal boundaries and needs and enables the hospital staff to provide more compassionate and sensitive care.

Leslie is a 67-year old woman admitted to the hospital for a medical procedure. To prepare her, a male nurse entered her room to shave her and start her intravenous medication. Leslie was very uncomfortable with a male nurse, but instead of calmly requesting a female nurse, she became agitated and began yelling at the hospital staff. Once the staff understood her discomfort with the male nurse, they exchanged duties and had a female nurse prepare her for surgery.

Being Admitted to the Hospital

"Healing is a matter of time, but it is sometimes also a matter of opportunity."

--Hippocrates

Admission to the hospital occurs several ways:

- as a direct admission, with a physician's order for a planned surgery, procedure, or treatment;
- as a direct admission, with a physician's order, secondary to sudden illness or an accident;
- through the emergency department for an acute illness;
- through outpatient services.

Most hospitals feature several admissions offices. For **direct admissions** during regular business hours (approximately 6 a.m. to 7 p.m.), you will usually be directed to the main admissions office.

If you are admitted through the **Emergency Department**, (ED) the emergency admissions personnel will first verify your personal information, medical insurance, and emergency contact information. This department is open 24/7 and located by the entrance to the ED. Once admitted to the emergency department, the ED doctor will need medical information and may consult with your primary care physician doctor regarding your medical history, condition, medications, former procedures, and treatment. If you previously received treatment in the hospital, the ED admissions office will request your medical records from the hospital's medical records department or, as this is the day of computerized records, the ED physician will access your electronic records on the computer. If needed, the ED physician can also contact other hospitals, physician offices, urgent care centers and community clinics to obtain copies of your medical history.

If admission is due to a **scheduled outpatient procedure**, you will register at the **outpatient services admissions office** or through the emergency department admissions desk. Some hospitals will use the ED admissions for both emergencies and outpatient procedures, especially after-hours.

If admission to the hospital is for **an outpatient procedure**, admission may be categorized as outpatient observation (OBS) or, if you meet the acute care criteria, as inpatient (IP.) Physicians can monitor a patient as an outpatient in an acute care environment for 24-48 hours. If the patient meets inpatient criteria, their admission status can change to inpatient. During the outpatient admission, you will receive a physician evaluation, treatment, and monitoring. As Medicare and many insurance companies enforce strict guidelines for acute care hospitalization, the physician will use the observation time to determine if you need hospital admission for observation or acute medical care.

Medicare patients are billed for outpatient observation bills under Medicare Part B, not under Medicare Part A, which covers hospital admission. This means that you are obtaining an outpatient service and will be responsible for outpatient co-payments and deductibles. Under original Medicare guidelines, your outpatient hospital stay does *not* count toward the required 3-night inpatient stay needed to qualify for skilled nursing care in a skilled nursing facility. Under Medicare managed-care programs, the 3-night inpatient requirement for skilled nursing care may not be necessary.

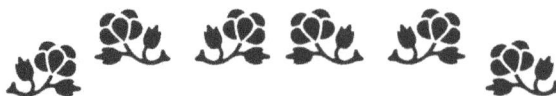

The Admissions Interview

(personal information, advanced directive, durable power of attorney for health-care, living will, durable general power of attorney, organ donor card, Physician Orders for Life-Sustaining Treatment form (POLST))

The hospital admissions staff needs to verify your personal information. Be patient, because they prioritize for emergencies. In the emergency department, the admissions staff gathers the information when you check in or at the bedside. Normally, the admissions clerk verifies the following information

- your full name and address;
- your home and cell telephone numbers;
- your birth date;
- your place of employment, if applicable;
- your Social Security number;
- your spouse's name and place of employment;
- your next of kin;
- an emergency contact in the family or a close friend;
- known allergies and medications;
- your physician's name;
- your presenting medical problem;
- your insurance policies and numbers.

The admissions staff prefer to see your Medicare, Medicaid, or insurance card. They will copy both the front and back of the card and should immediately return the documents to you. If you bring a copy of your cards, be sure to make a copy of both sides of the card. They will also need to see a photo ID card (i.e. a driver's license.) Bring the following information to your admissions interview or, if you do not have this available, have a family member or friend, bring it to the hospital.

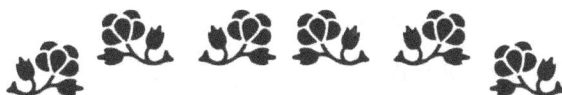

- ➢ photo Identification card*;
- ➢ medical and insurance cards;*
- ➢ list of medications and dosages (or bring the bag of medications with you);
- ➢ copy of Social Security card;
- ➢ advanced directives*;
- ➢ Physician Orders for Life-Sustaining Treatment (POLST)*;
- ➢ durable power of attorney for healthcare*;
- ➢ living will*;
- ➢ durable power of attorney *;
- ➢ organ donor card *;
- ➢ guardianship papers*;
- ➢ other pertinent legal documents*.

*This is important: *Retain the original documents for your files. Give copies to the hospital admissions office for your medical record, your primary care physician's office, your personal attorney, and any involved healthcare facility or community agency.*

Of course, in a sudden emergency, you may not have all this information available. Your family or friends can bring it to the hospital. Sometimes emergency staff will ask permission to look through your wallet to find an emergency contact person or medical card. However, if you are unable to respond and have an emergent condition, staff may do this without permission. Security hospital staff members store personal items in a secure location until either the patient or a family member can take responsibility for them.

On admission to the hospital, you or someone in your family, your conservator or guardian, or the person with a healthcare power of attorney will sign the *Conditions of Admission* form and other documents. By signing this standard form, you are consenting to:

- medical treatment and/or surgical procedures;
- general nursing care;
- secure storage of your personal belongings–the hospital is not liable and can hold your belongings in a hospital-based safe;
- participation in a teaching programs at hospitals that have educational programs for healthcare professionals;
- release of information that gives the hospital and/or treating physician or healthcare access to your medical record, including alcohol and drug abuse, and communicable disease related information;
- access of your medical record by third parties such as specialists, and

independent contractors, insurance companies, worker's compensation programs, government agencies, quality assurance programs utilization review committees and more;

- access of your medical record by medical auditors;

- financial agreement to pay for services rendered by the hospital and/or physicians and/or healthcare providers.

Review the *Health Insurance Portability and Accountability Act* (HIPAA) enacted by the United States Congress in 1996. Although it serves several purposes, the most relevant one for patients informs them of their rights regarding protection of privacy and confidentiality of personal healthcare information. For a summary of the HIPAA guidelines, go to http://www.hipaasurvivalguide.com/

The Advanced Directive and Other Legal Forms

(also called a living will, durable power of attorney for healthcare)

"Life is not measured by the number of breaths we take but by the moments that take our breath away."

--Anonymous

An advanced directive is a legal document completed by people before they face a serious medical condition, terminal illness, end-of–life, or permanent comatose state. When you are unable to communicate, the advanced directive directs the physician and healthcare professionals by expressing your wishes for medical care. The advanced directive does not expire and remains in effect until you change it. You may change or cancel this document at any time. The advanced directive varies from state to state. Therefore, it is important to review and possibly redo your advanced directive if you change states. With this document, you may:

- **appoint a healthcare representative** to direct your care if you are not able to competently make decisions;

- **complete healthcare instructions regarding life support,** tube feedings, and other limits of healthcare. *Life support* refers to the physician's use of medical procedures or devices such as ventilators to sustain life. *Tube feedings* include any food and water artificially supplied through medical means;

- **choose to receive treatment,** follow physician recommendations, or you may choose not to receive any treatments if close to death, permanently unconscious, if suffering from an advanced progressive illness, or if suffering extraordinary permanent and severe pain, and using life support or tube feedings would only postpone death;

- **request a Code status** be ordered by your physician. A **Do Not Resuscitate (DNR)** order means no resuscitation in the event of cardiac or respiratory arrest. **Do Not Intubate (DNI)** means that you do not want the physician to insert a flexible plastic tube into your trachea to protect your airway and provide mechanical ventilation. **Full Code** means hospital staff uses all medical means to sustain life. To request or change your code status, talk with your primary care physician.

- **A durable power of attorney for healthcare** enables you to appoint a healthcare representative to make medical decisions for you if you are unable to do so. These forms are usually available at the hospital admissions office.

- **A living will** is a binding legal document that expresses your wishes not to prolong life using extraordinary means or devices during terminal illness or a lasting comatose condition. It helps establish the no code status in the event of cardiac or respiratory failure when death is impending and certain. When the physician writes a No Code order, there will not be an attempt to resuscitate you if you experience cardiac or respiratory failure.

- **A general durable power of attorney** allows you (the principal) to appoint someone to act on your behalf and handle your real or personal property without advance notice or approval. These powers continue to exist if the courts declare you incompetent, disabled or incapacitated. The power of attorney can also be limited (a limited power of attorney) to specific transactions and responsibilities, such as the payment of your bills. You will not lose your right to manage your affairs. This device simply allows you to choose another person to help you with these matters. A general power of attorney form is available at many stationary stores or you can download one from an on-line website. Be sure an on-line power of attorney is upheld as legal in your state. For financial matters, contact the bank for financial power of attorney forms so someone or a bank representative can help you write checks, pay bills, and handle general financial issues.

- **An organ donor card** expresses your wishes to donate your organs at the time of death. There is no age requirement and no cost to your family. It is available at the time of admission or anytime through the Department of Motor Vehicles.

Piecing Together Quality Long-term Care" A Consumer's Guide to Choices and Advocacy can help you find acopy of your state's advance directive forms. Go to http://www.caringinfo.org/stateaddownload.

If you have questions about **Organ Donation**, talk with the hospital representative or go to http://organdonor.gov/about.asp

If you have any questions or concerns regarding the documents listed above, consult an attorney. Free legal advice is available through senior service agencies and state or county legal-service offices. A hospital social worker or spiritual care counselor may be able to help you understand these documents.

Please note: Each state adheres to different rules for advanced directives, a durable power of attorney for healthcare, and a living will. If you move to another state, it is important to complete the above forms again while you can still make these decisions.

Physician Orders for Life-Sustaining Treatment (POLST)

(also called Medical Orders for Life-sustaining Treatment (MOLST))

The POLST form, a voluntary physician order sheet was newly developed in the early 1990's in Oregon, for people with serious health conditions, advanced age, facing end-of-life decisions or residing in a long-term care facility. Other states adapted the POLST form, calling it MOLST or Medical Orders for Life-sustaining Treatment. It is used to specify to your physician and other healthcare providers your preferences (or if you are unable to participate, your legally designated decision-maker can accurately convey your preferences) and desires to avoid or receive life-sustaining treatment.

The POLST (or MOLST) improves the quality of patient care by increasing your understanding of your medical condition, prognosis, and clarifying the benefits and liabilities of life-sustaining treatment. It is useful in various healthcare settings, including hospitals, emergency care, physician offices, long-term care, assisted living facilities, adult care homes, and home healthcare and hospice agencies. Without the POLST form, emergency personnel are required to provide full treatment and resuscitation. Although the POLST is an excellent way for you to state your medical wishes, it is not available in every state.

At this time 10 states have endorsed programs – Washington, Oregon, California, Idaho, Colorado, Tennessee, North Carolina, West Virginia, Pennsylvania, and New York. Fourteen states are in the process of developing the POLST or MOLST programs.

You, your family, guardian or conservator, your physician, or a healthcare provider may initiate the bright pink POLST form. Your primary care or attending physician must sign it, but you can modify or cancel it at any time. You will need the doctor to initial any and all changes. The oringinal form should stay with you whenever you transfer or discharge from a healthcare setting. Provide updated copies to your physician's office, appropriate healthcare providers, hospitals, skilled nursing facilities, home healthcare and hospice agencies, and a member of your family.

The POLST form contains five sections. You can designate your treatment preferences in each by choosing active treatment, no treatment or placing limitations on the treatment you receive from your physician.

- **Section A: Resuscitation** means that if *there is no pulse and no breathing* you want the physician to revive you, regardless of your condition. You can choose Resuscitation or Do Not Resuscitate (DNR.)

- **Section B: Medical intervention,** including emergency medical care, means *there is evidence of a pulse and/or breathing.* You can choose comfort measures, limited intervention, advanced interventions or full treatment. Your physician will discuss with you and your family what each of these categories means in relation to your medical care.

- **Section C: Antibiotics** will be administered unless you place a limitation on their use.

- **Section D: Artificially administered fluids and nutrition** or the use of feeding tubes/IV fluids is designated if you become unable to take fluids or nutrition by mouth.

- **Section E: Basis for physician orders** states whom you discussed the orders with, summarizes the orders, and is signed and dated by your physician.

For information about the **Physician Orders for Life-Sustaining Treatment** (POLST) in your state, go to http://www.ohsu.edu/emergency/research/polst/

The Role of the Physician

(primary care physician, hospitalist, intensivist, attending physician)

Physicians who deliver medical care to patients range from primary care physicians to doctors employed by hospitals to specialists. Primary care physicians (PCP's) provide day-to-day medical care in a private office and occasionally will see patients in the hospital; hospitalists give medical care in a hospital setting; attending physicians offer care in a hospital, clinic, or in their private office. Specialists provide specialty care in a hospital or in their private office. They can serve as the primary physician or as an expert consultant requested by your hospital physician. All these physicians may confer with other physicians, make recommendations and referrals, request services, write orders for medical care, and prescribe medication and durable medical equipment for home use. For continuity of care, it is important for the physicians working with you to share medical information and coordinate a plan of care.

- The **primary care physician,** (PCP) the doctor chosen by you, coordinates your medical care and services. Your primary care physician can refer you to a specialist. Although primary care physician's years ago typically examined patients in their offices and in the hospital, times have changed. In the 21st century, few primary care doctors visit |patients admitted to a hospital. Increasingly, a doctor hired by the hospital, called a hospitalist treats these patients.

- **A hospitalist** is a physician who specializes in hospital medicine. Many hospitals use "hospitalists" to examine and treat patients admitted to the hospital. These physicians have received degrees as Doctors of Medicine in internal medicine, family practice, pediatrics or osteopathic medicine. An emerging service begun 10 years ago, it is now common to find a hospitalist providing care to patients rather than their primary care physicians. Hospitalists also serve indigent patients without insurance or a primary care physician as well as patients with insurance, but without a primary care physician. Hospitalists evaluate and treat patients during their stay in the hospital. Once you leave the hospital, your primary care physician again becomes your primary doctor. If you do not have a primary care physician, the hospitalist can refer you to a community clinic for follow-up medical care. Alternatively, a social worker can help you find a primary care doctor.

- **An intensivist** is often a pulmonologist, who specializes in the care and treatment of critically ill or injured patients within the intensive care unit.

- The **attending physician** (AP) any doctor other than a primary care physician or hospitalist who provides your medical care in the hospital includes specialists, surgeons, and other physicians consulted about your medical care.

When you are discharged from the hospital, your primary care physician should continue to monitor your progress, consult with the attending physician or hospitalist, receive medical information and reports, and provide follow-up care.

If you transfer from the hospital to a skilled nursing facility and your physician does not have privileges at the skilled nursing facility, your physician should make a telephone call (Dr.-to-Dr.) to a *house doctor* at the facility. The house doctor at the skilled nursing facility becomes responsible for writing orders for medical care during your stay at the skilled facility. The house doctor or your primary care physician (or sometimes attending physician) is required to evaluate your condition in the nursing facility once a month. If the house doctor determines that you require additional medical care, the nursing facility can arrange transportation to your primary care physician's office for a medical appointment or to an emergency department for evaluation and treatment.

The Role of Medical Social Workers, Case Managers, and Discharge Planners

The social worker/case manager/discharge planner function as your liaison between the physician, the hospital staff, the nursing homes and other community housing, the insurance companies, and community and government agencies. They can:

- explain advanced directives;
- assist with admission to skilled nursing facilities, adult care homes, and other alternatives;
- contact insurance companies for necessary pre-authorizations;
- make referrals to local, state, and government agencies;
- help you set-up in-home care services;
- assist with transfers to home or another setting;
- provide counseling to patients and families;
- discuss end-of-life care;
- secure financial assistance to help pay for medications, transportation, housing.

In some hospitals, the case manager handles all of the above. In other hospitals, the social worker may be responsible for counseling services, mental health assessments, and drug and alcohol evaluations while the discharge planner may be responsible for helping your family arrange your discharge from the hospital.

- **If you were living alone prior to hospitalization**, it may be necessary to contact community agencies for in-home support, home healthcare services and essential durable medical equipment and supplies. Often a family member or friend will offer to stay with you in your home or will have you stay in their home until you are able to resume independent living. A medical social worker, case manager or discharge planner can help arrange this care.

- **If you were living in a retirement community, assisted living facility, or an adult care home,** it may be necessary to increase help in your residence or alert the residence management that you will have increased care needs following hospitalization. Many facilities will send a nurse or admissions person to the hospital to assess your medical needs. If your medical care needs exceeds what the facility is capable of providing they may suggest hiring a private caregiver or recommend that you receive a temporary higher level of care before returning to the facility. In an adult care home, the caregiver must be able to provide the higher level of care. Some facilities cannot care for a person who has extensive medical needs. In these settings, you may be eligible for home healthcare and hospice care services.

- **If you are unable to return safely to any of these settings,** you may need to consider other options, such as a skilled nursing or rehabilitation facility. The discharge planner can act as a liaison between you, your physician, and the skilled or rehab facility, contacting appropriate facilities on your behalf, faxing them relevant medical information, contacting insurance companies for pre-authorizations, checking insurance benefits, and setting up transfer transportation.

- **If nursing home placement for skilled nursing care or an intensive rehabilitation program** is a reasonable option, it is important that you consult with your physician, the medical social worker, case manager, or discharge planner about applying to facilities or programs in your area.

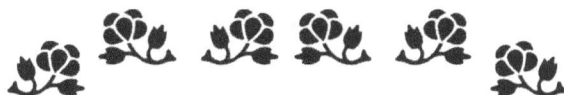

Paying for Your Hospitalization

"The great secret that all old people share is that you really haven't changed in 70 or 80 years. Your body changes, but you don't change at all."

-- Doris Lessing

As healthcare coverage in the United States is changing very rapidly, it is necessary to verify your insurance coverage and benefits whenever you obtain medical care. If treatment in a hospital would cause financial hardship for you, meaning you have limited or no income or assets and no insurance and are concerned about the cost of hospital care, call the hospital financial or business office to discuss your situation. They can guide you through the Medicaid application process and discuss ways for you to meet your financial obligations.

If you require emergency medical care, do not delay getting medical care due to your lack of finances. By delaying medical care, you may exacerbate your medical condition, resulting in a more serious problem and a more lengthy and expensive hospitalization.

On a Tuesday morning, Barbara, a 61-year old woman presented to the emergency department (ED) with a complaint of chest pain. In the emergency department, she told the ED physician, "Since Friday, I feel like I have an elephant sitting on my chest." After the emergency department physician diagnosed an acute heart attack and recommended hospital admission, I asked Barbara why she delayed coming to the hospital. She replied, "I lost my job. I'm losing my home. I have no insurance and I have no money." Barbara stayed in the hospital over 2 weeks, receiving tests and cardiac procedures. A financial counselor helped her apply for state Medicaid program and complete a financial assistance application to help pay her bill for her hospitalization.

Most people admitted to a hospital carry some type of insurance policy: original Medicare, a Medicare HMO or Managed-care Policy, Medicaid, Medicare supplemental, a Medigap policy, Veteran's benefits or a private insurance policy. In addition, there are many people without any health insurance. They may earn low wages and cannot afford medical care; they work, but do not receive healthcare benefits through their employer; they are self-employed and find the monthly cost of insurance prohibitive.

As a **Medicare beneficiary**, you may receive medical services under the original Medicare fee-for-service program or through a Medicare managed-care or HMO plan. If you receive limited income and are disabled or suffer from a serious illness or chronic condition that renders you unable to work, you may qualify for state **Medicaid** assistance. If you qualify for Social Security Disability, then, after 2- years, you may receive Medicare benefits. If you are experiencing financial hardship, hospital financial office counselors can work out a reasonable payment plan with you and sometimes reduce the hospital bill.

Original Medicare Part A - Hospital Insurance, 2014

- **Deductible:** an amount paid each year by a health insurance plan enrollee before benefits begin. It is not synonymous with co-payment.

- **Co-payment:** a fixed fee that subscribers to a medical plan must pay for their use of specific medical services covered by the plan.

- **Premium:** The amount paid or payable, often in installments, for an insurance policy. (The Free Dictionary)

Medicare Part A hospital insurance pays for a semi-private room and board, general nursing care, and inpatient hospital services and supplies for the first sixty days of hospitalization. If you carry a supplemental policy, it may pay the deductibles and co-insurance payments not covered by Medicare Part A.

Medicare Part A pays for **Hospice care in the hospital** as long as the doctor certifies the need for end-of-life care. It pays all expenses except a small fee for inpatient respite care and some outpatient medications. A patient can receive up to five days of covered care per hospital admission, which provides family members with respite care or a break in caregiving. Usually a patient facing end-of-life care transfers from the hospital to home with 24/7 caregivers, to a residence such as a Level 3 adult care home or an assisted living facility that can provide the necessary 24/7 care, or to a skilled nursing facility with Medicare Part A hospice benefits. Be aware that Medicare Part A hospice benefits in a skilled nursing facility do *not* pay for costly room and board.

If you are receiving hospice care in a hospital with a designated hospice room or unit, the hospital can transfer you to that unit. If the hospital layout does not include a designated unit, you may transfer to an inpatient hospice program in the community, a skilled nursing facility or receive outpatient hospice services in your home. In your home, you will receive additional support from family, friends, and caregivers. *(Please note: Medicare does not pay for room and board in a skilled nursing facility. Medicare will pay hospice nurses to visit in a skilled nursing facility. In some states, Medicaid does pay for limited end-of-life comfort care in a skilled nursing facility.)*

Lifetime Reserve Days - Original Medicare means additional days that Medicare will pay for when you are in a hospital for more than 90 days. You are entitled to 60 reserve days that can be used during your lifetime. For each lifetime reserve day, Medicare pays all covered costs except for a daily co-insurance ($608 in 2014.) (Reprint from Medicare and You, 2014)

Part A – Hospital Insurance Deductibles and Co-insurance, 2014

In 2014, for each benefit period, you will pay:

Inpatient Hospital deductible	$1,216 for days 1-60
Inpatient Hospital co-insurance	$304 per day for days 61-90
	$608 per day for days 91-150
	(Lifetime Reserve Days)
Inpatient Mental Health deductible	$1,216 for days 1-60
	$304 for days 61-90
Inpatient Mental health co-insurance	$608 for days 91 + per each lifetime reserve day
	Limited to 190 days in lifetime
	Beyond lifetime reserve days, you pay all costs
Skilled Nursing Facility co-insurance	$0 for days 1-20
	$152 per day for days 21-100
	All costs for additional days

--Data from Medcare.gov website: http://www.medicare.gov/your-medicare-costs/costs-at-a-glance/costs-at-glance.html

Original Medicare Part B - Medical Insurance

Medicare Part B medical insurance does not pay for inpatient hospitalization. It does pay for outpatient hospital services, outpatient treatment, and therapies, home healthcare services, durable medical equipment and medical bills submitted by Medicare eligible physician services. In 2014, for most people, the standard Medicare Part B monthly premium will cost $104.90. (In 2014, there are no changes in Part B-Medical Insurance Premiums and Deductibles.) People with high adjusted gross income may pay higher premiums for Medicare Part B. For those receiving Social Security Railroad Retirement benefits or Civil Service benefits, the Medicare Part B premium may be deducted from your benefit payment.

You also pay a monthly premium determined by your modified adjusted gross income filed on your individual or joint tax return. In 2013 and 2014, for individual incomes of $85,000 or less and joint incomes of $170,000 or less, expect to pay the standard monthly premium of $104.90; for individual incomes over $214,000 and joint incomes over $428,000 expect to pay a monthly premium of $335.70. For detailed Medicare cost information for 2013 and 2014, go to http://www.medicare.gov/your-medicare-costs/costs-at-a-glance/costs-at-glance.html#collapse-4809

For information about **Social Security Railroad Retirement benefits**, go to http://www.socialsecurity.gov/retire2/railroad.htm or call 1-877-772-5772

For more information about **Civil Service benefits**, go to http://www.socialsecurity.gov/retire2/fedgovees.htm

A $147 deductible per year is charged for Medicare Part B services and supplies before Medicare begins to pay its share. After paying your deductible, you are responsible for 20% of the Medicare-approved services. If you carry a supplemental health insurance policy, it may cover the 20% portion of the charges.

Outpatient hospital services, treatment and therapies are benefits covered under Medicare Part B. You are responsible for 20% of hospital charges. Your supplemental policy may pay your deductible.

For **partial hospitalization for mental health services**, you can expect to pay 40% of the Medicare Part B-approved amount for services you receive from a qualified professional and 20% for each day of your stay in a hospital outpatient department or community mental health center. For **outpatient mental health services,** you can expect to pay 20% of the Medicare Part B approved amount that includes visits to your doctor for diagnosis monitoring, and treatment of your condition. If you receive counseling or psychotherapy, you can expect to pay 35% of the cost to visit your physician in his office. You are also responsible for a co-payment in a hospital outpatient setting.

For **a complete list of services and supplies** covered and non-covered, go to www.MEDICARE.gov or call 1-800-Medicare (1-800-633-4227)

Applying for Medicare Parts A or B

To apply for Medicare Part A or Part B, it is necessary to contact the nearest **Social Security Office**. Staff can help determine if you meet the requirements for receiving or buying into a Medicare insurance policy. It is important to remember that Medicare eligibility requirements, monthly premiums, and hospital deductibles change. In addition, the Social Security Office can direct you to helpful brochures and information. To apply for Medicare on-line go to http://www.socialsecurity.gov/medicareonly/.

If you have questions about your eligibility for Medicare Part A or Part B, or if you decide to apply for Medicare, please visit or call your local *Social Security Office* at 1-800-772-1213. If you are diagnosed with a disability or receive low- income, ask if you are eligible to waive or receive assistance with some of the Medicare premiums. There is a limited open enrollment period, usually between mid-October and early December, when you can sign up for Medicare benefits.

Determining Original Medicare Eligibility

To be eligible for government Medicare benefits, you must meet certain requirements. You must be:

- **65 years of age or older** and a legal United States resident or 65 years of age or older with permanent legal citizenship for at least 5 years and 10 years at a job that pays into the Medicare system;

- **under 65 years of age**, and

  - ➢ receiving Social Security Disability Insurance (SSDI) or;

  - ➢ receiving Railroad Retirement Board Disability benefits, for at least 24 months, or;

  - ➢ with a diagnosis of Lou Gehrig's disease (also called ALS or amyotrophic lateral sclerosis), or;

  - ➢ with a diagnosis of permanent kidney failure with dialysis or transplant or other specific conditions.

Medicare Advantage Part C - HMO's and Managed-care Programs

Medicare Advantage managed-care or HMO plans are government subsidized healthcare programs that provide benefits within their own network of hospitals, and care by their own network of preferred providers, which includes physicians and other health professionals. They were created to help reduce the cost of healthcare and increase the number of benefits to our nation's elderly. Under a Medicare Advantage program, you will receive medical care by a primary care physician, within the network, that you select. Medicare pays these plans a fixed monthly fee for each enrollee to their plan. There are different types of Medicare Advantage plans that include:

- **Health Maintenance Organization Plans** (HMO) that employs staff to provide treatment to enrollees;

- **preferred provider plans** (PPO's) that contracts with community physicians and healthcare providers to provide care to enrollees;

- **special needs plans** (SNP's) are for underprivileged poor and very ill people with complex medical care needs who are eligible for both Medicare and Medicaid benefits;

- **private fee-for-service** plan (PFFS) enrollees can see any provider that is authorized to provide medical services as long as the provider also accepts the plans terms and conditions of payment. Payment rates may vary due to the provider's specialty and location. No prior authorization should be required. As the rules and charges for out-of-pocket expenses change each year, carefully check the plan details.

To qualify for a Medicare managed-care program you must:

- be age 65 years or older or disabled and collecting Social Security Disability Income for 24 months;

- reside in the area serviced by the managed-care program;

- carry both Medicare Part A and Part B;

- not be diagnosed with permanent kidney failure at time of enrollment.

If you sign up for a Medicare Managed-care program, you will:

- receive your medical care from an in-network physician, nurse practitioner or physician assistant;

- require a referral/ and/or pre-authorization to visit a specialist or out-of-network physician. Managed-care programs may restrict medical care visits or increase fees for out-of- network physicians;

- need prior authorization or pre-approval for some types of services, procedures, and medical procedures *(You may not need prior authorization under the Medicare fee-for-service plan)*;

- receive more prescriptions for less costly generic medications;

- see some limits on your healthcare benefits.

In addition, a Medicare Advantage plan may use stricter guidelines than private pay insurance for what constitutes emergency care or the need for initiating or continuing rehabilitation or skilled nursing care.

(Please note: Some Medicare Advantage managed-care programs use stricter guidelines than original Medicare and may authorize shorter stays in hospital or nursing facilities or may not authorize treatment by a specialist outside the managed-care program area. They also may adhere to different guidelines such as not requiring a person to have a three-night inpatient hospital stay, as required by original Medicare, to receive care in a skilled nursing facility.)

Check with your managed-care plan about its policy for receiving emergency care outside your local area, as some plans will try to transfer you back to your service area for necessary follow-up care, often at your own expense. The out-of-network area hospital treating your medical emergency can usually negotiate a contract with the managed-care plan administrators to keep you until they judge your condition as medically stable for a safe transfer to a participating Medicare Advantage facility. If you require air or ground ambulance transportation to another hospital, be sure to establish who pays for this potentially expensive transportation.

While vacationing 300 miles from his home, a car swerved off a roadway and hit Sam. The ambulance brought Sam to the nearest hospital emergency department. The ED physician admitted Sam to the out-of-network hospital with a fractured pelvis, multiple rib fractures, a concussion, and several contusions and abrasions. During his hospitalization, he was unable to walk or move and deemed medically unstable for transfer. Nonetheless, personnel from his Medicare Advantage plan requested that Sam transfer to an in-network hospital by commercial airline at the family's expense. When told he was not medically stable for transfer, especially by commercial airline, his Medicare Advantage representatives requested his transfer by medical air ambulance, again at the family's expense, at a cost of more than $4000. After many days of negotiation with the treating hospital, the Medicare Advantage insurance plan finally agreed to allow Sam to stay and receive the necessary medical care until he could be safely transported to an in-network facility.

Medicare Supplemental and Medigap Policies

Developed by the *National Association of Insurance Commissioners*, these policies cover the "gaps" or "holes" in your original Medicare benefits. Standard Medigap policies range from basic benefit packages to packages with additional options, plans that span from Plan A to Plan J. States are required to offer Plan A, but are not required to offer additional Medigap policies.

Medigap policies also pay for specific services not covered under Medicare. Some policies pay the Medicare deductible and co-insurance payments. Medicare supplemental policies may limit benefits or exclusions for specific medical conditions. Medigap policies do not work with Medicare Advantage managed-care plans.

To choose a Medigap policy, review the official U.S. government handbook from the **Centers for Medicare and Medicaid, 2014: Medicare and You**. To view this official Medicare handbook on-line, go to http://www.medicare.gov/pubs/pdf/10050.pdf

Veteran's Benefits

"The provisions of the Affordable Care Act (ACA) upheld by the U.S. Supreme Court will not affect the current role the Department of Veterans Affairs (VA) has in the lives of America's Veterans. We will continue to provide Veterans with high quality, comprehensive health care and benefits they have earned through their service. VA health care does not change as a result of the ACA." -- United States Department of Veteran Affairs

The Department of Veteran Affairs serves over 8.3 million veterans in 152 medical centers spread throughout the United States. It is a large and complex program and can be difficult to navigate. To receive veteran benefits, it is necessary to apply to the Department of Veteran Affairs. You are eligible for inpatient hospital care and outpatient services if:

- you are active military, naval or air service and separated (leaving active duty) from the service under any condition other than dishonorable;

- you served active duty in combat operations after November 11, 1998;

- are an active duty service member;

- you are a family member of a veteran and can receive benefits under specific circumstances. Contact the nearest Veteran Affairs office to determine your eligibility;

- you are a former member of an allied armed forces during World War 2.

If you receive veteran's benefits, and do not retain Medicare or private insurance coverage, the hospital must contact the nearest *U.S. Department of Veterans Affairs* to authorize inpatient medical treatment. Although the VA may agree to pay for the care you receive in a non-VA facility, the VA may prefer to transfer you, with your agreement, to a VA facility for continued treatment. For service-connected veterans, the VA usually provides transportation for a transfer from the acute care hospital to the Veteran's hospital.

For information on **applying to the United States Department of Veteran Affairs**, go to http://www.va.gov/healthbenefits/apply/

To locate a **VA Community-based Healthcare Center**, go to http://www2.va.gov/directory/guide/division_flsh.asp?dnum=1

Medicaid

"The Affordable Care Act fills in current gaps in coverage for the poorest Americans by creating a minimum Medicaid income eligibility level across the country. Beginning in January 2014, individuals under 65 years of age with income below 133 percent of the federal poverty level (FPL) will be eligible for Medicaid. For the first time, low-income adults without children will be guaranteed coverage through Medicaid in every state without need for a waiver" (excerpt from Medicaid.gov)

The Affordable Care Act is changing the way states determine eligibility for Medicaid benefits. Although under the Affordable Care Act, most Americans will have some form of insurance, at this time, many people remain without insurance. Individuals with no insurance and limited income and limited assets can apply for Medicaid insurance, the benefits of which can help pay for your hospitalization. If you are hospitalized and uninsured, talk with the hospital financial assistance office about how to apply for this program. Often, the financial counselor can help you begin the process of applying for benefits. Eligibility and benefits vary from state to state, so it is important to contact the nearest *State Area Agency on Aging Office* or *Senior and Disabled Services Office* to obtain their Medicaid guidelines and an application.

Private Insurance Plans

For people who purchase their own health insurance, private insurance companies offer a wide assortment of programs and benefits. It is important to compare several insurance policies. Look at co-payment and deductible fees, office visit fees, prescription coverage, outpatient and inpatient benefits, and vision and hearing benefits. Also, check for a cap on the number of visits. Determine if the insurance company requires pre-authorizations for procedures, hospitalizations, skilled nursing facility care, and rehabilitation services. Check the referral process for seeing a specialist. Be sure that the insurance company lists your current primary care physician as a preferred provider.

If you utilize alternative medicine treatments, such as acupuncture, chiropractic services, massage therapies and others, be sure to check the policy coverage for these benefits

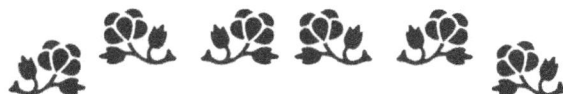

Programs to Help You
Pay Your Medicare Benefits

(Qualified Medicare Beneficiary (QMB), Specified Low-Income Medicare Beneficiary (SLMB), Qualifying Individual (QI), and Qualified Disabled and Working Individuals programs (QDWI.))

The **Qualified Medicare Beneficiary program (QMB)**, pronounced "quimby", can help qualified low-income Medicare Parts A and B beneficiaries pay their healthcare costs by paying Medicare deductibles, monthly premiums, co-payments and co-insurance amounts. You must be eligible for Medicare Part A, even if you have not enrolled in the program. Your income must make you ineligible to qualify financially for the state Medicaid program. Medicaid is a state- regulated program, so the income limits will vary.

U.S. Department of **Health and Human Services LIHEAP** Clearinghouse lists the 2013/ 2014 HHS Federal Poverty Guidelines. Go to http://liheap. ncat.org/profiles/povertytables/FY2014/popstate.htm

People eligible for Medicare Part A may benefit from the **Specified Low-Income Medicare Beneficiary (SLMB)** program. Designed to help qualified individuals with incomes slightly greater than (not more than 20 percent) the national poverty level, this program requires the state to pay the Medicare Part B monthly premium. You are responsible for the deductibles, co-insurance, and any other charges not covered by Medicare.

The **Qualifying Individual** (QI) program helps pay for Medicare Part B premiums only. The Qualified Disabled and Working Individuals program helps pay for Medicare Part A premiums.

As each state administers its own program, it is necessary to contact the nearest *Department of Health and Human Services Office* to apply for these programs. Bring your proof of residency, Social Security card or proof of the number, proof of citizenship (birth certificate), proof of income and assets, (bank statements, tax return) and a copy of your insurance cards. *(Please note: The monthly income limits for these programs change each year.)*

For information on **Medicare Assistance Programs,** go to http://www. medicare.gov/navigation/medicare-basics/medical-and-drug-costs.aspx

Insurance Hints

It is important to be familiar with your hospital insurance coverage. By reviewing your healthcare insurance policies, you can identify areas with coverage gaps. Be sure that your insurance pays the following benefits:

➢ hospital deductible;

➢ coverage for extended hospitalization;

➢ co-insurance in case of lengthy hospitalization;

➢ outpatient health services;

➢ skilled nursing facility co-insurance coverage for days 21–100;

➢ prescription drug coverage;

➢ hearing and vision care;

➢ alternative medicine *(chiropractic, acupuncture, naturopath and more)*;

➢ end-of-life care benefits.

Watch out for policies that have:

• **exclusions for specific medical conditions**. If you have a pre-existing medical condition with a strong probability that you will need medical treatment, do not sign any contract that states it will not pay for medical care related to that specific condition. Exclusion policies for pre-existing conditions are currently changing under the new *Affordable Healthcare Act*;

• **managed-care plans with strict guidelines that can override** some of your original Medicare benefits;

• **duplicate coverage** of benefits;

• **inadequate policies**. Do not cancel your policy until you can replace it with another policy. You do not want to find yourself in an "insurance gap," without medical coverage;

- **limits on benefits**. Some Medicare supplement policies (not Medigap policies) have limits on what they pay for specific benefits. This allowable amount may be less than the Medicare approved amount for hospital outpatient services or services provided by your physician.

Do not be pressured into buying a policy. Take the time to check with the *Medicare Hot Line* or the *National Association of Insurance Commissioners*. Use only a reputable company. Read the entire policy and write down your questions.

Remember, these are only guidelines. To include all the information necessary to understand Medicare, Medigap, and Medicare supplemental policies more completely, you must read the available booklets and talk with knowledgeable professionals in the insurance and healthcare field.

For **Medicare** information, call 1-800-633-4227 or go to

http://www.medicare.gov/navigation/help-and-support/contact-medicare.aspx

Be aware that **Medicare is currently undergoing many changes** that will affect eligibility and benefits in all areas of healthcare. Check for updates at: http://www.medicare.gov/

Planning Your Discharge from the Hospital

"Don't take anything for granted. No one knows everything–don't be afraid to ask questions." Seanette, Hospital Medical Unit Clerk

When your physician decides you are ready for discharge from the hospital, you may receive as little as a one-day warning. Your physician will evaluate your medical condition each day, and if he decides that you are medically stable and no longer require acute hospital care, he may recommend discharge from the hospital. Although most hospital discharges are straightforward, others can be more complex. When you consider all the changes you will experience in the hospital, it is easy to see why some people do not quickly bounce back to their usual activities. Consider the number of tests, procedures, and surgeries you receive in the hospital. Think about the amount of time you are inactive, in bed, or in a chair. Think about the changes in your diet, mobility, and the changes in your ability to perform your activities of daily life. As each hospitalized person responds to medical procedures differently, it is necessary to anticipate increased care needs and supervision following hospitalization. All these variations from normal, everyday life can affect the amount of time it takes for recovery from a hospitalization

Although each person's time in the hospital varies, each medical diagnosis has a standard pre-determined length of stay. Assuming no complications arise, your physician should be able to anticipate and communicate your discharge date. You may be able to return to your previous living situation or home, or you may need increased care at your place of residence, an assisted living facility, adult care home, and an inpatient or outpatient rehabilitation program in a skilled nursing facility.

When you are close to discharge from the hospital, speak with a social worker, case manager, or discharge planner about your discharge plans. They will review your medical record and, with help from your family and information from hospital staff and your physician, discuss all the reasonable care options. The social worker can provide you with helpful information and clearly lay out all the discharge options. If you require home healthcare, durable medical equipment and supplies, or information and referrals to community and government agencies and programs, the discharge planner can guide you to these resources. To provide the most relevant options, the social worker will ask questions about your current living situation, including:

- the layout of your residence;
- the number of stairs inside and access to the bathroom;
- access to the bedroom area;
- safety features in the home;
- medical equipment in the home or residence;
- your care needs and preferences;
- available financial resources;
- availability of help from family, neighbors, and caregivers;
- the names of community agencies or caseworkers working with you.

If needed, the social worker can act as a liaison between you, your family, your physician, and active community agencies.

Appraising Your Living
Situation And Care Needs

After leaving the hospital, you may need a different living situation or increased care and supervision for a shorter or longer period. To determine the appropriate living situation and care needs, consider the following questions:

- Where did you live prior to hospitalization?

- Do you feel you can safely return to this living situation?

- Do you feel some in-home supervision or assistance would be helpful?

- Are you interested in exploring an alternative living situation while you recover from your hospitalization?

- Prior to hospitalization, how would you describe your general physical health?

- Prior to hospitalization, did you receive any assistance with personal or medical care?

- Prior to hospitalization, did you receive care from a registered nurse, physical therapist, or home healthcare agency?

- Prior to hospitalization, how would you describe your mental health?

  - alert and oriented;
  - can make your own decisions;
  - good memory;
  - easily follows directions;
  - disoriented;
  - cannot make your own decisions;
  - poor memory;
  - have difficulty following directions.

- How would you describe your current mobility?

  - walk independently;
  - use cane or walker;

> - use standard wheelchair;
> - use electric wheelchair or scooter;
> - frequent falls;
> - balance problems;
> - bedridden;
> - unable to walk.

- Which living situations would you consider at discharge from the hospital?

> - home alone with no support;
> - home alone with caregiver support;
> - home with friends or family;
> - retirement community;
> - assisted living community;
> - adult care home;
> - skilled nursing facility;
> - other_____

- Is your monthly income adequate to private pay for services in your home or placement in an alternative living situation?
- What coverage does your healthcare insurance and/or long-term care insurance policies provide?
- Do you receive Veteran's benefits?

Ask to speak to a hospital discharge planner, social worker, or case manager to gather resource information, ask for help with placement if you need it, and for arrangement of care, support, and medical supervision and supplies in your home.

Receiving Care in a Skilled
or Intermediate Nursing Facility

*(also called 'sniff', healthcare centers, skilled rehabilitation
facilities, intermediate care facilities)*

It is common to hear someone say to a family member, "Please, promise you will never send me to a nursing home." The phrase "nursing home" brings up images of a place people go to die or end up, forsaken by family and friends. However, nursing homes also play an essential role in healthcare as temporary and sometimes long-term care medical facilities for people recuperating from a long-term illness, injury, accident, surgery, or hospitalization.

The decision to enter a nursing facility may follow a recommendation from your physician. Although you may plan to return home following a hospitalization, it is not always the best choice. Your physical condition and the physical layout of your home can make it difficult for you to resume your normal activities of daily life without assistance from family, friends, or a caregiver.

As many admissions to a skilled nursing facility occur immediately after a hospitalization, medical professionals – social workers, discharge planners, or case managers – are available to help you navigate the admission process. By reviewing your medical record and insurance information, they can determine your eligibility for services and benefits in a nursing facility under Medicare, Medicaid, or private insurances. Be aware that families may have little time to gather information and visit nursing facilities before the discharge date. By visiting the skilled nursing facilities with a family member or friend, you will benefit from different viewpoints and observations.

To find and compare skilled nursing facilities in your area, go to www. medicare.gov/NHCompare/home.asp

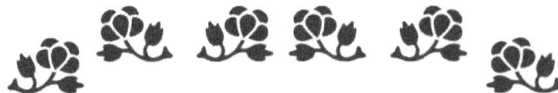

Imagine this scenario

You live alone. You have recently undergone surgery and are lying in a hospital bed recovering, feeling every ache and pain. You are not thinking clearly due to after affects from anesthesia and new and different medications. The nurses are helping you with your daily activities of life, as they are difficult for you to do. You are feeling dizzy and weak, experiencing balance problems, and very slowly walking 10 feet with contact guard assistance (a therapist or nurse has a hand on you to ensure your safety.) Getting in and out of the bed requires moderate assistance from the hospital staff. You are afraid of falling. You have a bandage over a wound that is still open and draining and requires sterile dressing changes three times a day. The pain from your surgery is still not resolved. You are beginning to recognize that returning home will be difficult for you. You will need help getting up in the morning, going to bed at night, getting to the bathroom, and performing your activities of daily life such as getting dressed and preparing meals. Your pain management continues to limit your recovery. Your dressings require bandage changes multiple times during the day. The doctor enters your room and informs you that you are doing well and he plans to discharge you the following day. A social worker meets with you to discuss your options. You can choose to:

- return home with assistance from family;

- return home alone with a part-time or full-time hired caregiver;

- return home alone with a referral for a home healthcare nurse, and therapist;

- transfer to a skilled nursing facility to receive physical therapy, wound care, and pain management;

- transfer to an adult care home that can help you with your care needs until you can return home. A home healthcare nurse and a physical therapist can visit you in the adult care home to help with wound care and physical therapy.

Realizing that returning to your home may place you at-risk for injury, you inform the social worker that your family is not available to help you and that you do not have funds to hire a private caregiver or receive care in an adult care home. She suggests going to a skilled nursing facility for short-term skilled care: physical therapy for strengthening, to increase your mobility and decrease your fall risk. In addition, you will receive wound care and dressing changes and pain management by registered and licensed practical nurses. As you have stayed in the hospital as an inpatient for 3 overnights and have a skilled need, your original Medicare benefits will help pay for this stay. *(Under some Medicare Managed-care plans, the three overnight stay as an inpatient is not required. Be aware that outpatient admission does not count toward the 3-night hospital stay.)*

Most people admitted to a nursing facility stay for a short time, returning to their previous living situation or if needed, an alternative living arrangement. A social worker/discharge planner employed by the nursing facility can help make these arrangements, locating alternative housing, making referrals to community and government agencies, ordering necessary durable medical equipment for the home, and arranging transportation home.

Although some people do become permanent long-term residents at a nursing home and eventually pass away at the nursing facility, it is important to remember that the majority of people receive medical care and services and are then discharged. More often, a stay in a nursing facility functions as the interim step between hospitalization and returning home.

It is important to remember that a nursing facility resident can change their mind if they decide receiving care in the nursing home care does not benefit them or offer the appropriate environment for recovery. Other options, such as home healthcare, private-duty nursing, and in-home support from community and government agencies are available to help provide care in the home. Alternatives to living in a nursing home depend upon your medical, physical, and emotional needs and include living with family or friends and living in an assisted living facility or adult care homes.

If your illness is considered complex and includes some neurological component, and if you are capable of some rehabilitation potential, that is, the ability to regain some or most of your physical abilities, it is strongly recommended that you consult with your physician regarding rehabilitation therapy programs in a hospital or a private rehabilitation center.

Deciding If You Need Care in a Skilled Nursing Facility

To gather the information necessary to make an informed decision about receiving care in a nursing home facility, it is important to talk with a healthcare professional. They will be able to guide you to appropriate nursing facilities and provide information about the different levels of care, the medical criteria for skilled nursing care, the advantages and disadvantages of receiving care in a skilled nursing facility, the types of insurance benefits through Medicare, Medicaid, and supplemental policies, private pay rates, and admission procedures. They can also act as a liaison between you, the doctor, hospital staff, nursing home staff, and community agencies.Gathering the necessary information to make decisions regarding care in a skilled nursing facility can be a lengthy and time-consuming process. You should know:

- your medical condition, including your skilled care needs;
- the doctor's treatment recommendations;
- admission procedures;
- the levels of care available in a nursing facility;
- original and managed-care Medicare requirements and benefits for skilled nursing care;
- Medicaid requirements and benefits for skilled nursing care;
- private insurance requirements and benefits for skilled nursing care;
- how to evaluate a nursing facility;
- patient's rights and responsibilities.

Looking at Your Medical Condition

"Nobody grows old by merely living a number of years. People grow old only by deserting their ideals. Years may wrinkle the skin, but to give up interest wrinkles the soul."

-- Douglas MacArthur

When you are recovering from a serious illness, surgery, prolonged hospitalization, or living with a debilitating chronic condition, you recuperate at your own pace. Insurance companies do not ask you how you feel or what you feel able to do. They review your medical record and talk with utilization review case mangers about your condition. They look for specific physical diagnoses, medical conditions and procedures. If you have any of the following medical issues, you may want to consider going to a skilled nursing facility where you can receive skilled nursing care and rehabilitative therapies.

- change in your ability to walk;
- paralysis;
- amputation care;
- daily dressing changes;
- seizures requiring monitoring;
- intravenous therapy (IV);
- severe or uncontrolled pain;

- ➢ leg, arm, or body cast;

- ➢ difficulty with speech or swallowing;

- ➢ temporary or permanent tubes;

- ➢ tube feedings;

- ➢ total parenteral (intravenous) nutrition (TPN);

- ➢ loss of consciousness;

- ➢ oxygen therapy;

- ➢ tracheotomy care;

- ➢ new medications requiring injections or monitoring;

- ➢ weakness from an extended illness;

- ➢ severe weight loss;

- ➢ insertion of a breathing tube *(Few skilled facilities can provide this care.)*

Each nursing facility will review the medical needs of every patient *before* they accept a patient for admission. Some facilities adhere to very strict guidelines and do not accept patients with very complicated medical issues. Others provide clinical training to their staff to prepare them to handle the more complex patient. Examples of complex medical care can include tracheotomy care, intubations, total parenteral nutrition (TPN) for patients that are unable to take nutrition through the mouth (trained family members can perform this procedure in the home.) Sometimes, a combination of medical care needs creates eligibility for medical coverage in a skilled nursing facility. As Medicare requirements are changing and becoming stricter, it is important to work with a healthcare professional when applying for skilled care.

Admission Requirements in a Skilled Nursing Facility

"A man is not old until regrets take the place of dreams."

-- *John Barrymore*

To receive care in a nursing home with original Medicare Part A coverage, you must meet all of these eligibility requirements. In addition, the skilled nursing facility must participate in the federally managed Medicare program.

1) **The physician must admit you to the hospital as a full inpatient admission for at least three overnights**, not counting the day of discharge. *Please note: If your physician admits you as an outpatient and your admission status changes to an inpatient, the outpatient days do <u>not</u> count as full regular admission days.* If you are undecided about receiving care in a skilled nursing facility, under Medicare, you have thirty days from the time of discharge, after a three-night inpatient stay at the hospital, to receive care at a skilled nursing facility. For example, if you discharged more than thirty days before, you would need readmission to the hospital for a three-overnight stay before you can use the skilled nursing care benefits in a nursing facility. *(Please note: Original Medicare requires the 3-nights inpatient stay, but <u>some Medicare managed plans do not require the three-night inpatient stay. Pre-authorization may be required.)</u>*

2) **Your physician must certify that daily skilled nursing care is required.**

3) **You must require a skilled nursing care or rehabilitation service** that only a skilled nursing facility can provide.

4) **You must require skilled nursing care on a daily basis** for a condition treated or occurring while you were a patient in the hospital.

Levels of Care in a Skilled Nursing Facility

Three basic types of nursing facilities provide medical care, personal care and assistance, and supervision: hospital-based skilled-plus nursing units, community-based skilled nursing facilities, and intermediate care nursing facilities. Each type of facility has specific eligibility requirements, insurance benefits, and admission procedures. This section will outline the levels of care and basic information you should know when considering placement in a skilled nursing facility. The five levels of care are:

1) Skilled-plus care in a hospital-based nursing facility;

2) skilled nursing care in a community-based nursing facility or retirement community –based Medicare-approved healthcare center;

3) intermediate care;

4) terminal care/comfort measures;

5) custodial care.

Hospital-based Skilled-plus Nursing Units and Transitional Care Units (TCU)

Some hospitals maintain a skilled-plus or transitional care unit within the hospital complex. For patients who no longer meet the acute or critical level of care provided by a hospital, but still require a high level of medical care, these units can provide a continuity of medical care within the hospital. In some cases, the patient's medical care needs may exceed the amount of skilled nursing care available at a community or retirement-based skilled nursing facility or health care center.

The primary care physician or hospitalist is instrumental in determining if your medical condition warrants skilled-plus care. The physician may conclude that you require skilled medical care, a high degree of monitoring and medically necessary services and supplies essential to the diagnosis and treatment of your illness or injury. A patient receiving care in a skilled-plus facility must receive at least two types of skilled treatments at least three times daily. You will usually need pre-authorization or approval from the insurance company *before* a transfer to a skilled-plus or transitional care unit. If a designated admission person works on the skilled-plus unit, they may review your medical record to determine if your care needs are appropriate.

Insurance companies review the prescribed treatment, services, and physician recommendations to determine the availability of a different and lower cost mode of medical treatment. Skilled-plus care in a hospital costs less than receiving acute care and inpatient rehabilitation, but more than medical care received in a community or retirement-based skilled nursing facility. As these specialized units are not always available in a hospital, talk with your physician about skilled care within the hospital or within your community.

Appropriate Diagnosis for Treatment in a Skilled-plus/Transitional Care Unit

A skilled-plus care unit may be appropriate if you have a serious or complicated illness. Listed below are a few skilled-plus care diagnoses:

- **infectious diseases** such as AIDS, Hepatitis B, staphococcus infection, active tuberculosis, and other contagious conditions;

- **multiple skilled needs** such as a comatose condition, severe pressure ulcers, contractures, tracheotomy care, tube feedings, intravenous feedings, oxygen and respiratory treatments, and complex sterile dressing changes, and conditions requiring highly technical equipment, such as ventilators;

- **Other diagnoses**, such as stroke, congenital deformity, amputation, major multiple trauma, fractures, brain injury, polyarthritis, and rheumatoid arthritis, and neurological disorders, such as multiple sclerosis, Parkinson's disease, and polyneuropathy.

Advantages and Disadvantages of Skilled-plus Care

The advantages of placing a patient in a hospital-based skilled nursing unit or TCU include:

- a higher level of skilled care;
- an extension of the continuum of medical care begun in the hospital;
- an alternative to comprehensive inpatient rehabilitation units;
- lower cost than a rehabilitation unit;
- access to doctors and emergency care;
- access to x-rays, scans, test procedures, and lab work;
- simple transfer to skilled-plus unit, eliminating need for ambulance transportation;
- a smoother and easier transition for the patient.

The disadvantages of placing a patient in a TCU include:

- higher cost than a skilled nursing facility.

Community-based Skilled Nursing Facilities and Retirement Community–based Healthcare Centers

This type of nursing facility offers several levels of care: skilled nursing care, intermediate care, end-of-life care/comfort care, and custodial care. The medical services considered covered or non-covered may vary in each type of nursing facility. **Covered care*** refers to Medicare, a federal health insurance program for people sixty-five and older and disabled people, that pays for specific skilled medical care ordered by the doctor and provided by the skilled nursing facility. **Skilled nursing care** is medical care that requires the services of skilled health professionals, such as a registered nurse, physical therapist, or speech therapist, to provide necessary medical services and therapies. In addition to Medicare, private insurance policies, Medicaid, and the Veteran's Administration (VA) will also pay for skilled nursing care. **Non-covered care or custodial care** refers to care and services not covered by the Medicare program. Private health insurance policies and the VA do not pay for custodial care in a skilled nursing facility. Medical care and services provided in a skilled nursing facility can include:

- **Skilled observation:** Professional medical staff appraises a person's medical condition to determine his skilled care needs. Short-term Medicare and Medicaid benefits can cover this service.

- **Foley catheter care**: If catheter care is the primary reason for nursing home care, it is a non-covered service. However, if catheter care requires irrigation and considerable medical care due to a diagnosis such as bladder cancer, it may be covered.

- **Wound care/dressing care**: If you require extensive wound care, dressing changes at least three times daily, and the services of a professional registered nurse, it may be covered. As wounds have several stages, the depth, drainage, and skin condition of the wound determines the need for wound care.

- **Decubitus/bedsore care:** Large, deep, and draining bedsores that require the services of a professional registered nurse are covered care. They must be: multiple stage 2 on the trunk of the body, similar to a shallow crater, blister, or abrasion; stage 3, which presents as a deep crater; or stage 4, which shows extensive damage to tissue, muscle, bone, tendons, or joints.

- **Diabetic observation**: For people with unstable diabetic conditions, insulin-dependent and receiving injections, this can be considered a short- term covered service that requires medical supervision.

- **Teaching and administering insulin/diabetic care**: For new diabetics or insulin users, who require medical supervision and instruction, this is a covered service until the family or person is able to perform competently the necessary care. Medicare covers this care only once.

- **Teaching and administering intramuscular and subcutaneous injections:** Conditions that require a skilled professional to administer or teach the individual or family how to administer medication can be a covered or non-covered service. It is necessary to talk with the admissions staff at the nursing home to determine if this is a covered service.

- **Administering intravenous feeding:** This service requires the skills of a professional registered nurse and is a covered service.

- **Teaching ostomy/ileostomy care:** For people who have new or complex ostomies, teaching and care is considered a covered service.

- **Teaching/administering tube feedings:** For a person, who requires medical supervision and instruction, this is a covered service until the family or person is able to perform the necessary care competently. Nasogastric tube feedings may receive one hundred days of coverage. New gastro tubes may only receive fourteen days of coverage.

- **Teaching/administering tracheotomy care:** For people requiring medical supervision and instruction, this is a covered service until the family or person is able to perform the necessary care competently. Daily suctioning must also be required.

- **Teaching and administering respiratory/inhalation treatment:** For people with an unstable respiratory condition that requires medical supervision and teaching or high oxygen needs, this is a covered service until the family or person is able to perform the necessary care competently. Medical nebulizer treatments needed four times daily may also be covered. Non-covered care includes patients with chronic respiratory problems, such as emphysema. They can receive treatments at home with the assistance of a home healthcare agency.

- **End-of-life Care:** If you have 6 months or less to live, you can receive hospice care from a certified hospice program while receiving end-of-life care in a skilled nursing facility. However, be aware that Medicare Part A does _not_ cover room and board for hospice care in a skilled nursing facility. *Comfort care* (also called palliative care) places emphasis on the relief of symptoms and pain control, and only covers a limited number of days. It is not considered a skilled service. If you have a skilled need that is unrelated to a terminal diagnosis, Medicare may pay for this skilled care. Medicaid may pay for hospice care in a skilled nursing facility. Be aware that Medicaid benefits differ in each state. *(See section on Hospice Care.)*

- **Insert/maintain feeding tube / gastrostomy tube:** For people requiring medical supervision and teaching, this is a covered service until the family or person is able to perform the necessary care competently.

- **Suctioning care/teaching:** For people, who require medical supervision and teaching, this is a covered service until the family or person is able to perform the necessary care competently.

- **Ventilator support:** Although this is a covered service, it can be difficult to find a facility to provide adequate medical care and support. Hospital case managers and social workers can help you find an appropriate facility.

- **Physical therapy:** This therapy is a covered service for people who are recovering from long-term illnesses that requires some physical restoration. People may have diagnosis including strokes, fractured hips, femurs, amputation, and other specific fractures, some neurological disorders, and multiple traumas and extensive hospitalization resulting in physical deconditioning. Therapists work to increase your mobility, decrease your fall risk, general strengthening, and improve your ability to transfer safely from a bed to a chair. You must receive physical therapy on a daily basis five times per week.

---

1. *Remember to stretch before exercise. Three times for 30 seconds will help prepare for exercise.*

2. *Exercise will help to slow the aging process. We can become more fit by regular exercise. I plan to exercise 7 days a week. You don't have to plan for time off. It will happen if the goal is 7 days a week, then you will be sure to get more sessions in.*

3. *Our bodies are adaptable but you should start out gradually to prevent injury. The process is slow but you will improve your functional ability with a commitment to regular activity. Functional activity translates into more time-spent doing things that you like to do.*

4. Be smart and listen to your body. If you are sore after an exercise, you may be doing it wrong or doing it with too much intensity.

-- Todd, MPT, Hospital Physical Therapist

- **Deferred therapy**: To receive coverage for deferred therapy, you should be unable to bear weight on your legs or torso for six weeks. After receiving three to five days of covered Medicare benefits for physical therapy, the nursing facility may move you to an intermediate care unit with room and board through private pay. Therapy would continue with coverage at 80 percent under Medicare Part B. After six weeks, you may move back to the skilled care unit with Medicare benefits for physical therapy. The 30-day rule for Medicare benefits for skilled nursing care after hospitalization is exempt as long as your physician writes orders for *"deferred therapy related to weight-bearing status."*

- **Restorative therapy:** If you require therapy for less than twenty days that utilizes a skilled therapist, Medicare covers the therapies. When a rehabilitation aide provides restorative therapy, Medicare HMOs and managed-care policies may not cover this therapy. The *restorative aide program* is not chargeable to Medicare or reimbursable through private pay.

- **Occupational therapy**: This treatment is a non-covered service unless your physician orders other specific therapies. When used in collaboration with physical therapy, a skilled service, it is usually covered.

- **Speech and language therapy**: This therapy is a covered service when skilled medical care and supervision are required.

- **Social work and case management services**: The social workers in nursing homes provide an invaluable service by helping families understand insurance requirements, providing counseling, arranging transportation to home, ordering necessary durable medical equipment, making referrals for assistance to community and home healthcare agencies, and helping you set up in-home services when you are discharged. This non-covered service is usually provided free of charge.

Please note: Some Medicare managed-care programs may not pay for care usually covered under original Medicare. In addition, Medicaid, a joint federal and state regulated program for people with low-incomes and limited assets, sometimes pays for medical care considered non-covered by Medicare. As the Affordable Care Act progresses, expect additional changes in Medicare policies.

Getting Admitted to a Skilled Nursing Facility

"A healthy attitude is contagious but don't wait to catch it from others. Be a carrier."

–Tom Stoppard

When you decide to transfer to a nursing home, the hospital case manager, discharge planner or social worker acts as a liaison between you, the hospital, and the nursing facilities admissions office. She will review your medical care needs, insurance information, and fax relevant sections of your medical record to the skilled nursing facility, fax relevant medical information, ensure physician follow-up care, arrange wheelchair or gurney transportation, and prepare you and your family for the nursing home transfer.

You or a designated family member will meet with an admissions coordinator or social worker at the skilled nursing facility and complete an admissions contract and personal information sheet. Bring your insurance cards and any pertinent financial information. Make copies of the following information. <u>Never give the original unless directed to do so</u>. This information may include:

- Medicare card;
- Medicaid card;
- other insurance cards;
- living will;
- advanced directives;
- POLST (Physician Order for Life Sustaining Treatment);
- power of attorney for healthcare decisions;
- power of attorney or guardianship papers;
- name, address, and phone number for your primary-care physician;

- emergency contact information;
- list of medications.

The nursing facility needs to know the name of the physician responsible for following your medical care, writing orders and prescriptions. This physician needs privileges at the nursing home to provide this care. If your primary care or hospital physician does not have privileges at the nursing home, your doctor will need to contact a physician who has privileges at the facility, the designated medical doctor or the medical director of the nursing home. It is important to remember that specialists such as cardiologists, pulmonologists, and surgeons, usually do not visit and provide medical care to a patient transferred from a hospital to a nursing facility. They may continue to see you in their office.

Many people stay in a skilled nursing facility for a short time while they receive skilled nursing care and therapies. They expect to complete their rehabilitation and then return home or to their previous living situation. However, sometimes, a person needs a longer stay or long-term care. The goal of long-term care is not to cure an illness, but to support and care for a person with a chronic ailment, illness, or trauma with their daily activities of life. An intermediate care facility, assisted living, adult care home, or family, friends, and hired caregivers, can provide long-term care with support from home and community-based programs.

SkilledNursingFacilities.org provides ratings, information, articles, and blogs on 15,100 United States nursing facilities. Go to http://www.skillednursingfacilities.org/blog/life-in-nursing-homes/federal-regulations-nursing-homes/

Licensing in a Skilled Nursing Facility

The *Healthcare Financing Administration* certifies approximately sixteen thousand nursing homes that receive Medicare and Medicaid funds. The state survey or inspection report, published every twelve to fifteen months and based on unannounced visits to the nursing facility describe patient care, safety, health, quality of life, incident reports, and the list deficiencies in the last state survey The report should be displayed or available upon request for your family to read. If the nursing home is reluctant to show this report, contact the local state ombudsmen program.

Long-term Care Ombudsman Programs

An ombudsman is a volunteer or a person hired by the state to advocate and investigate complaints filed by a nursing home resident or by a concerned family member, friend, or visitor on behalf of a nursing-home resident. *An ombudsman is not a legal representative.*

Established by the Older Americans Act in 1975, the state requires that ombudsmen regularly visit nursing facilities, talk with residents, investigate complaints, and gather information. They keep records of the initial complaints and results of the investigation. Although ombudsmen cannot recommend a nursing facility to you, they can provide your family with helpful information. Look for posted information on the ombudsman program near an exit or elevator.

For a listing of **State Ombudsman Programs**, access to a National Nursing Home Guide, rating reports, and resident rights, go to http://www. iqnursinghomes.com/

Insurance Benefits for Skilled Nursing Care

(Original Medicare, Managed Medicare Policies, Medicare Supplemental Insurance, Medigap policies, Medicaid, Private Pay)

In the past, there was one type of Medicare plan. Now a person may select their Medicare program from many options. In addition to the original Medicare program, you can sign up for Medicare through a managed-care program. This section will discuss some of the differences between original Medicare and Medicare managed-care programs.

Original Medicare Benefits in a Skilled Nursing Facility

In the past, most people age 65 and older, or younger than age 65 receiving Social Security Disability, dialysis, or in need of a kidney transplant, received Medicare benefits. There was only one Medicare program. Now, insurance companies offer Medicare managed-care programs that differ from original Medicare. Under original Medicare, *you must stay three overnights as an inpatient in a hospital before you can receive Medicare benefits for treatment in a skilled nursing facility.* Or, if you recently discharged from a hospital stay of three nights or more, you have 30 days to enter a skilled nursing facility and receive original Medicare benefits for your skilled care needs. If you meet the original Medicare requirements for skilled nursing care in 2014, you will receive the following coverage

- original Medicare covers the costs for the first 20 days in the skilled nursing facility at 100 percent;

- original Medicare covers the next 80 days in the skilled nursing facility except for a daily co-insurance of $152 for days 21–100. *(Please note: This co-insurance changes every year.)*;

- After 100 days, you are responsible for all costs. Some long-term care insurance policies provide additional skilled nursing facility benefits, extending the coverage beyond.

If there is a change in your medical condition during your stay in the skilled nursing facility and you no longer meet the requirements for skilled nursing care, further Medicare benefits may cease, and not cover the remainder of your nursing home stay.

If you are receiving medical care in a skilled nursing facility, and it is determined that you require hospitalization, the facility must keep your bed as long as Medicare pays for the bed. You must let the nursing facility know that you plan to return to the nursing facility after your hospitalization. Often, a hospital social worker or case manager will contact the nursing facility to provide medical updates, enabling it to anticipate a readmission date. If the nursing facility is unable to hold your bed, the hospital social worker/discharge planner will help you find another skilled facility.

Medicare Advantage / Managed-care / HMO's

A managed-care policy differs from original Medicare benefits. Some Medicare Advantage managed-care programs do *not* require an inpatient hospital stay of three inpatient over-nights as required by original Medicare. As Medicare managed-care programs require pre-authorization, prior to your admission to a skilled nursing facility, the hospital case managers or discharge planners (or a person designated to obtain pre-authorizations) may need to contact the managed-care program and share your medical information to receive approval for treatment. A managed-care case manager will review and evaluate your medical needs to determine if you are eligible for skilled nursing care, and, if approved, will authorize your stay. As each Managed-care program is different, it is important to review your policy if you are considering care in a skilled nursing facility.

Medicare Supplemental Insurance

(also called Medigap insurance)

A private Medicare supplemental insurance or Medigap policy complements original Medicare benefits by covering the "gap" between expenses not covered or partially covered by original Medicare. It can help pay for deductibles and co-insurances not covered by original Medicare. A deductible is the amount you must pay before Medicare begins to pay for covered services. Co-insurance is the Medicare- approved amount you are responsible to pay for services.

Each Medigap policy provides different benefits, so it is important to look at your insurance policy or contact your insurance agent or program to determine your supplemental benefits. Be aware that Medigap policies are *not* compatible with private Medicare Advantage managed-care policies.

In a skilled nursing facility, these Medigap policies may pay the daily co-insurance (days 21-100) if you meet the Medicare eligibility requirements for benefits. Or some policies may pay a specific amount on admission to the nursing facility and/or a percentage of the charges not covered by Medicare.

For example, in 2014, the daily co-insurance after twenty days in a skilled nursing facility is $152 per day. Under original Medicare, you would be responsible for paying this amount effective Day 21, or a Medigap policy could pay the daily co-insurance as long as you continue to meet Medicare requirements for skilled nursing care.

Medicaid Benefits

Designed for people who are elderly or disabled and have low-income and limited assets, the Medicaid program differs state to state, with different requirements for financial eligibility and medical care. To determine if, according to state guidelines, you qualify for Medicaid benefits in a skilled nursing facility, it is necessary to contact the local *State Area Agency on Aging or Disabled Services.* They can direct you to the nearest office for assistance completing a Medicaid application. Or if you are in a hospital or skilled nursing facility, the social workers, case managers, or discharge planners can help you contact the appropriate department or agency to complete an application.

To receive Medicaid benefits, the nursing facility must participate in the Medicaid plan. A good nursing facility will talk with your family about Medicaid *before* you face financial difficulties and will accept the Medicaid payments when it becomes necessary. It is important to note that since Medicaid pays a much lower reimbursement rate to the nursing facility, some nursing homes are reluctant to accept Medicaid patients or have long waiting lists for Medicaid patients. *(Please note: Each state has its own Medicaid program and eligibility and benefits will vary from state-to-state.)*

Private Pay Costs

You can pay privately for care in a skilled nursing facility if you have used up your Medicare and supplemental insurance benefits and do not financially qualify for Medicaid benefits. The national average daily cost per person for care in a skilled nursing facility is about $200 per day and the average monthly cost is about $6,083, based on double room occupancy. The costs of care will differ state-by-state and even within the same city, depending upon a variety of reasons that may include:

- the cost of living in the state. States with a higher cost of living may charge more than states with a lower cost of living;

- costs related to staffing at the skilled nursing facility;

- costs dependent on the type of services received i.e. a private room will cost more than a shared room;

- costs related to your daily care such as nursing care, prescription medication management, meals and special diets, phone services, laundry services, and equipment and supplies.

SkilledNursingFacilities.org provides detailed information. Go to http://www.skillednursingfacilities.org/articles/nursing-home-costs. php

When a resident depletes their financial resources, they may become eligible for long-term care under the state Medicaid program. Again, be sure the nursing home accepts Medicaid and will help you pursue eligibility for the Medicaid program when your funds are exhausted.

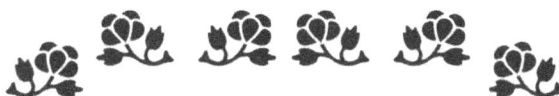

Long-term Care Insurance

These policies sometimes provide additional skilled nursing facility benefits. In addition, they may provide benefits for lower levels of nursing home care, such as intermediate care, care in an assisted living facility, an adult day care center, or care in a private home. Purchasing long-term care insurance when you are older and have pre-existing medical problems can be expensive. Many policies are offered so it is best to research them carefully before you decide which one to purchase.

Veteran Benefits

"The secret of health for both mind and body is not to mourn for the past, not to worry about the future, or not to anticipate troubles, but to live the present moment wisely and earnestly."

-- Siddhartha Gautama Buddha

For skilled nursing care services, the Veteran's Administration may use fee-basis, a fixed charge for a single event, or contract out to pay for a veteran's care in a skilled nursing facility. To be eligible for care in a skilled nursing facility:

- **You must have a service-connected disability.** This means that you are receiving money or healthcare services at a Veteran facility for an injury sustained while in the military service. You should be receiving compensation for this injury since discharge from the service. The greater percentage of service connection (50% or higher), the more Veteran's benefits are available. Occasionally a veteran with a non-service connected disability can receive services.

- **You must receive pre-authorization from the Veteran's Affairs Office to receive benefits**.

To verify you are receiving your entire **Veteran benefits**, contact your nearest Veteran Affairs Office or call the **VA National Computer Base** at 1-800-827-1000.

Worker's Compensation Programs (WC)

Each state runs its own program and may have different allowable amounts of compensation and services. If you have recently applied for WC because of a work-related injury, it is necessary to contact your local claim office regarding skilled nursing facility benefits. Contact the personnel office at your place of employment.

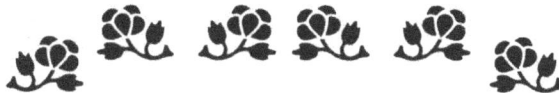

SUMMARY OF INSURANCE COVERAGE and BENEFITS IN A SKILLED NURSING FACILITY, 2013

	SKILLED-PLUS CARE	SKILLED NURS-ING CARE	INTERMEDIATE CARE	CUSTODIAL CARE	END-OF-LIFE CARE
HOSPITAL-BASED	X				X
COMMUNITY-BASED		X	X	X	X
ORIGIANL MEDI-CARE You must meet Medicare require-ments for care	Medicare Part A pays 100 % for 20 days. Pays 80% for 80 days. You pay $152 co-insurance per day	Medicare Part A pays 100 % for 20 days. Pays 80% for 80 days. You pay $152 co-insurance per day	X	X	May pay for end-of-life care depending on care needs
MEDICAID Federal and state program for persons with low-income and assets	Must be Medic-aid recipient to receive benefits. Payment var-ies from state to state.	Must be Medic-aid recipient to receive benefits. Payment var-ies from state to state.	Must be Medic-aid recipient to receive benefits. Payment var-ies from state to state.	Does not pay for custodial care, but Area Agency on Aging may be able to provide free or low cost services in other setting.	Must be Medic-aid recipient to receive benefits. Payment var-ies from state to state.
MEDICARE SUPPLEMENTAL	May provide ad-ditional benefits	May provide ad-ditional benefits	Does not pay for intermediate care	Does not pay for intermediate care	May pay for end-of-life care
MANAGED-CARE/ HMO'S	Eligibility and benefits deter-mined by insur-ance program. Pre-auth may be required.	Covers skilled care based on its guidelines; may override original Medicare benefits if it is your pri-mary insurance	Does not pay for intermediate care	Does not pay for custodial care	May have stricter eligibility guidelines than original Medicare. May not pay for end-of-life care. Check individual policy.
LONG-TERM CARE INSUR-ANCE	May pay for care after Medicare benefits have been exhausted.	May pay for care after Medicare benefits have been exhausted.	May pay for some intermediate care services	May pay for limited custodial care in the home, adult care home, or assisted living facility.	May pay for limited end-of-life care.
VETERANS AF-FAIRS Must meet eligi-bility guidelines for VA	Federally regu-lated. May pay all costs if approved by the VA. Check with the VA re-garding benefits.	Federally regu-lated. May pay all costs if approved by the VA. Check with the VA re-garding benefits.	Federally regu-lated. May pay all costs if approved by the VA.	Does not pay for custodial care but may help with supportive services	May pay for limited end-of-life care.
PRIVATE PAY	If you have no insurance or don't meet the requirements for skilled-nursing care, you may be able to private pay.	If you have no insurance or don't meet skilled nurs-ing rules, you may be able to private pay.	You may private pay for this care	You may private pay for this care	You may private pay for end-of life care

Intermediate Care Nursing Facilities

"Intermediate care facility" means a facility that provides, on a regular basis, health-related care and services to individuals who do not require the degree of care and treatment that a hospital or skilled nursing facility is designed to provide, but who because of their mental or physical condition require care and services above the level of room and board that can be made available to them only through institutional facilities." -- Source: Oregon Legislature

When a resident at a skilled nursing facility receives skilled nursing care and therapies, they retain the potential for reasonable improvement in their condition. Those receiving intermediate care do not possess rehabilitation potential. On the continuum of care, intermediate care falls between care provided by a skilled nursing facility and an assisted living facility or adult care home. It is an excellent alternative for people with senile dementia, Alzheimer's disease, mental health challenges, or psychological conditions. A licensed nursing facility staffed with registered and licensed practical nurses and certified nurse's aides can provide intermediate care to residents.

State licensed intermediate-care facilities provide routine nursing care to people requiring medical supervision and assistance with the daily activities of living, such as bathing, dressing, grooming, toileting, and personal care. Residents may have difficulty with transfers, getting in and out of bed or a chair. Or they may be confused and disoriented, unable to remember who they are, where they are, or the time of day. They may not recognize close family members and friends. Because of safety issues, this confusion may lead to a need for 24-hour supervision. There may be additional fees for physical and occupational therapies and an activities program. Be aware that some facilities may hesitate to accept a patient with behavior or severe cognitive problems if they place other patients or staff at-risk.

Intermediate care services in a skilled nursing facility are one of the lower levels of care. Not covered by Medicare, some states will provide Medicaid benefits to pay for intermediate care. The facility nursing staff can provide the following non-skilled nursing care:

- routine foley catheter care and incontinence issues;
- medication management, excluding IVs and insulin injections;
- physical therapy three times weekly;
- occupational therapy three times weekly;
- general skin care, simple dressing changes;

- assistance with feeding at mealtimes;

- basic oxygen / respiratory care;

- behavioral issues;

- assistance with the activities of daily living, including personal hygiene, bathing, grooming, and dressing.

Original and managed-care Medicare and private insurance policies do *not* pay for intermediate care. Each state determines its Medicaid benefits and may provide coverage for intermediate care, a lower level of care than skilled care.

Custodial Care

Custodial care is general care and assistance for the activities of daily living, such as eating, dressing, bathing, grooming, and personal hygiene, as well as supervision that prevents personal harm. This is not medically necessary care as an unskilled person can provide this assistance. Medicare benefits and private insurance companies do not cover this care. The United States Department of Veteran Affairs may have special programs that provide custodial care to veterans living in the community. Medicaid and some long-term care insurance policies provide limited benefits for this care.

When a nursing facility provides custodial care, it is considered a private pay service. People with Alzheimer's disease who display mental confusion and disorientation, wander, and require 24-hour supervision are considered candidates for custodial care. Some nursing facilities have a secure locked Alzheimer's unit designed to ensure safety by preventing afflicted residents from wandering or inadvertently injuring themselves. Medicare and private insurances do not pay for this care.

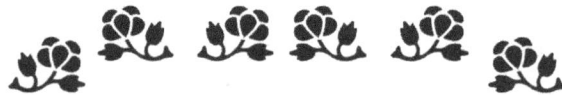

What to Bring To a Skilled Nursing Facility

Each nursing facility has a list of items to bring with at the time of admission. Use this checklist to guide you in packing:

- ➤ 4 changes of clothing for day and night;
- ➤ non-skid washable slippers or slip-on shoes;
- ➤ one-week supply of socks and underwear;
- ➤ bathrobe;

- ➤ one to two sweaters / light jacket / sweatshirt;
- ➤ personal toiletries;
- ➤ a touch of home such as a favorite photograph.

Hints:

- Sweatshirts and sweatpants with an elastic band are easy to pull on and take off. They do not have zippers or buttons are very comfortable.

- Bring permanent press clothing, as nursing facilities usually do not iron clothing.

- Do not bring delicate fabrics or favorite clothing as items can be lost or damaged.

- Family can choose to do personal laundry instead of using the laundry service available at the nursing facility.

- Mark your name on clothing and personal items with a permanent marker or label.

- Check with the nursing facility to see if they allow you to bring incontinence diapers (depends) or other medical supplies. It is often less expensive to have family provide these items.

Questions To Ask at a Skilled Nursing Facility

Visit several nursing facilities before making a decision. Bring a friend with whom you can share your impressions. Every person will notice different details about the facility. Trust your instincts even if you are unable to pinpoint why you feel the way you do.

You can visit a nursing facility anytime you wish during regular working hours, usually 8 a.m. to 5 p.m. If you are interested in speaking with the admissions coordinator or a social worker, call in advance to set up an appointment. If you are interested only in visiting the facility, drop in and ask for a tour. Most facilities should be able to accommodate you. Use this questionnaire to keep track of your observations and responses to your questions. The following nursing home checklist will help you evaluate the nursing facilities you visit. When you walk into a nursing facility, look at the general appearance of the residence.

Outside Area

- Do the grounds look well maintained?
- Are the walkways paved?
- Is the residence taller than one story?
- Are there ramps along the curb for easy wheelchair access?

Inside Area

- Do you detect an odor in the nursing facility?
- Does the nursing facility seem clean?
- Is the nursing facility equipped with air-conditioning?
- Do you see a security guard stationed inside the door?
- Does the lobby area seem empty or do you see residents sitting around?
- Are the hallways wide enough to accommodate a walker or a wheelchair?
- Are the hallways equipped with handrails?
- Are elevators easy to access?
- Does the facility allow smoking?
- Is there a designated smoking area?

- Can you easily access a public telephone or does your room include a private telephone? Is there an extra charge for a room telephone?

- Are fire exits clearly marked and easily accessible?

- Can you easily access a mailbox and purchase postage stamps?

- Does the atmosphere seem formal or informal?

- What is the policy regarding standard/non-standard visiting hours?

Watch for:

➤ bad odor;

➤ safety hazards;

➤ residents who are not dressed or groomed residents who remain in their rooms;

➤ residents who are restrained or tied in chairs *(The law strictly limits the use of restraints, especially for convenience of nursing staff.)*

Rooms

- Are private rooms available?

- How many residents can reside in a room?

- Will you need to share a room?

- Will you be paired with a compatible roommate? *(This is an important question. If you are alert and oriented, you do not want to share a room with a confused or disruptive patient. You do not want to share a room with a patient with an infectious disease.)*

- Can residents provide their own furnishings?

- Are rooms equipped with handicap features such as emergency call buttons and grab bars in the bathroom?

- Does each bed include a privacy curtain?

- Does each room include a window or view?

- Does the facility allow pets to visit or stay with residents?

- Does the facility policy specify who can/cannot visit, such as small children?

Nursing Care

- What levels of care are available in the nursing facility?
  - ➢ skilled nursing care
  - ➢ intermediate care
  - ➢ end-of-life care
  - ➢ custodial care

- What therapies are available to residents?
  - ➢ physical therapy
  - ➢ occupational therapy
  - ➢ speech therapy
  - ➢ respiratory therapy
  - ➢ wound care therapy
  - ➢ other_____

- Does the facility allow residents to self-administer their own medication?

- Is medication management available to resident who have difficulty taking their correct medication at the proper time of day?

- Does the facility have a policy for re-filling prescriptions? *(The state can require that a pharmacist prepare all medications in individual doses and place them in a bubble pack. Self-medication must be kept in a locked box or secure area.)* Are prescriptions refilled:
  - ➢ on the premises
  - ➢ by a local pharmacy
  - ➢ by a mail order pharmacy
  - ➢ by family

- Do staff members maintain health and medication records for each resident?

- If a resident experiences a change in health, is staff available to provide additional assistance?

- Is staff available to help with the activities of daily living, such as bathing, grooming, personal hygiene, feeding at mealtimes, housekeeping, laundry, transfers, and mobility?

- Can a resident hire a private-duty caregiver to provide additional care?

- Does staff encourage family involvement?

- Can family supply medical supplies, such as incontinence diapers?

Nursing Home Staff

- Do staff members act in a professional manner? Can they answer your questions?

- How does the staff determine each resident's care needs?

- What is the resident-to-staff ratio?

- How many registered nurses are on duty during each shift?

- Does the facility maintain a care plan for each resident?

- Does staff help coordinate services with community agencies, such as home healthcare and medical-equipment companies at time of discharge?

- Do you feel comfortable with the staff?

- Is there a house physician on the facility's staff?

- How often does the physician visit the facility?

- Can your primary care physician continue to provide medical treatments to you in the nursing facility?

- Is there a private place in the facility for exams by your physician?

Staff should be:

- affectionate;
- cheerful;
- pleasant;
- courteous;
- respectful;
- warm;
- encouraging;
- helpful;
- honest;
- responsive to calls for assistance.

Watch for:

- disgruntled staff;
- excessive complaining by staff;
- yelling at residents;
- excessive time before staff responds to call light;

> ➤ impatient staff;

> ➤ bad attitude displayed by staff.

Activities

- Does the facility staff include an activities director?

- Is there a posted schedule of activities?

- Are activities: flexible ___ required ___structured ___ optional___

- Are religious services observed at:
  the facility___ a local church___ synagogue___ mosque____

- Are community volunteers active at the facility?

- Does the nursing facility provide a library?

- Is there a beautician or barber who visits regularly?

- Is there a massage therapist who visits regularly?

Watch for:

- no scheduled activities;

- a very part-time activities director;

- residents sitting around with nothing to do.

Transportation

- Does the facility own a wheelchair van?

- Does the facility provide transportation to medical appointments?

- Is there a small fee for transportation services?

Cost

- What services are included in the monthly fee?

- What services are not included in the monthly fee?

- Are there any hidden fees?

- If the medical care needs of a patient change, does this affect the monthly fee?

- If a resident changes his level of care or decides to leave the facility, what is the refund policy? Does the facility accept Medicaid payments? *(This is an important question. Some facilities do not accept Medicaid. Others accept Medicaid payments but may be reluctant to accept their low reimbursement rate. They may have a lengthy waiting list for accepting new Medicaid residents.)*

- What is the policy regarding residents if their funds run out? *(This is an important question. Some facilities may discharge or evict a resident unable to pay for care. Others may try to work closely with you to prepare for reduced funds. Look for a facility that will help you apply for Medicaid and financial assistance through a state agency.)*

- Will the facility help a resident apply for Medicaid?

- Does the facility accept long-term-care health insurance?

Nursing Home Resident Bill of Rights.

Federal regulations require all nursing facilities to have written policies describing the rights of nursing home residents. The nursing home must list and give all new residents a copy of these rights. Resident rights include (but are not limited to):

- Respect: You have the right to be treated with dignity and respect.

- Services and Fees: You must be informed in writing about services and fees before you enter the nursing home.

- Money: You have the right to manage your own money or to choose someone else you trust to do this for you.

- Privacy: You have the right to privacy, and to keep and use your personal belongings and property as long as it doesn't interfere with the rights, health, or safety of others.

- Medical Care: You have the right to be informed about your medical condition, medications, and to see you own doctor. You also have the right to refuse medications and treatments. -- Medicare.gov

---

Rehabilitation Programs

"The goal of the rehabilitation program is "to restore the rights, authority, dignity and former capacity "to an individual by using the skills of an interdisciplinary team of physicians, healthcare professionals, therapists, family, friends, and community."

-- Western Unabridged Dictionary

Most people take for granted that they will be able to get up in the morning, brush and floss their teeth, brush and comb their hair, shave, button their shirt, tie their shoes, and put on a skirt or a pair of pants. They assume they will be able to prepare breakfast, set the kitchen table, and eat their meal with a fork and knife. After breakfast, they may expect to walk, bike, or drive a car to work, run errands, exercise, or cook dinner and clean their house. When an unexpected medical event or crisis occurs, an accident, injury, or a severe illness, it can quickly turn a person's life upside down. It can affect their ability to perform these normal, everyday activities and may dramatically change their life and the lives of their family and friends. Independence can rapidly give way to partial or complete dependence on others. The future, once clear, may now seem confusing and frightening.

Each individual enters a rehabilitation program for similar reasons: their ability to function, that is, to think, perceive, feel, cope, move, behave, or manage in their daily life, has dramatically changed. Each person may experience unfamiliar and unsettling emotions that affect their ability to reason and to make rational decisions. New physical limitations can occur. Control of movement in arms, legs, and upper body and bodily functions, including bowel and bladder control may be compromised or lost. Activities once taken for granted may become difficult or impossible to perform. However, with comprehensive rehabilitation, training, and education, a person can relearn living skills and develop new skills to help adapt.

When You Need a Rehabilitation Program

Treatment in a rehabilitation program can benefit many medical conditions and can begin at any point on the continuum of care. This means you can enter a rehabilitation program:

- during or following an acute care hospitalization when you are medically stable;

- from a sub-acute or skilled nursing facility;
- from home.

You may benefit from a rehabilitation program if:

- you are experiencing difficulty with mobility and balance or recognize deterioration in your physical abilities;
- you are experiencing increased difficulty thinking rationally and making decisions, or are suffer from significant memory impairment. To participate in the program, you must be able to follow some directions and commands;
- you display impaired learning, but retain the ability and potential to learn;
- you area affected by neurological complications or cognitive deficiencies that could benefit from constant and consistent intervention;
- you are recovering from a recent illness, accident, injury, or debilitating chronic illness;
- you experience difficulty maintaining adequate nutrition as a result of difficulty swallowing;
- you experience difficulty functioning with the activities of daily life due to a significant nerve or sensory loss;
- you are at-risk at home and may need home safety modifications that require an evaluation and the expertise of skilled rehabilitation staff;
- you are at-risk of being placed in an institution or other setting;
- you suffer from complicated lower or upper extremity orthotics needs;
- you require nursing care needs at a higher level of care than can be provided in a sub-acute setting;
- you have daily physiatry (non-surgical treatment of pain or disability) needs;
- you exhibit low endurance for physical activity or are severely deconditioned (*You may be referred to a skilled nursing facility to build up your strength before being admitted to a rehabilitation program.*)

Some of the diagnoses eligible for treatment in a rehabilitation program include:

- cerebrovascular accident or stroke;
- major multiple traumas;
- debilitating arthritis;
- spinal cord injury;
- neurological conditions;
- congenital or hereditary deformities;
- severe orthopedic conditions;
- brain injury or trauma;
- chronic illnesses such as multiple sclerosis;
- Parkinson's disease;
- cognitive or mental changes;
- amputation or loss of a limb;
- Amyotrophic lateral sclerosis; (ALS or Lou Gehrig's disease);
- Huntington's chorea.

What Your Family Should Know about Rehabilitation Programs

Because most people who need rehabilitation are already in a hospital, sub-acute, or skilled nursing setting or have lived with a chronic illness, the transition to a rehabilitation program should be smooth. If you are living at home but experiencing increasing difficulty managing everyday activities, make an appointment with your physician to discuss the feasibility of admission to an inpatient or outpatient rehabilitation program to improve your life skills and ability to function.

To gather the information necessary to make an informed decision about rehabilitation programs, it is important for you to talk with your physician, therapists, and a medical social worker or case manager. These healthcare professionals can begin the process needed to determine if admission to a rehabilitation program is appropriate. They can also verify insurance information and review the benefits for inpatient or outpatient rehabilitation, home health nursing care, durable medical equipment, and more. The more information you can gather about available rehabilitation programs, the clearer the guidelines for admission will be. Here are some considerations:

- Does your current medical condition or event justify care or treatment in a rehabilitation program?
- What are your doctor's treatment recommendations?

- To what extent does the rehabilitation program include family involvement?
- What types of rehabilitation centers are located near you?
- What are the eligibility requirements for admission to the rehabilitation program?
- What are the specific insurance benefits for treatment in a rehabilitation program?

Choosing a Rehabilitation Program

"Your body hears everything your mind says."

-- *Naomi Judd*

To gain optimum benefits from a rehab program, family involvement and participation play an important role. Therefore, it is necessary to consider where the program is located. If you live in a major metropolitan area, you likely can choose from a range of facilities and programs. If you reside in a smaller city or town or a rural area, your options may be more limited. If you require specialized treatment, it may be necessary to travel to another state for a comprehensive rehabilitation program. Your physician, therapists, and case managers are familiar with programs and can assist and guide you to an appropriate program that is geared to your disability and medical care needs. Look for:

- an accredited rehabilitation program;
- a physician familiar with rehabilitation programs;
- a comprehensive program that meets your recovery needs;
- a rehabilitation facility approved as in-network by your insurance company;
- rehabilitation staff members who are compassionate, flexible, and well trained.

The *Joint Commission of Accredited Hospital Organizations (JCAHO)* offers accreditation to rehabilitation programs affiliated with hospitals. In addition, many rehab programs seek accreditation with the *Commission on Accreditation of Rehabilitation Facilities (CARF.)* CARF is a private, nonprofit organization that establishes standards of quality care in rehabilitation facilities. Rehabilitation facilities that seek CARF accreditation must meet these strict standards and guidelines. Programs that receive accreditation earn a certificate of accreditation and are included in the *Directory of Accredited Organizations.*

To find an accredited provider, go to the **Commission on Accreditation of Rehabilitation Facilities** Go to: http://www.carf.org/providersearch.aspx

Joint Commission on Accreditation of Healthcare Organizations (JCAHO): To find accredited and certified health care organizations, go to http://www.jointcommision.org/

Commission on Accreditation of Rehabilitation Facilities (CARF): For additional accreditation information, at http://carf.org/aging/

Preparing for Admission to a Rehabilitation Program

Before you can be admitted to a rehabilitation program, you must:

1) obtain a referral from your primary care physician, a hospitalist, a specialist, neurologist or physiatrist (a physician who specializes in physical medicine and rehabilitation);

2) meet the criteria for admission;

3) review your insurance benefits and, if needed, obtain pre-authorization for treatment *(Before admission to a rehab program, an admissions coordinator may verify your insurance benefits, and if you are accepted to the program, obtain pre-authorization from your insurance company.);*

4) consider and plan a post-rehabilitation discharge arrangement for care *(Social workers and the rehabilitation team will work with your family to make these arrangements.)*

Admission is not black and white; it is flexible and allows for extenuating circumstances. Many programs require active participation of at least 3 hours daily. If you are not able to meet this requirement, some programs will encourage a stay in a skilled nursing facility to build up your endurance before admitting you into the more intensive rehabilitation program. Because participation in a rehab program is more costly than care in a skilled nursing facility, insurance guidelines for admission are growing more stringent, necessitating rehab programs to justify the need for admission to a rehabilitation program rather than a skilled nursing facility.

Getting a Physician Referral

To enter a rehabilitation program, it is necessary to get a referral from a primary care physician, a specialist, or a hospitalist. Or a referral may be made by a neurologist or physiatrist actively involved in treatment, who then recommends admission to a rehabilitation program. A physician-to-physician call with a request for a physiatrist consultation begins the process. When the rehabilitation staff members receive the referral, they may send team therapists to meet you and evaluate your physical and cognitive capabilities. The admitting rehabilitation physician decides if your rehabilitation needs are appropriate for the program and must determine that you can actively participate in the program. Once admitted into the rehabilitation program, the physiatrist or neurologist may become your attending physician. A hospitalist or primary care physician may provide medical care for non-rehabilitation medical issues. Upon discharge from the program, your regular primary care physician may resume responsibility for your basic medical care.

Meeting the Admission Criteria

To enter a rehabilitation program, there must be *a defined rehabilitation need*, that is, not only one medical need, but also a comprehensive group of needs that require the skills of the rehabilitation team and skilled nursing care. You must possess the endurance and tolerance to participate actively in the daily program, sometimes for as long as three hours or more. If you do not have the endurance to participate, sub-acute or skilled nursing care can start you with a less rigorous rehabilitation program. After receiving therapies at a skilled nursing facility, a person can transfer to a more intensive rehabilitation program.

If a rehabilitation program is considered reasonable, necessary, and appropriate for your medical needs, expect an evaluation by the rehabilitation team. This team may consist of a physiatrist, registered nurse, neuropsychologist (or neurologist), physical therapist, occupational therapist, a speech-language (or communication-disorder) therapist, and a medical or rehab social worker.

Prior to admission to the rehabilitation program, the rehabilitation admissions coordinator or intake person will verify your insurance benefits and receive, if necessary, pre-authorization , for your stay. You will also provide personal and medical information. You may need to sign a release of information, which gives the rehabilitation staff permission to access and review your most recent medical transcript - a history and physical, consultations, medications, therapy notes, x-ray and lab reports and other significant information. It is important to have your family bring or make copies of the following information:

- medical and insurance cards;

- copy of Social Security card;

- organ donor card;

- living will*;

- advanced directives*;

- Physician Orders for Life-Sustaining Treatment (POLST)*; power of attorney for healthcare* *(This document allows the staff to know whom to contact for health care decision you may not be able to make.)*;

- a durable power of attorney for finances*;*(This document allows staff to know whom to contact when financial matters need to be addressed.)*

- guardianship papers*;

- other pertinent legal documents*.

- list of current medications and dosages;

This is important: Retain the original documents for your files, and give copies to the admissions office your primary care physician, your attorney, and any involved healthcare facility or community agency.

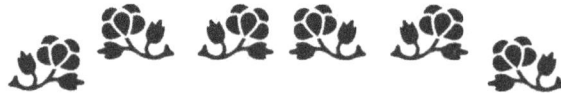

Entering the Rehabilitation Program

"A good life is when you assume nothing, do more, smile often, dream big, laugh a lot, and realize how blessed you are for what you have."

-- Unknown

Once you are admitted to the rehabilitation program, you enter a new environment. Although similar to a hospital in many ways, the treatment program differs from an acute care hospital setting. In a hospital, they emphasize the treatment of an acute medical problem. The nurses do everything for the patient. In a rehabilitation program, the expectation is for you to do as much as you can. Here, the emphasis is on restoration or giving the patient an improved or compensatory level of functioning. The goal is to make you as independent as possible within realistic expectations.

On admission, you will usually meet with a social worker or nurse case manager. She will interview you extensively, asking about medical history and problems, current abilities, family history and support system, family dynamics, the physical living situation, including steps outside and within the home and bathroom accessibility, transportation assistance, the splitting of household chores, vocation and education, interests and activities, finances and insurance, family and patient goals and expectations, and other practical considerations. In addition, she will ask about anticipated problems or other considerations that might affect the discharge plan. Your family is encouraged to play an active role in this discussion.

You will participate in a strenuous therapy program three to six hours daily. Basic activities taken for granted for many years will present new challenges. Walking, standing, sitting, buttoning shirts, tying shoelaces, dressing, grooming, holding utensils, speaking, thinking, reasoning, remembering, visualizing, and comprehension may present difficulties when you begin the program.

A daily schedule of activities, therapies, and appointments will be posted in a general living area or by the door to your room. This enables staff, visitors, and family to plan their day around important therapy sessions and meetings. Although schedules change, usually a brief phone call to the rehabilitation unit can confirm any modifications.

The rehabilitation team shares their patient evaluations and assessments at weekly, biweekly, or bi-monthly case conferences, after which realistic individual goals and a tentative and flexible discharge date, are set. The typical length of a rehabilitation program varies from region to region and program to program. Programs can range from three days to several months with an average length of stay of three to six weeks. Goals and lengths of stay are usually flexible and can change depending on your progress or lack of progress.

Family Involvement

Family involvement, support, and encouragement are instrumental for a successful rehabilitation program. The extent of family involvement will differ with each individual patient. Most families are unfamiliar with the specific objectives and goals of rehabilitation programs. They may not understand that participation in the program does not guarantee full restoration of your previous functioning and quality of life. They may not understand how the medical event or condition affected, and will continue to affect, the physical body, and they may not be aware of the cognitive or psychological changes that can occur.

It is common for patients with new and severe limitations to feel frustrated, discouraged, depressed, helpless, angry, confused, disorganized, or agitated. If these feelings remain during participation in the rehabilitation program, they can directly affect your ability to relearn coping skills, adapt, and adjust to any new limitations. It is important to maintain realistic expectations: You may not completely recover all your lost capabilities. However, any progress you make moves you from dependence on family, caregiver, or community toward increased independence

A positive family interaction will enable you to cope more easily with your disability and encourage you to work harder in the rehabilitation program. The more hopeful and realistic your family is about recovery, the more empowered you will feel. The more your family compliments your progress—even if it is in small steps—the more confident you will feel about your progress.

Your family can be your advocate and intermediary. Family participation in caregiver training and rehabilitation education is essential. The sooner the training begins, the greater the comfort level your family will have providing any necessary help or care.

Programs and Classes

A team of healthcare professionals with a multitude of skills develops your comprehensive treatment plan. The plan provides consistency, continuity, and momentum geared toward helping you progress to a higher level of functioning by the time you are ready for discharge from the program. The rehabilitation staff will work with you on improving your basic life skills, including meal preparation, adaptation skills, community socialization, and activities of daily living (ADL's.)

Each rehabilitation program assigns different names for specific treatment programs. Although these programs and life skills may seem trivial to a healthy person with two functioning arms, two functioning legs, and no cognitive problems, imagine the difficulty a person in a wheelchair may have reaching a countertop, preparing a meal, or using a wall telephone. Imagine shopping for goods that are several feet higher than your reach.

When cognitive, reasoning, and organizational skills are not adequate, how do you make appointments, write a shopping list, manage your finances, or communicate?

After his stroke, Carl entered a rehabilitation program. Although he was able to communicate verbally, he had difficulty performing more than one task at a time. In one of his life skills classes, he helped place postage stamps and a return address sticker on an envelope. To the surprise of his family, Carl experienced difficulty placing the stamp in the upper right hand corner and the return address in the upper left corner. He placed the stamps in many incorrect places on the envelope. Until his family witnessed his inability to multi-task, they were unaware of this cognitive problem. It provided his family with a more realistic insight on Carl's abilities.

- **Meal Preparation** can include planning and preparing a simple or complex nutritious meal, preparing a shopping list, food budgets, and using appropriate assistive or adaptive devices. Meal preparation may involve social interaction skills, organizational and coordination skills, the ability to focus and remain focused on a task, the ability to solve problems, develop an increased awareness of safety issues and strengthen stamina. Practice sessions with an occupational therapist in a kitchen setting in the rehabilitation facility may reinforce the individual's capabilities to perform simple daily tasks.

- **Adaptation Skills** help you relearn and adapt to performing common everyday tasks. There is emphasis placed on improving your range of motion, strength, coordination, balance, and endurance. You will learn how to adjust and compensate despite cognitive, perceptual, or sensory losses, including hearing, seeing, and touching.

- **Community Socialization** programs focus on developing social skills. You may need to learn how to interact appropriately with staff, family, and other patients and behave appropriately in public situations. You will also learn how to rebuild relationships, maintain social boundaries, recognize emotions, and accept and acknowledge physical, emotional, and personal losses. This program may be offered in individual and group settings.

- **Activities of Daily Living** classes focus on relearning basic living skills: doing household chores, preparing meals, dressing, selecting clothes, grooming, toileting, managing simple finances, following a budget, writing a check, and balancing a checkbook. If you are unable to perform some of these tasks, staff can recommend that a family member obtain a power of attorney for finances so they can assist you with your personal finances.

- **Exercise Classes** will help you work on strengthening muscles and improving joint flexibility, endurance, range of motion, and mobility.

- **Pool/Aquatic Classes** utilize water exercises to benefit those unable to stand on their own. It can help increase muscular strength and joint flexibility. Water therapy helps decrease anxiety and defensive, edgy, and excitable behavioral tendencies. Be aware that not all rehabilitation programs have pools on their premises.

- **Pet Therapy classes** may use dogs, cats, birds, and sometimes horses for pet therapy. As you interact with the animals, they strengthen your social skills, increase your endurance and whole body movement, and decrease feelings of depression and isolation. You can develop a sense of responsibility and boost your own senses and orientation to the real world as you provide pet care.

- **Peer Counseling Programs** can arrange for former patients to talk with current patients who are experiencing similar problems. Sometimes talking with someone who has already been through the program helps allay fears and concerns regarding the ability to participate in the program or about your future. For example, a patient who has had a traumatic amputation of his leg may feel hopeless and depressed following surgery. Seeing a former amputee patient walk into his room on two legs, using prosthesis, can give the rehabilitation patient hope and motivation. Peer counselors should participate in a training program before speaking with patients and should respect confidentiality.

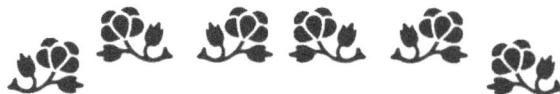

Ed is a 69-year old man who recently had surgery for an infected leg. A below-knee amputation was performed. Ed felt very depressed, showed no motivation in physical or occupational therapies, and lay in his bed, refusing to get dressed or participate in his care or therapy program. He shared that his life was over if he could not walk. With Ed's permission, the medical social worker talked with Pauline, a former patient who had similar surgery two years before and had resumed her normal activities with the help of a leg prosthesis. She asked Pauline if she would be comfortable meeting with Ed to talk about her rehabilitation. When Pauline walked into his room and lifted her pant leg to show Ed her prosthesis, Ed began to talk about his feelings. The next day, Ed participated actively in his therapy sessions, stating that he now felt motivated as he realized he would be able to walk again.

- **Sexuality Classes** offered by the rehabilitation program enable a patient to express concerns and ask questions about this important issue. Following a major accident, injury, or disability, you may want to know: What can I do? What has changed? In many rehabilitation programs, a staff member discusses these vital issues privately with the patient. Group sessions, held with other patients and interested family members, are also used to discuss these matters.

- **Day or Weekend Passes** offered by some rehabilitation programs provide real life challenges within the rehabilitation complex, including a realistic post office or grocery store where you can practice your newly acquired skills. As you near your discharge date, you may be encouraged to use a weekend pass to go home. A home visit with a therapist can improve your confidence and self-esteem as you move toward increased independence. It may highlight specific problem areas and allow therapists and staff to focus on them prior to your discharge date. Most programs require a signed release form prior to the home visit.

A home visit can highlight potential difficulties such as getting into your home, climbing stairs inside your home, preparing meals, and more. If after a home visit you are not sure returning home is the right choice, a social worker or case manager may recommend hiring a caregiver or transitioning to a supervised setting, such as home with a family member, an assisted living facility or an adult foster care home. If a family member, friend, hired caregiver, or adult foster care home caregiver provides in-home care following the rehabilitation program, they will be encouraged to attend caregiver training and actively participate with you and the staff during therapy sessions.

Checking Insurance Benefits

Entering a rehabilitation program without insurance benefits can be expensive, which is why it is important to have your insurance benefits checked *before* you enter a program. Usually, a rehabilitation case manager, an admissions official, or a business office representative contacts the insurance company to verify your eligibility and benefits and obtain pre-authorization from the insurance company.

Rehabilitation benefits may be limited by the number of days (standard is thirty to sixty days, although short-term rehab programs are also offered), a monetary amount, or may have unlimited benefits determined by medical necessity. Medical necessity includes the medical care, services, and supplies essential to the treatment and diagnosis of an illness or injury.

Insurance companies may require pre-authorization and review the physician's prescribed treatment, services, and recommendations. They can recommend different treatment options with lower costs. The insurance company can recommend a preferred provider program or if they do not deem your medical condition as appropriate for an intensive rehab program, recommend a different option, such as receiving rehabilitation in a sub-acute or skilled facility, or through outpatient rehab, or home healthcare therapies.

Private Pay

Many programs charge more than one thousand dollars per day, which may include all therapies. Regardless of the method of payment, you must still meet all the criteria for admission to participate in the program. Pre-authorization may be needed. If you are considering private pay in a rehabilitation facility, talk with a financial counselor regarding the potential costs.

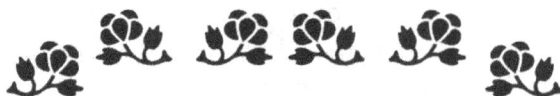

Original Medicare Parts A and B in a Rehabilitation Program

Treatment in an inpatient rehabilitation program falls under original Medicare Part A hospital benefits. A three-day inpatient hospital stay is not required prior to receiving rehabilitation services. If you meet all the admission criteria, in each benefit period, original Medicare Part A up to 100-days of rehabilitation at 100%. An admissions person should confirm your benefits before you are admitted to the program.

Outpatient rehabilitation therapies provided in a hospital fall under original Medicare Part B. Medicare Part B pays 80 percent of the approved amount after a patient pays the one-time annual deductible. *(Please note: Medicare eligibility and benefits may change under the Affordable Care Act.)*

Medicare Managed-care and HMO Programs

Many Medicare HMOs and managed-care programs maintain contracts with the rehabilitation facility and may consider them as in-network preferred providers. Or they may be willing to negotiate a rate with a facility that is out-of-network. As the cost for treatment in a rehabilitation program is more costly than care in a sub-acute skilled nursing facility, many managed-care programs may prefer to authorize more cost effective treatment in a sub-acute facility. Some policies require rehabilitation to start within a period of two consecutive calendar months per episode of care. Different illnesses or medical conditions can justify an additional 2-month benefit period. This benefit renews each calendar year.

Often managed-care programs require pre-authorization prior to admission to a rehabilitation program. In these cases, the rehabilitation admissions or intake person contacts the insurance company, shares and often faxes medical information, and obtains pre-authorization from the insurance company. This person acts as a liaison between the rehabilitation program and the insurance company, providing the insurance company with any necessary medical updates.

Check with your managed-care program regarding benefits for inpatient rehabilitation, sub-acute or skilled nursing care, outpatient rehabilitation programs and therapies, durable medical equipment and orthotics, and home healthcare services. Ask your managed-care program if it has contracts with any rehabilitation facilities in your area. In-network programs cost less than out-of-network programs. Ask your managed-care program if it prefers to admit patients who have rehabilitation needs to sub-acute facilities, hospital-based TCU's, inpatient or outpatient rehabilitation programs.

Medicaid Benefits
in a Rehabilitation Program

Medicaid pays a much lower reimbursement rate than Medicare, commercial or private insurance. Prior to admission to a rehabilitation program, pre-authorization or approval from the Medicaid program is usually required.

Medicaid pays most of the rehabilitation program fees for physician services, therapies, nursing care, orthotics, and medical equipment. It can cover outpatient services, supportive care at discharge from the rehab program, assist with payment of transportation, home healthcare services, durable medical equipment for home use, and homemaker support, which includes housecleaning, shopping, and meal preparation. As each state offers different Medicaid programs, it is important to check the Medicaid eligibility and benefits in your state.

Commercial/Private Insurance Policy Benefits

Because each individual commercial policy provides different benefits, it is important to review your policy carefully for coverage for inpatient rehabilitation services, outpatient rehabilitation services, and sub-acute or skilled nursing care services. Most commercial plans limit the amount of money paid out or the number of allowed treatments. In addition, check the coverage for home healthcare services and durable medical equipment, as these services provide continued medical supervision and treatment after the rehabilitation program. Pre-authorization is usually required. Check your insurance policy for:

- inpatient rehabilitation coverage;
- limitations on rehabilitation treatments;
- the number of days allowed for rehabilitation benefits for inpatient treatment;
- the out-of-pocket or co-pay cost to you, especially for outpatient therapies.

Veteran Benefits

If you are service-connected Veteran, you can contact the nearest U.S. Department of Veteran's Affairs for information about the rehabilitation programs offered by the Veteran's Administration. To locate this office, go to http://www.va.gov/

Long-Term-Care Insurance Polices

Some people purchase long-term care policies for extra coverage. Be aware that skilled nursing care (sub-acute care) falls under Medicare Part A, private insurance policies, and Medicaid. A long-term care policy should primarily provide benefits for care *not* covered under other policies, including custodial care, intermediate care, and non-skilled care. Look carefully at the premium to determine if it is worth purchasing. Check your policy to see if it helps pay for care in a rehabilitation center or for caregivers in your home *after* you have received your rehabilitation. Be aware that some long-term care policies provide limited benefits or benefits that do not cover the entire cost for hiring a private caregiver in the home.

What to Bring to the Rehabilitation Program

To participate in the rehabilitation program and therapy sessions you will need at least three sets of clothing including:

- loose-fitting clothes such as sweatpants, leggings, sweatshirts that are easy to get on and take off. Avoid zipper tops, because they may scratch or be difficult to manage, particularly if you are addressing an upper-body disability;

- front fastening bras;

- non-slip shoes and slippers;

- jacket for outside therapy;

- tennis shoes or comfortable flat nonskid shoes;

- sleep attire, such as bathrobe and pajamas;

- toiletries including toothbrush, razor, hairbrush, comb, and makeup;

- personal items, including glasses, dentures, hearing aids, pillows, important telephone numbers, or a picture of your family;

- leisure activities such as a book, puzzles, suduko.

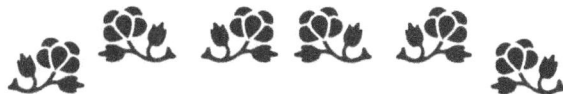

Do not bring:

- ➤ sentimental or personal items or anything that you would not want to lose;
- ➤ jewelry or other valuables;

- ➤ credit cards or cash;
- ➤ delicate clothing;
- ➤ dress shoes or clothing

Questions to Ask a Rehabilitation Facility

Admission

- How are patients screened for admission to the facility?
- Are there special admission requirements to enter the rehabilitation program?
- Is a physician referral required?
- Can a person be admitted from a hospital? From a skilled nursing facility? From home?
- Is the rehabilitation program for inpatients or outpatients or both?

Programs

- Are there specialty programs for brain-injury rehabilitation, spinal cord injuries, or strokes?
- How many hours a day is a person expected to participate in the rehabilitation program?
- What is considered an average length of stay in an inpatient rehabilitation program?
- How is an individual's rehabilitation program and goals determined?
- Are these goals reevaluated during a person's course of treatment?
- Who determines these goals?
- If a person does not meet these goals, are the goals revised?

Therapies and Services

- What therapies are considered part of the rehabilitation program?
  - ➢ physical therapy
  - ➢ occupational therapy
  - ➢ speech and communication therapy
  - ➢ other

- What services are considered part of the rehabilitation program?
  - ➢ nursing
  - ➢ nutrition
  - ➢ social work
  - ➢ psychologist
  - ➢ physiatrist
  - ➢ other

- How many hours a day is a person expected to participate actively with therapies and other rehabilitation services?

- What is the policy of the rehabilitation program is a person is unable or unwilling to participate actively with therapies and/or services?

- Does the program include facilities for practicing the activities of daily life such as a kitchen, dining room?

- Do therapists take patients on a home visit to evaluate potential needs of the patients in their homes?

Patients

- What is the average number of patients participating in the rehabilitation program?

- What are the most common types of limitations or disabilities found in these patients?

- What is the staff-to-patient ratio?

- Is smoking allowed? If yes, does the facility have a designated smoking area?

- What are the visiting hours?

- Do patients share a room or have a private room?

Staff

- Is staff specifically trained to perform rehabilitation services?

- Does staff help patients who require assistance with their activities of daily living, including help with eating at mealtimes?

- Is staff patient, helpful, kind, compassionate, and professional?

- Does staff participate in developing a care plan for each patient?

- Does staff help coordinate post-rehabilitation care with outside agencies?

Family

- What is your family's role in the rehabilitation program?

- Does family participate with any therapies or services?

- Is family or caregiver training provided to those responsible for post-rehabilitation program care?

- Is there a contact person that family can call with questions and to receive updates on a person's progress in the rehabilitation program?

- Are there written or on-line resources for family to read?

- Is laundry performed by the rehabilitation program or can family launder the patients clothing at home??

Cost

- Does Original Medicare provide benefits for rehabilitation programs?

- Do Medicare Advantage plans provide benefits for rehabilitation programs?

- Do private insurance plans provide benefits for rehabilitation programs?

- Is pre-authorization required from the insurance company? If yes, who obtains the prior authorization?

- Can a person private pay for the rehabilitation program? If yes, what is the approximate cost per day?

Discharge Services

- Does the rehabilitation team evaluate a person's home prior to discharge from the program?

- Who is responsible for this evaluation?

- If a person cannot return to their previous living situation, who will help him find a new and safe home?

- If in-home services and continued therapy are indicated, who helps set up these services?

- Will family be included in making discharge arrangements?

In-Home Medical Services

(home healthcare, hospice and end-of-life care,
home infusion services)

"If you don't learn to laugh at troubles, you won't have
anything to laugh at when you grow old."

-- Ed Howe

In this section, we will look at home healthcare, hospice and end-of-life care, and the less known, infusion or intravenous services administered at home or in an outpatient clinic. Most people are familiar with the concept of receiving medical care in a hospital, a doctor's office, or at an outpatient clinic. In a hospital, you are admitted to a medical or surgical floor where a physician visits you, evaluates your medical condition, and oversees treatment. Nursing and other hospital staff members implements the physician's orders, providing you with medical care in your hospital room. In your doctor's office or in an outpatient clinic, you register, meet your physician at the scheduled appointment time, and receive a medical evaluation and treatment. You leave the physician's office, maybe with a prescription to be filled at your pharmacy or a referral to see a specialist, and return to your home.

Sometimes options like going to the doctor's office or the hospital to get blood work taken or going to an outpatient setting for physical therapy are problematic due to a medical condition, lack of mobility, and difficulty with transportation. In these situations and others, having a visit in your home from a healthcare professional for your skilled care need can provide continuity of care, convenience, and less expense. While recovering from an illness or surgery it is often small things such as getting dressed, walking to the car, seeing the doctor in his office, and returning home, that become exhausting and difficult. Although seeing your doctor following a hospitalization is important, some of the recommended procedures like lab draws and therapies performed in the comfort of your home contribute to your rest and recovery.

Maryann, an obese 70-year old woman, was admitted to the hospital with respiratory failure and elevated blood sugars. During her hospitalization, a physical therapist evaluated her mobility and recommended in-home physical therapy to improve her walking, transfers from her bed to a chair, and to minimize her fall risk. At discharge, her physician ordered home healthcare, and a new home oxygen system due to her continuing shortness of breath. A new user of home oxygen, MaryAnn felt anxious and had many questions about using the oxygen in her home. A home healthcare registered nurse visited her home to provide continuity of care, educate her on the use of home oxygen and to help monitor her blood sugars. In addition, because MaryAnn had difficulty walking, a physical therapist visited her in her home to evaluate and treat her mobility issues.

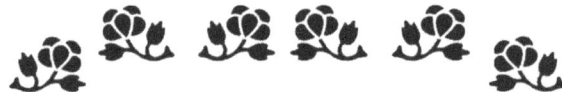

Home Healthcare Services

"Nursing encompasses an art, a humanistic orientation, a feeling for the value of the individual, and an intuitive sense of ethics, and of the appropriateness of action taken."

-- Myrtle Aydelotte, PhD, RN, FAAN

Home healthcare is reasonable and medically necessary skilled medical care you receive in your home, care that is provided by a Medicare-certified or approved Home Healthcare Agency. Home is where you live: it can be a private residence, family home, apartment, shared housing, houseboat, manufactured home park, retirement community, assisted living facility or adult foster care home. With visits from a variety of medical professionals, your home becomes the medical office, the rehabilitation room, and the place where you recuperate from a hospitalization, accident, injury, or chronic illness. Under the orders of a physician, healthcare professionals such as registered nurses, physical and occupational therapists, speech-language pathologists, home infusion specialists, licensed social workers, and home healthcare aides – treat you in your home. For people with a mobility issue, chronic illness or injury that makes it difficult to leave the home, these in-home services allow you to conveniently receive necessary medical care. Although medical social services and home healthcare aides are not skilled services, as long as you have a skilled need, they are available to you in your home.

This benefit falls under original Medicare Part B that covers outpatient services, physician services, home healthcare, and other medically necessary services and supplies. It is an excellent alternative for people who prefer or find it necessary to receive medical care in their home. Original Medicare Part B, Medicare Managed-care policies, Medicaid, and most private insurances will cover these services. If you are uninsured or have limited financial resources, many agencies offer patients the services of financial advocates and applications to financial assistance programs. They will work with you to ensure that you receive the necessary healthcare you require. There are three types of In-Home Services:

- Home Healthcare;
- Hospice or End-of-Life Care;
- Home and Outpatient Infusion Services.

For an excellent summary of Medicare benefits, go to **Medicare Consumer Guide** at http://www.medicareconsumerguide.com/?andallid=160163

Where Can I Receive Home Healthcare Services?

Not everyone who receives home healthcare services resides in their own private home. Some people live in retirement communities, assisted living facilities, or adult foster care homes. Home healthcare professionals can visit you in any of these settings. You cannot receive home healthcare services in the hospital or in a skilled nursing facility. However, to ensure continuity of medical care your home healthcare nurse can contact the social workers, discharge planners, or case managers at the hospital or nursing facility to request a physician order to receive home healthcare services at discharge. If you are already active with a home healthcare agency, your physician can write an order to resume home healthcare services.

When to Request Home Healthcare Services

To receive this Medicare Part B benefit from a Medicare-certified agency, you must be eligible for services. Eligibility includes a home healthcare services order from your physician, an intermittent skilled medical need, and a condition that renders you homebound. A registered nurse, or a licensed practical nurse, a physical or speech therapist can provide skilled care. A physician might order **Skilled Nursing Care** from a certified Home Healthcare agency when you have:

- a hospitalization needing follow-up treatment such as wound care, lab draws;

- a new, recent, or deteriorating diagnosis;

- a significant change in medication in the last 60 days *(this depends on the type of medication)*;

- new medication in the last 30 days *(this depends on the type of medication)*;

- a change in your primary caregiver, necessitating a transition period to teach skilled care to a new caregiver;

- an illness or injury that requires skilled nursing care provided by an registered nurse.

A physician might order **Skilled Physical and Speech therapies and continued Occupational therapies** for:

- a recent decline in your functional status such as walking, transferring, toileting;

- recent falls, fractures, or stroke;

- a home safety evaluation to maintain your current level of functioning;

- difficulty swallowing and/or speaking.

Advantages of Using Home Healthcare Services

In your home, you have the advantage of living in familiar surroundings, sleeping in your own bed, eating food that you or your family prepares, receiving visits and help from neighbors, family, and friends. The home healthcare nurse is your advocate and liaison with your primary care physician and can call him on your behalf for treatment recommendations and orders.

The home healthcare team will visit you in your home during scheduled appointments. Following a thorough assessment in your home by a registered nurse, the home healthcare team will provide medical care and therapies. In the comfort of your home, a registered nurse can provide your medical care and teach friends and family how to perform specific medical procedures such as wound care. A physical therapist can assess your daily physical surrounding and make recommendations regarding home safety. In addition, they can evaluate and treat problems with mobility, fall risk, and transfers. An occupational therapist can work with you on managing your activities of daily life in your home environment.

Your primary care doctor will continue to see you in his office for scheduled appointments. He will issue orders to the home healthcare nurse and other healthcare professionals visiting you in your home. If there is a change in your condition, the home healthcare nurse can contact your physician on your behalf or, if needed, recommend that you receive care in a local hospital emergency department.

Transitional care services through a home healthcare agency provide a bridge between home healthcare and hospice services. They are designed for homebound people with complex and advanced illness, who are actively receiving treatment.. These people may be eligible for hospice or end-of-life care services, but choose not to receive hospice. Healthcare professionals are available to help with symptom management, decision-making in relation to care goals, and spiritual and emotional support to you and your family. The home healthcare team will work with you and your family helping you transition from care to hospice care.

If you have questions about community and government resources, prescription assistance, require counseling services, caregiving assistance, and more, medical social workers can visit you in your home and help you to access these services. Home healthcare aides can help with basic unskilled care such as bathing, while you receive skilled care from the home healthcare agency.

Disadvantages to Receiving Home Healthcare Services

There are several disadvantages to receiving home healthcare services in your home. In a skilled nursing facility, rehabilitation services include therapeutic equipment not available in your home. Treatment can be 5-days a week, sometimes twice a day, whereas physical therapy in the home may only occur several times a week. This can sometimes delay recovery.

Nursing care in a skilled nursing facility is available 24/7; at home, the nurse will visit for an hour or two only, providing medical care ordered by your primary care doctor. Support staff will visit, perform their medical care or therapy, and leave. If your need for medical care exceeds these short visits, you may want to consider staying a short time in a skilled nursing facility and later, receiving home healthcare services in your home. On the other hand, if you are able to get into a vehicle with assistance, you may want to consider outpatient therapy at a local rehabilitation center, office or clinic.

Insurance Benefits for Home Healthcare Services

Original Medicare Part B Benefits

Home healthcare services fall under Medicare Part B and include any reasonable and necessary skilled nursing care, physical and speech therapies. To qualify for home healthcare services under Medicare Part B, you must meet the following requirements:

1). **You must obtain a referral from your physician** stating that you need skilled services in the home. To receive visits from a home healthcare professional, it is necessary to get a written order from your primary care physician, stating the services you will need, your diagnosis, and an ICD code number for the diagnosis. (ICD (International Classification of Disease) codes are used to classify diagnosis and document medical conditions.) Made on the day of discharge from the hospital, from an emergency department or directly from the doctor's office, this referral along with pertinent medical records, insurance information, and personal data is faxed to the home healthcare agency. The intake person at the home healthcare agency will then call you and schedule a visit in your home. If you do not have a primary care physician, some specialists or doctors working in community clinics can make a referral. The home healthcare agency requires a primary care physician they can work with to get orders, prescriptions, and medical guidance.

2) **You must demonstrate a skilled medical need** requiring a registered nurse, a physical therapist or speech language pathologist. Skilled medical needs include:

- ➢ nursing care;
- ➢ speech, language, and swallow therapy;
- ➢ respiratory and cardiac care;
- ➢ medication management;
- ➢ tube care (feeding, catheter, naso-gastric);

- ➢ physical therapy;
- ➢ home safety evaluation;
- ➢ self-care primary caregiver teaching;
- ➢ wound care.

3) **You must be homebound** and unable to leave your home easily due to an illness or injury. Leaving your home must require substantial effort, be for a short time, or necessary to receive medical care. You should need an assistive device, help from another person, or special transportation. Absences or times when you are not available for a visit from a home healthcare nurse are allowed if you are attending a licensed adult day care program for therapeutic treatment or a religious services.

4) **You must receive services from a certified or Medicare-approved home healthcare agency**. Medicare.gov has a resource finder that can help you locate an agency close to your home. Go to http://www.medicare.gov/HomeHealthCompare/search.aspx

5) By entering your state, county, zip code, or the name of an agency, you can easily gather contact information. If you cannot access a computer or are not comfortable using computers, contact your local hospital or look in the yellow pages under, "Home Health Care."

6) **Additional support services** are available as long as you are also receiving skilled services. These support services can include occupational therapy, consultation from a licensed medical social worker, or respiratory therapist, or caregiving assistance from a home healthcare aide. These are un-skilled services and covered by original Medicare only in conjunction with an already received skilled service.

For information on **Original Medicare Part B Home Healthcare Services,** go to http://www.medicare.gov/coverage/home-health-services.html

---

Medicare Advantage Plans - Part C

"This option provides several different alternatives to Traditional Medicare, each offered through many private insurance plans that Medicare approves and regulates. Every year Medicare gives each plan a set amount of money toward the care of each person enrolled in the plan, regardless of how much healthcare he or she uses, and you pay what the plan requires for each service. Each plan must provide at least the same services as Traditional Medicare, but may offer extra benefits."

-- Quote by AARP Bulletin senior Editor Patricia Barry in article, Deciphering Medicare by Deborah Moon, Oregon Jewish Life, November, 2012

Medicare Advantage Plans go by many names, the most common being Health Maintenance Organizations (HMO's) and Preferred Provider Organizations (PPO's.) They also are referred to as Private Fee for Service Plans (PFFS), and Special Needs Plans (SNP.)

Medicare-approved private companies administer preferred Provider Plans (PPO's.) In addition to covering original or traditional Medicare benefits, they also may provide extra benefits such as vision, hearing, dental, health and wellness programs, and prescription drugs. However, they use different rules than original Medicare. For example, you may

- pay additional out-of-pocket expenses;

- need a referral to see a doctor;

- need prior authorization for some services;

- use only in-network facilities, physicians, and suppliers approved by the plan;

- incur additional costs for seeing a healthcare professional out-of-network.

A private insurance company offers Medicare Private Fee-for-Service Plans (PFFS.) Each month Medicare pays a set fee-for-services for healthcare offered to its members. The insurance company, not Medicare, is responsible for determining the cost for your services and may set varying benefits and costs in a region. As not all Medicare private fee-for –service programs are offered in all parts of the United States, the insurance company decides which areas it will provide the plan and services.

Medicare Special Needs Plans (SNP) are intended people with both Medicare and Medicaid who require nursing care for a chronic or disabling condition such as diabetes, congestive heart failure mental health, or HIV/AIDS. Check with your individual policy regarding eligibility for home healthcare services.

Medicaid Programs

Medicaid is a joint Federal and state program for people with limited income and resources. It is possible to have Medicaid along with Medicare. As benefits under state Medicaid programs differ from state to state, it is necessary to contact your state Medicaid office to determine your eligibility and the benefits you can receive under the Medicaid program.

Medicaid recipients are assigned state caseworkers. The caseworker can help obtain pre-authorization to receive services and assistance. If eligible, Medicaid pays 100 percent of the cost for skilled home healthcare and hospice services. If you are in the hospital, the social worker, case manager, or discharge planner often works closely with the state caseworker to ensure that you receive the post-hospital care that you need.

Veteran Home Healthcare Programs

For veteran's without Medicare or Medicaid benefits, who are receiving their healthcare through the veteran system, the United States Department of Veteran Affairs may offer a home-based program or contract with local home healthcare agencies to provide veteran services. Contact your nearest U.S. Department of Veterans Affairs for information. If you are a veteran with a primary care physician and Medicare or Medicaid, a local home healthcare agency should be able to connect you with in-home services.

A home healthcare social worker shared the following twenty reasons for receiving home healthcare. After visiting people in their homes for many years, she appreciated the role of the home healthcare professionals, including their ability to provide continuity of medical care in the home, advocacy and support to her clients, and problem-solve to keep people in their homes and out of the hospital. Here are the twenty reasons to obtain home healthcare following a hospitalization.

Twenty Reasons for Home Care

by Val J. Halamandaris

There is no question in my mind that home care is the wave of the future. There is growing public demand for healthcare services that are available to the public in their own homes. The reasons for this trend are complex. They have to do with tradition, with technology, and with cost effectiveness.

1) **It is delivered at home.** There are such positive feelings that all of us associate with being home. Our home is our castle, our refuge from the storm. When we are not feeling well, most of us ask to go home. When we are feeling well, we enjoy the sanctity of our residences and the joy of being with our loved ones.

2) **Home care represents the best tradition in American healthcare.** Home healthcare agencies were started as public agencies to seek out the poor and the needy who otherwise would go without care. No one was turned away. This is still true for most of America's home healthcare agencies.

3) **Home care keeps families together.** There is no more important social value. It is particularly important in times of illness.

4) **Home care serves to keep the elderly in independence.** None of us wants to be totally dependent and helpless. With some assistance, seniors can continue to function as viable members of society.

5) **Home care prevents or postpones institutionalization**. None of us wants to be placed in a nursing home unless this is the only place where we can obtain the 24-hour care that we need.

6) **Home care promotes healing.** There is scientific evidence that patients heal more quickly at home.

7) **Home care is safer**. For all of its lifesaving potential, statistics show that a hospital is a dangerous place. The risk of infection, for example, is high. It is not uncommon for patients to develop new health problems as a result of being hospitalized. These risks are eliminated when care is given at home.

8) **Home care allows a maximum amount of freedom for the individual.** A hospital, of necessity, is a regimented, regulated environment. The same is true of a nursing home. Upon admission to either, an individual is required to surrender a significant portion of his rights in the name of the common good. Such sacrifices are not required at home.

9) **Home care is a personalized care.** Home care is tailored to the needs of each

individual. It is delivered on a one-to-one basis.

10) **Home care, by definition, involves the individual and the family in the care that is delivered.** The patient and his family are taught to participate in their healthcare. They are taught how to get well and how to stay that way.

11) **Home care reduces stress.** Unlike most forms of healthcare, which can increase anxiety and stress, home care has the opposite effect.

12) **Home care is the most effective form of healthcare.** There is very high consumer satisfaction associated with care delivered in the home.

13) **Home care is the most efficient form of healthcare.** By bringing health services home, the patient does not generate board and room expenses. The patient and/or his family supply the food and tend to the individual's other needs. Technology has now developed to the point where almost any service that is available in a hospital can be offered at home.

14) **Home care is given by special people.** By and large, employees of home healthcare agencies look at their work not as a job or profession but as a calling. Home care workers are highly trained and seem to share a certain reverence for life.

15) **Home care is the only way to reach some people.** Home healthcare has its roots in the early 1900s when some method was needed to provide care for the flood of immigrants who populated our major cities. These individuals usually did not speak English, had little money, and did not understand American medicine. The same conditions exist now to some extent because of the new wave of immigrants and the large number of homeless individuals who roam our streets.

16) **There is little fraud and abuse associated with home care.** Other parts of the healthcare delivery system have been riddled with fraud and charges of poor care. There have been few, if any, major scandals related to home care.

17) **Home care improves the quality of life.** Home care helps not only add years to life, but life to years. People receiving home care get along better. It is a proven fact.

18) **Home care is less expensive than other forms of care.** The evidence is overwhelming that home care is less expensive than other forms of care. Home care costs only one tenth as much as hospitalization and only one fourth as much as nursing home placement to deal with comparable health problems.

19) **Home care extends life.** The US General Accounting Office has established beyond doubt that those people receiving home care lived longer and enjoyed living.

20) **Home care is the preferred form of care, even for individuals who are terminally**

ill. There is a growing public acceptance and demand for hospice care, which is home care for individuals who are terminally ill.

--Reprinted from CARING Magazine, Vol. IV, No. 10 (October 1985.)

Questions to Ask a Home Healthcare Agency

Accreditation

- Does the Joint Commission on Accreditation of Healthcare Organizations accredit the home healthcare agency?

- Is the agency Medicare-certified? *(The home healthcare agency should be accredited by the JCAHCO and be Medicare-certified.)*

Staffing

- Once a referral is made to the home healthcare agency, how long will it take home healthcare services to begin in the home?

- What staff training and instruction are required by the home healthcare agency?

- Is staff closely supervised?

- What is the average caseload or number of patients seen by individual home healthcare staff each day?

- Does the agency seem flexible when scheduling home visits?

- Is there a waiting period for any of the services or therapists?

- What are the staff's daily working hours?

- Does the agency have twenty-four-hour emergency staffing?

- How many visits from home healthcare staff should I expect? Is there a maximum number of visits?

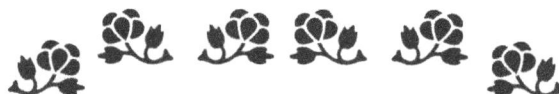

Services

- What professional staff is provided by the home healthcare agency?
  - ➢ registered nurse;
  - ➢ speech therapist;
  - ➢ physical therapist;
  - ➢ occupational therapist;
  - ➢ respiratory therapist;
  - ➢ certified nurse's aide;
  - ➢ medical social worker;
  - ➢ dietician.

- Will the home healthcare agency help or provide necessary medical equipment and supplies?

Billing

- Does the home healthcare agency handle all Medicare and insurance billing?
- Does it accept Medicaid payments?
- Does it have a contract with the U.S. Department of Veteran Affairs to provide services to veterans?
- Does it have a sliding scale for people with no insurance?

Communication

- Will the home healthcare agency contact your physician for a referral, medical orders, or prescriptions?
- Is the home healthcare staff easy to talk with?
- Do staff members patiently answer your questions and, explaining medical terms you may not understand?
- Does the home healthcare agency view itself as a liaison between you and your doctor? If not, how do its representatives see their role as health care professionals?
- How do you feel when you speak with someone for the agency on the telephone?

Hospice Care Services / Comfort Care / Palliative Care

"No one should feel compelled to choose between care that extends life and care that provides comfort."

-- Harvard Women's Health Watch

Everyone is entitled to death with dignity and without pain. When you choose hospice services due to an advanced illness or a terminal condition, you will no longer receive active treatment and will receive palliative or pain-relieving treatment. You can enter a hospice program after your primary care physician and a member of the hospice team certify that you have 6 months or less left to live and are nearing your end-of-life.

Goals of Hospice, Comfort Care, and Palliative Care

There are several terms used to describe the goals of end-of-life care. It is important to know the differences between these terms.

The goal of **hospice care** is to offer physical, emotional, and social support to the patient and family during the final six months of life.

The goal of **comfort care** is to relieve the symptoms of a serious illness and to make a person as comfortable as possible. Its purpose is not to cure the disease or aggressively treat the illness. Many settings are appropriate for comfort care. A physician referral is necessary to initiate this program.

The goal of **palliative care** is to relieve suffering and symptoms of a serious illness regardless of life expectancy. It can improve quality of life during any stage of illness. A physician referral can initiate palliative care at any time during a serious illness. It does not offer cure or a prolongation of life. Cancer patients and those with a serious disease may benefit from palliative care, not as a cure, but as a treatment to relieve pain, nausea, loss of appetite, shortness of breath and other uncomfortable symptoms.

Hospice services provide comfort and support to the terminally ill and their families and caregivers. These services are provided by medical professionals - your primary care physician, a hospice physician or doctor specializing in palliative care, hospice nurse, social worker, spiritual counselor, certified home healthcare aide, homemaker, pharmacist, bereavement counselor, hospice volunteers - all specializing in end-of-life care and support. Using compassionate and palliative care, the hospice team works to prevent suffering, improve pain control and medical management, provide emotional and or spiritual support, educate family about the dying process, and enhance the remaining quality of life.

Most hospice programs begin with a referral from a physician, social worker or registered nurse or a request from a family member to discuss hospice services. Many hospice referrals begin in the hospital or a physician's office with the physician writing an order for a hospice consultation. Once receiving the referral, a hospice intake worker meets with the family and explains the program, outlines the services and answers any questions. It is important for the family to think about what they are realistically able to provide in terms of support and caregiving. Will the person receiving hospice care:

- return home with support and caregiving from family and/or friends;

- stay in the hospital in a room designated for end-of-life care;

- be transferred to an private community- based hospice program;

- be transferred to a skilled nursing facility for end-of-life comfort care;

- be transferred to a skilled nursing facility for hospice care;

- be transferred to an adult foster care home specializing in terminal care;

- be transferred to an assisted living or memory care facility which can either allow your family to provide care or hire private caregivers;

After receiving a referral, the hospice intake worker reviews your medical record and speaks with you and your family. Discussion covers end-of-life services and building a comprehensive discharge plan. If you return to your home, you will need 24/7 support and care by family and friends. An evaluation of your care needs dictates which durable medical equipment, such as a hospital bed, home oxygen, wheelchair, bedside commode, hi-rise toilet seat, shower stool - the hospice program needs to order and have delivered to your home. A call to your insurance carrier confirms your hospice benefits. A visit to the home by the registered nurse is scheduled, pain medications ordered, and transportation home arranged. The hospice professional works closely with your primary care physician and other medical professionals involved in your care

You must consent to receiving the hospice benefit and treatment. Once you sign up for hospice care, the focus of your care will be on comfort and pain management. Being on hospice will not shorten or prolong your life. You will complete a DNR or Do Not Resuscitate and DNI or Do Not Intubate form, which helps you express your wishes for end-of-life care. If your state uses POLST or MOLST forms, this may also be completed. If you do not have an advanced directive or have questions about it, talk with your physician, hospice professional, spiritual counselor, or social worker. This form is important if you wish to prevent unnecessary resuscitation efforts by paramedics responding to a 911 call. However, it is *not* required to receive hospice services.

If you suffer from an illness unrelated to your terminal diagnosis, Medicare Part A will continue to pay for medical treatment *not* related to your terminal diagnosis. However, if you require hospitalization or aggressive treatment, you will need to consult with the hospice team regarding any medical treatment that is not end-of-life comfort care.

Where Can I Receive Hospice Care?

"It's heavy, but also it's sort of the philosophy of Hospice that it's not about death. It's about life. When you're able to confront the realities of death, you're able to live life as long as you can."

-- Landon Adams

In- Home Hospice Care: A team of hospice professionals visit you in your home, assess your care needs, provide necessary durable medical equipment, manage pain, respiratory, and end-of-life medical needs. These services can be provided in your own home, a friend or family member's home, a retirement community, assisted living facility, adult care home, or in a skilled nursing facility. Be aware that original Medicare pays for hospice care in a skilled nursing facility, but does not pay for the daily room and board.

Inpatient Hospice Care in the Hospital and the Community: If you are in the hospital for medical treatment and your primary care physician determines that you would benefit from hospice services, he can write a referral for a hospice team member to talk with you and your family. Usually, a person will start the hospice referral here while in the hospital and then discharge to their home. However, some hospitals or communities offer an alternative, an independent not-for-profit residential community hospice facility or a room within the hospital dedicated to caring for a hospice patient. This setting is excellent if you have persistent pain issues or require palliative medical procedures best performed in a hospital. Most hospitals work closely with a hospice program and, for a limited period, can designate a bed for hospice care under original Medicare Part A.

Skilled Nursing Facilities: These nursing facilities can provide end-of-life or comfort care and often will designate a room for terminal care. However, be aware that Medicare pays for comfort care for a limited time, no more than 7 days. If you wish to have a hospice team involved in your care at the skilled nursing facility, Medicare does *not* pay for the room and board at the skilled facility. This is private pay and can be quite expensive. Medicare does cover visits from the registered nurse and other hospice staff. Some State Medicaid programs will pay for hospice care at a skilled nursing facility. Check with the *State Area on Agency on Aging* regarding Medicaid benefits in your state.

Respite Care: Hospice programs offer respite care to patients and their families and caregivers. Too often caregivers suffer from "burnout" from providing care 24/7 to their loved one. This can result in the caregiver becoming ill or being unable to continue caring for their family member. Respite care gives a break to the family or caregiver by providing up to 5 days of care in a Medicare–approved inpatient facility (hospice inpatient facility, hospital, skilled nursing facility) one time in each benefit period. You may be responsible for a small co-payment, about 5%. Respite allows the caregiver to catch their breath, recharge their batteries, and re-approach caregiving with love and compassion.

Crisis Care: If you are experiencing constant and uncontrolled pain or other symptoms related to your terminal condition, the hospice team can offer short–term crisis care. An increase in services can include daily visits from a registered nurse, a certified home healthcare aide and a licensed vocational nurse.

MedlinePlus:
Go to http://www.nlm.nih.gov/medlineplus/hospicecare.html

American Cancer Society:
Go to http://www.cancer.org/treatment/findingandpayingfortreatment/ choosingyourtreatmentteam/hospicecare/hospice-care-toc

International Association for Hospice and Palliative Care:
Go to http://www.hospicecare.com/home/

What Hospice Services are Available?

Hospice care and services include:

- **physical care** provided by Registered nurses (RN's) and case managers who work closely with you and your doctor to develop a plan of care. RN's provide skilled nursing care; home healthcare aides can help with the activities of daily living;

- **physical, occupational, and speech therapies** that can help with range of motion exercises, transfer training for patient and caregiver, swallowing difficulties;

- **respiratory therapy services** for people who rely on oxygen and breathing treatments. Hospice respiratory therapists are available for consultation and home visits;

- **home infusion services or home intravenous therapy** for relief of pain and other symptoms. *(See section on Home Infusion services at the end of this chapter as it is not exclusively for hospice patients and more commonly used to treat infections requiring long-term intravenous antibiotics.)*

- **dietary counseling** offered by nutritionists to help you plan meals at a time when your appetite may be diminished or when there are changes in how food tastes because of medications or palliative treatments;

- **emotional, spiritual, and bereavement counseling for patient, caregivers and family** provided by medical social workers and hospice chaplains;

- **medications for comfort and pain and symptom management,** which are usually ordered by the hospice team. You may be responsible for a small co-payment (5%) for these outpatient drugs. Doctors may use "standing orders" for hospice medications to control pain. The physician can change these orders if needed. These medications are sometimes referred to as 'rescue medications';

- **durable medical equipment and supplies** which are ordered by the hospice team to ensure your comfort at home;

- **homemaking services** to help you maintain your home when you are no longer able to perform these activities;

- **24/7 availability from the hospice team** to ensure there is always someone available to talk with you and provide medical guidance;

- **integrative health programs** which are alternative medicine programs offering acupuncture, Chinese medicine, aromatherapy, and massage and energy therapies. These programs aim to reduce pain, manage symptoms, alleviate depression and anxiety, and increase quality of life.

At The Integrative Palliative Medicine Program at Scripps Green Clinic in San Diego, I recently observed a nurse use the Healing Touch, an energy medicine, on an elderly hospice patient. The patient was very uncomfortable in any position, restless, and had labored breathing. Less than 30 minutes after receiving the Healing Touch, his body and breathing relaxed, and his head fell sideways into a comfortable position on his pillow. He slept in this peaceful position until his death less than 24 hours later.

To locate **Healing Touch** resources and practitioners in your area, go to http://www.healingtouchprogram.com/

Hospice Insurance Benefits

"A medical prognosis with a life expectancy of six months or less if the disease runs its normal course, as certified by a physician."

-- Medicare Hospice regulations

Under the periods of care, if you meet the Medicare requirements for hospice care, you are entitled to (2) 90-day periods followed by an unlimited number of 60-day periods. For each of the 60-day periods, it is necessary for your physician and the hospice team to recertify your condition as terminally ill.

If your health improves, you go into remission from your illness or you decide you do not want to continue hospice services, you can stop them at any time. Contact your hospice case manager or registered nurse or your physician and request the termination of hospice services. Although many people benefit from hospice, it is not for everyone. Even if you stop services, you can restart them with a new referral if you change your mind. Some discharge situations follow:

- You can remain in the hospice program until your time of death;

- You have received the benefits from the program for an extensive time and your prognosis has improved;

- You can voluntarily leave the hospice program;

- If you are admitted to a hospital that does not have a contract with the hospice agency, hospice may withdraw their services. These services can be restarted following hospitalization;

- The hospice program can dismiss you from receiving hospice services if they determine that your home situation places the hospice staff in an unpredictable or harmful position, or if you are non-compliant with hospice guidelines.

Original Medicare Benefits for Hospice Care

Medicare benefits for hospice services fall under Medicare Part A or hospital insurance. Be sure to check your insurance benefits for hospice care if you have a Medicare managed- care program. To qualify for hospice care you must:

- have your doctor or a hospice medical director certify that you are terminally ill or have less than 6 months to live *(A nurse practitioner cannot certify care for hospice);*

- sign a statement stating that you accept hospice services instead of the usual Medicare hospital benefits;

- sign up for hospice services with a Medicare-approved hospice program.

What Original Medicare Hospice Care Does Not Cover

As the emphasis of hospice care is on comfort and pain control, once you are on hospice Medicare does not pay for any treatments or prescription drugs designed to "cure" your terminal illness.

It is important to contact your hospice team before seeking any medical care. If you go to the emergency department at your local hospital, are admitted for inpatient care, or receive ambulance transportation for care related to your terminal illness without prior approval from hospice, Medicare may *not* cover these services. Remember, you can still receive medical care for illness not related to your terminal condition. If you need medical care, it is important to contact your hospice team and allow them to make arrangements. Medicare can refuse to pay for services not set up by your hospice provider.

Medicare Part A pays for palliative end-of-life care such as chemotherapy or radiation therapy to provide temporary pain relief or alleviate symptoms but not necessarily affect a cure. Medicare coverage can include care for pain management using injections or intravenous medication, nutrition, and skin care.

If you request aggressive or extraordinary measures to prolong life, you may *not* qualify for Medicare benefits under end-of-life care. In a skilled nursing facility, Medicare may pay for a limited time (up to 7 days) for comfort care without hospice services. If hospice is involved, Medicare does *not* cover room and board for hospice care, although hospice services are covered. Medicaid benefits will vary state-to-state. Some Veterans Hospitals will offer end-of-life care or they may contract out to a skilled nursing facility in the community to provide this service. Check your policy for specific information on end-of-life care. Some long-term care policies can provide limited coverage for end-of-life care.

Medicare Advantage Plan
Hospice Benefits (HMO's, PPO's)

Private insurance companies issue Medicare Advantage Managed Plans that contract with Medicare to provide Medicare Parts A and B benefits. You usually pay a deductible and co-payments. As many of these plans are offered and each one delivers different benefits, it is important to read the home healthcare and hospice care section of your policy carefully.

Medicaid

Medicaid benefits cover hospice care in most states. Usually you will need to meet eligibility conditions similar to those required by Medicare for hospice care. As each state regulates their Medicaid program, it is necessary to contact your state Medicaid agency for information regarding benefits. Alternatively, contact a local hospice agency, as they will be able to discuss Medicaid benefits with you.

The **Center for Medicare and Medicaid Services** publishes this official government booklet with extensive information about Medicare and Medicaid benefits.
Go to http://www.medicare.gov/Pubs/pdf/02154.pdf

Private Insurances

Each policy will differ in its benefits for end-of-life care. Read your benefits booklet and call your insurance company to verify your benefits. Be sure to check benefits for: home healthcare, hospice care, respite care, durable medical equipment and supplies, (as you may need a hospital bed and other supplies), prescription benefits, and hospice care in a skilled nursing facility, hospital, or private not-for-profit hospice facility.

Veteran Benefits

For information on hospice benefits available through the U.S. Department of Veteran's Affairs, contact your nearest veteran's office. Some veteran facilities will provide hospice and end-of-life care in their inpatient infirmary. Other VA facilities may contract with local skilled nursing facilities and adult care homes. For information on veteran benefits, go to http://www.va.gov/

Private Pay

Private paying for hospice care can be very expensive. If you are approaching end-of-life care with a low-income, it is important to apply for Medicaid. Applications for end-of-life care are often fast-tracked through the Medicaid system. Getting assistance from a hospital social worker or financial assistance representative can help you navigate this complex process.

Organizing Your Affairs During Your Final Days

"We are not victims of aging, sickness, and death. These are part of scenery, not the seer, who is immune to any form of change. This seer is the spirit, the expression of eternal being."

-- Deepak Chopra

Supportive services to you and your family are available through the hospice social worker. She can provide you with information about funeral homes, cremation and burial, and death certificates. Organize your important papers before your final days. Have your family review them with you. Be sure the surviving spouse or a designated family member has authorization to handle any financial issues. Be sure you have the following papers in order:

- durable power of attorney;
- burial arrangements *(The mortuary will usually take care of the death certificate)*;
- living will;
- bank and investment accounts;

- insurance policies *(life, health, long-term care, mortgage or loan, auto);*
- location and access to your safety deposit box;
- military discharge papers;
- Social Security and Medicare information;

Be sure to order and keep several copies of the original death certificate, as many institutions and government agencies will need an original death certificate to complete their paperwork. Banks, insurance companies, investment firms, and pension offices may need this documentation especially if you hold a joint account or if the account is in the name of the deceased. A Social Security Death Benefit and one-time payment of $255 is payable to the surviving spouse if they lived with the beneficiary at time of death. Even if they no longer resided together at the time of death, the spouse may be eligible to receive the deceased beneficiaries Social Security benefits. Be sure to notify the following business, community, and government agencies:

- banks;
- credit card companies;
- pension and retirement funds;
- insurance companies;
- investment accounts;
- Social Security *(notify of death, apply for widow's benefits and social security);*
- Department of Motor Vehicles;
- attorneys;
- financial advisor.

For more information on **Social Security Death Benefits** go to:

What to Do When a Beneficiary Dies:
Go to http://www.ssa.gov/pubs/deathbenefits.htm

Survivor's Benefits:
Go to http://www.ssa.gov/pubs/10084.html

Understanding the Benefits:
Go to http://www.ssa.gov/pubs/10024.html

Questions to Ask a Hospice Program

- What region does the hospice program cover?

- Is the hospice program state-licensed?

- Is the hospice program Medicare–certified?

- Does the hospice program accept Medicaid?

- Does the hospice program accept other insurances?

- What services does the hospice program provide?

  - pain management;
  - comfort care;
  - palliative care;
  - crisis care;
  - respite care;
  - medication management;

  - help with adl's;
  - counseling for patient and family;
  - pastoral or spiritual care;
  - medical equipment and supplies;
  - volunteer assistance.

- Are there services that hospice does not offer?

- Is there a family member or friend available to help with caregiving? If not, will the hospice program help arrange in-home caregiving?

- What is the caregiver's role when working with hospice?

- How often does a hospice staff member visit the home? How long do they stay?

- If a crisis occurs after regular business hours (8 a.m –5 p.m.), is there a number you can call to get help? Will a hospice member visit your home after hours, if needed? Is hospice staff available 24/7?

- Are there any fees for hospice care? If yes, what are the charges?

- If respite care is needed, does the hospice program utilize the services of a local skilled nursing or assisted living facility?

- Does the hospice program also run an inpatient hospice unit?

- Will the hospice program help my family with making the final arrangements?

- Are bereavement services provided by hospice staff? If not, who provides bereavement counseling and support?

Home and Outpatient Infusion Services

(also called Home or Outpatient Intravenous (IV) Therapy)

In the past, a person requiring intravenous (into a vein) therapy would stay in the hospital until the treatment was completed. Now, teams of healthcare professionals under the direction of a physician can visit you in your home, in a physician's office or at an outpatient clinic, to treat you with IV therapies. These therapies treat infections, cancer, pain, AIDS and more. As these therapies are administered through a special line (peripheral, central, PICC) or pump, it is important to work with your IV team. Learning how to self-manage your care constitutes a primary teaching component you, your family, and caregivers will receive from a registered nurse.

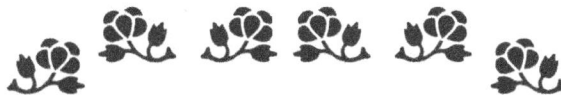

When to Use Home Infusion Services

Home infusion or IV therapies can include:

- anti-inflammatory and steroid therapies;
- antibiotic antiviral, and antifungal therapies;
- cardiovascular therapies;
- chemotherapies;
- enteral therapy (nutrition through tubes);
- HIV therapies;
- hydration and electrolyte replacement;
- immunotherapies;
- infusion pump management;
- pain management;
- peripheral and central line management;
- PICC line placement *(For long-term IV access)*;
- post-transplant therapies;
- prenatal and women's health therapies;
- total parenteral nutrition (TPN).

Advantages to Using Home Infusion Services

Receiving home infusion therapy where you live brings many advantages. Instead of remaining in a hospital, your treatment is delivered in the comfort of your home. The team of healthcare professionals come to you, teach you about your treatment, and then continue to offer support, in some cases, 24/7. Alternatively, if you are active and easily mobile, you can choose to travel to an office to receive your treatment as an outpatient.

If your physician recommends that you receive home IV therapy, a staff member, sometimes a nurse or a case manager will arrange an evaluation for a peripheral, central or PICC line. A specialist places this line before you are discharged from the hospital or arranges for you to receive it in an outpatient setting. The lines allow easy access for the infusion treatment.

Paying for Home Infusion Services

A specialist will check your insurance to obtain pre-authorization, and determine your co-payment, and any other costs associated with the treatment. Factors that help determine the coverage provided by the insurance plan includes the type of medication, the dosage amount, and the number of times each day the infusion is necessary. Some of the drugs used for home infusion cost significant amounts. Luckily, many of the pharmaceutical companies offer financial assistance for these medications. Often, the prescription is faxed to a local pharmacy to determine the cost of the medication prior to you being set up with infusion services. A social worker or case manager can help you access these financial assistance programs.

When your physician orders home infusion services so you can receive medication such as intravenous antibiotics, in your home, a referral is faxed to the infusion agency. As insurance policies vary, with some providing coverage for the medication and others just for the infusion services, it is necessary to receive prior authorization from the insurance company.

At this time, there is a new bill in Congress that seeks Medicare benefits for home infusion therapy. Not only does Medicare Part D cover the drugs used in treatment, but under the new bill, it will add Medicare Part B coverage for the nurse's visits, and the medical equipment and supplies necessary to provide the patient with comprehensive medical treatment.

There are times when the option of receiving home infusion therapy is not the right type of treatment. If you do not have a clean place to live, strong support from family or friends, or the mental or physical ability to manage the treatment when the nurses are not present, consider receiving the treatment in a more supervised setting such as a skilled nursing facility.

Questions to Ask when Receiving Infusion Services

- Does the infusion team work closely with my physician?

- Can I receive infusion service in my home? At an outpatient clinic?

- Do my insurance benefits provide coverage for infusion services in my home? In an outpatient clinic?

- How do these two options differ? Is there a difference in the cost?

- Does a registered nurse administer the infusion? At my home? In the outpatient clinic?

- Can I administer the infusion myself? Do I need to designate a friend or family member to help me?

- Will my insurance benefits pay for the services of the infusion team and all the necessary infusion pumps and medication?

- Is scheduling for receiving infusion services flexible?

- Will I need pre-authorization from Medicare or my insurance company?

- Who is responsible for receiving pre-authorization?

- Are there any activities I will not be able to do while receiving infusion services?

- Are there red flags that may indicate a problem or infection, that I should be aware of when I am receiving this treatment?

- If I run into a medical problem, is there an infusion services staff person available on-call?

"You and I are essentially infinite choice-makers. In every moment of our existence, we are in that field of all possibilities where we have access to infinity of choices."

– Deepak Chopra

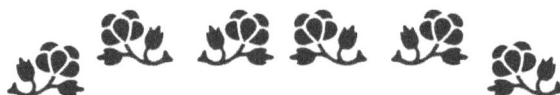

Appendix A

The Wisdom of Experience:
An Insightful Collection of Knowledge

"One starts to get young at the age of 60."

– Pablo Picasso

Or, as my spouse of over 35-years says, he will soon turn 30, with 30-years of practice. It is hard not to notice the changes in the world around us, or when we look closer, the changes within ourselves. We approach each day with the enthusiasm of our youth, while realizing that the days are flying past us faster and faster. We count the years and cannot believe that so many have passed. Life happens just as age happens. We control what we can and learn to accept what we cannot change. The *Wisdom of Experience* is an insightful collection of knowledge gathered from family, friends, colleagues, and strangers eager to share their wisdom with others. Some wisdom is original; others shared favorite sayings, poems, and lessons learned from their lives. We begin with wisdom from our oldest old, the fastest growing age group in the United States.

"We all have this incurable disease. It's called Aging."
"Energy is a lot like money. You have to spend it to use it."

--Joe, age 89, retired physicist and photographer, San Diego, CA. Joe aged in place in his home until his death in 2011.

A letter expressing the joys of living in a retirement community:
"As for living our older years in a CCRC - Continuing Care Retirement Community - I can't rave enough about our quality of life, the things that are offered to us, the care we receive, the "no hassle" life we live. In fact this is really a Life-Fulfilling community!! Most of us still do community services, involvement in our surroundings and staying connected. We are like a big family - as we care for each other, we take courses all year round, we have our own theater which is a performing arts center on our campus. We have fully equipped

business/computer center, club and game rooms, a cozy library and up to the minute sight enhancement machines which help the visually impaired.

In a nutshell, this is a hassle free way of life. We can't even change a light bulb --- maintenance comes and does that for us. Also, we have transportation - free - to go to doctors appointments, shopping in the nearby malls and to the airport. Since we live in a small home, we do not have to have meals in the dining room if we dont wish to do so. We have no minimum, as the people in the main buildings do. However, if at 4 p.m. I don't feel like cooking, we can go to the dining and have a delicious dinner at reasonable prices. Also, if we do not feel well take-out and delivery are available.

Our fitness center is a joy!!! My husband goes every day to walk on the treadmill. I go every day to water aerobics. We also have two hard true tennis courts - and they're well used - by me also!! "Have a positive outlook."

I cant begin to tell you how fortunate we are to be here at this stage of our lives. We dont think of this as an old folks home!" We live on a campus, dine in a beautiful dining room with a huge varied menu, play all sorts of games: bridge every day, trivia, bingo, dancing in the thistle bar/lounge, lectures on all sorts of subjects most days, and live performances in our large comfortable theater. All I can say, it is like living on a cruise ship and we couldnt be happier.

What can I say -- we are living life to the fullest with so many amenities to insure good health and vitality. This is called a life fulfillment facility - and so it is! We have nurses on duty 24/7 and they are there for us constantly. Should we need long-term care, we have a health center with full time nursing care. Of if we need assistance dressing etc. we have an assisted living facility."

--Maje, age mid-80's, retired and active, living with her spouse in a continuing care retirement community in Sarasota, Florida.

"Where you live doesn't matter--
If you keep breathing, you will find the perfect spot."

--Bicky, age mid-80's, Pittsburgh, Pennsylvania, in the process of moving to Florida with her spouse.

Collection of wisdom and thoughts from a Women's Bridge Group and Book Club

"Keep spirits up."

"Don't ever say, "in my day" when speaking to younger people."

"Be kind to yourself – no one else will be as kind to you. Learn to say no. Take care of yourself."

"You need a lot of gold for the Golden Years."

"Screw the Golden Years."

"You need to socialize, to read, to have hobbies."

"Volunteering is important. Being with people is important, and it gives you gratification."

"Learn to make adjustments."

"I got older, my friends may have noticed, but I didn't. Grandson's prom date cancelled. I said, "It's ok, I'll go with him." A few days later, his mother said, "You don't have to worry, he has a date. You can stop looking for the prom dress.""

"We always thought that my grandmother made it to 86 because she looked forward to the next happy family occasion and "skipped" from one to another."

--Women's groups, ages 80-90's, Washington D.C.

"As I grow older, every day is precious to me. I try to build in at least one satisfying or fun experience into each day. It might include a half hour walk in a beautiful park, a long visit on the phone with an old friend from afar, bringing flowers to a person who underwent recent surgery, a cup of coffee with a neighbor, or simply making space in a closet for a seasonal change of clothes."

"I like to think that I "go with the flow" and accept the lifestyle and mores of the current generation."

"People are more important to me than a perfectly clean house or a gourmet dinner on the table."

"A broken cup or vase is just that, nothing more. I don't fret over spills or losses of things. Family, friends, and the world of people are what really concern me."

"Aging is liberating, too. I can be myself and choose my activities and my friends. I do as much as my energy allows and my days are full and my spirit happy!"

"I hope to stay in my home as long as possible. It makes me feel more independent, alive, and involved in the city in which I live. I like to be surrounded by people of all ages and varied backgrounds."

-- Marge, age 80's, artist leading active and independent life-style, San Diego, CA

"Do it – traveling while you're younger and can do it."
-

- Barbara, age 83, retired, currently a hospital volunteer in Medford, Oregon. Barbara and her spouse traveled the USA for 12 years in an RV.

"My advice is to find the thing you love to do, the thing that you can't imagine not doing, and work at it with a passion. Challenge yourself! Dare!"

"When I thought about "retiring" when I was 65 years old, I was quite joyful. All I could think of was that now I could finally spend as much time as I wanted playing the cello. I hope to be playing til the day I die, whenever that may be."

--Barbara, age 78, retired, cellist, Portland, Oregon

I would like to share my favorite poem.
My Get-Up-And-Go Has Got Up and Went
By Anonymous

Old age is golden, or so I've heard said,
But sometimes I wonder, as I crawl into bed,
With my ears in a drawer, my teeth in a cup,
My eyes on the table until I wake up.

As sleep dims my vision, I say to myself
Is there anything else I should lay on the shelf?
But, though nations are warring, and Congress is vexed,
We'll still stick around to see what happens next!
How do I know my youth is all spent?
My get-up-and-go has got up and went!
But, in spite of it all, I'm able to grin
And think of the places my getup has been!
When I was young, my slippers were red;
I could kick up my heels right over my head.
When I was older my slippers were blue,
But still I could dance the whole night through.
Now I am older, my slippers are black.
I huff to the store and puff my way back.
But never you laugh; I don't mind at all:
I'd rather be huffing than not puff at all!
I get up each morning and dust off my wits,
Open the paper, and read the Obits.
If I'm not there, I know I'm not dead,
So I eat a good breakfast and go back to bed!
How do I know my youth is all spent?
My get-up-and-go has got up and went!
But, in spite of it all, I'm able to grin
And think of the places my getup has been!

--Harold, age 76, retired "over the road" driver, and miner, Oregon.

"Take care of your body—it's the only one you have—and it will be good to you if you're good to it."

"Take care of your mind—it's even more important than your body."

" Remain open to life, and try to experience something new every day. If you do these things, the joy you have in your relationships will follow naturally."

"I always wanted to write novels, which I'm doing, having completed three and started a fourth."

"I also hike daily, although health issues have slowed me down, and I play bridge three times a week. My independence and privacy are top priorities."

-- Addie, age 70, retired technical writer and journalist, now writing fiction, Ashland, Oregon

---

"Age gracefully. Be stylish don't wear high heels, you'll wobble, miniskirts are out too they always were difficult to sit down in let alone getting up, don't wear lots of cheap perfume and most of all refrain from showing off too much cleavage, even if you're proud to have some after 50+ years. Wear a smile you'll always look charming and met some interesting people waiting in line."

"Accept aging. Keep a journal of absurd situations you've gotten yourself into ... learn to laugh at yourself."

"Wisdom: There is something true about this. You do accumulate wisdom but being wise is when to know when to share this with your loved ones."

-- Linda, age 66, retired in Sonoma, CA.

"Enjoy the moment"

"Elderly is a state of mind."

"Be willing to be vulnerable so you can help others find joy."

-- Lavon, age 66, emergency room nurse, Yreka, CA.

"The most important lesson of life for me is to remember to keep the big picture, that is, my Soul's perspective, on everyday life so that I don't fall asleep and forget what really matters. Books such as Victor Frankl's Man's Search for Meaning, Schultz's Your Soul's Plan and Newton's Journey of Souls have had a profound impact on my ability to do this. Also, a daily spiritual practice that allows me in some way to access my personal guide and/or Soul essence helps to guide me throughout my day so that I don't get lost in the minutia and duality of earthly plane existence. What matters most in life to me are my relationships with family, friends and even enemies, who are sometimes my greatest teachers. When I finally came to accept that I had chosen my life's greatest challenges, I was empowered to learn how to deal with them in the way that would most benefit my soul and others who might follow a similar path. Remember, only love is real."

-- Susan, age 62, self-employed court reporter, Phoenix, Oregon

---

"If you don't know where you're going,
You probably won't get there."

-- Jim, age 62, research director, Alexandria, Virginia

"Many people today wonder where they will live when they get old. Long Term Care will be outside their budgets, and affordable options will probably be unappealing. We need to reconsider how we manage the needs of an aging population and find creative solutions that honor body and soul.

-- Marybeth, writer, age 62, Oregon.

"An ounce of prevention is worth a 100 lbs. (not 1 lb) of cure"

"I've never heard anyone say on their death bed that they wished they had worked more. Laugh more—and when you do work, do your best work. And for your book the phrase that comes to my mind—which it good advice to myself is, Laugh more. Have more fun. It may not fix you but it will make you feel better. It is all about attitude."

--Andy, age 62, university professor, Colorado

"A stitch in time saves nine."

"Don't be pennywise, pound foolish."

"Use that rainy day fund for which you have so carefully saved. If not now, when?"
"Ditto if you have long-term care insurance. Otherwise the insurance company is the big winner."

"If your kids want you to conserve your money for their inheritance instead of encouraging you to use it appropriately to meet your care needs, they do not deserve an inheritance."

-- Syl, age 60, home health and hospice social worker for 24-years, Oregon

"Be kind and empathetic at all times.
Judging others wastes your time & energy.
Be NONJUDGEMENTAL.
Practice this BASIC and Essential communication Rule to deal with conflict.
State
1) How you feel about a situation using I statements.
2) What the situation is
3) What behavior you prefer
(i.e. I feel angry and hurt when anyone yells at me. I respond better when a person uses a calm voice.)

As much as possible, travel & experience other cultures. Start young & don't buy into "barriers" (i.e. time, money, fear.) Consider it education, just not in a classroom.

Learn how to use your BREATH to bring yourself to your CENTER, especially when chaos is all around you.

Everything you need to know in life is within you. Take the time to be Quiet, to ask & to listen."

-- Laurie, age 59, R.N, MSN, Oregon

"Very few problems have simple answers. When you hear politicians telling you, "the problem is too much government" or "the problem is taxes are too high" or "the problem is too much regulation" the real problem is that they don't understand all the problems."

- Jeff, age 59, small business owner, High Point, North Carolina

A woman's perspective

"Take responsibility for your own life from an early age (females, especially), and don't ever depend on another person or a relationship to support you or fulfill all your needs. Only you can make yourself happy, and only you care that much about you to do the best for you. A relationship should be out of desire, not necessity, or ultimately, it breeds resentment."

"Buy life insurance while you're young and healthy, and when children come along, buy more. If you wait, your health may change and you may become ineligible for a policy."

-- **Susan, age 59, retail customer service, North Carolina**

"As far of wisdom of experience here is one: when you visit with your senior loved ones, let them be the host, don't offer help; it's the best way to learn where they need help the most."

-- **Hanna, age 49, Director, Riverview Apartments Inc. Pittsburgh, Pennsylvania**

If you would like to share your Wisdom of Experience,
Go to http://www.whenyougetolder.com

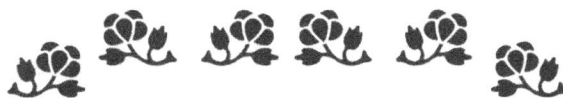

Appendix B

Quick Website Resources Guide

Adult Day Care

> **National Adult Day Services Association:** http://www.nadsa.org

Alzheimer's disease

> **Aging Parents & Elder Care:** http://www.aging-parents-and-elder-are.com/Pages/Checklists/Alzheimers_Chklst.html
>
> **The Alzheimer's Association:** http://www.alz.org/index.asp
>
> **The Music and Memory website:** http://www.musicandmemory.org
>
> **U.S. News with content developed with the Cleveland Clinic:**
>
> http://health.usnews.com/health-conditions/brain-health/alzheimers-disease/managers#13

Assisted Living

> **Assisted Living Facilities.org:** http://www.assistedlivingfacilities.org/
>
> **Assisted Living Federation of America:** http://alfa.org/alfa/
>
> http://www.alfa.org/alfa/Consumer_Corner.asp
>
> **Assisted Living Source:** http://www.assistedlivingsource.com/
>
> **Medline:** http://www.nlm.nih.gov/medlineplus/assistedliving.html
>
> **National Center for Assisted Living:** http://www.ahcancal.org/ncal/Pages/default.aspx

Caregiving Support and Programs

> **Administration on Aging Caregiver Programs:** http://www.aoa.gov/aoa_programs/hcltc/caregiver/index.aspx
>
> **CaregiverList:** http://www.caregiverlist.com/RequestServices.aspx

Helpguide.org: http://www.helpguide.org/elder/caring_for_caregivers.htm

LIVHOME: http://www.livhome.com/

Medicare.gov Caregiver Support: http://www.medicare.gov/campaigns/caregiver/caregiver.html

Community Movements

Ashby Village, Berkley, California: http://www.ashbyvillage.org

Gramatan Village, Bronxville, New York: http://www.gramatanvillage.org

Supporting Active Independent Lives, Madison, Wisconsin: http://www.sailtoday.org

The Village to Village Network: http://www.vtvnetwork.org/

Chevy Chase at Home: http://www.chevychaseathome.org/

Cooperative Housing

CoHousing: http://www.cohousing.org/directory/view/6355

The Senior Cooperative Foundation: http://www.seniorcoops.org/index.php

Durable Medical Equipment

A1 Wheelchair Ramp Guide: http://www.a1-wheelchair-ramps.com/info/ada-wheelchair-ramps-html

Handi-RAMP: http://www.handi-ramp.com/ramp-plan.htm

Medicare Coverage of Durable Medical Equipment and Other Devices: http://www.medicare.gov/what-medicare-covers/part-b/durable-medical-equipment.html

Medicare list of services and supplies: http://www.MEDICARE.gov

RampsPlus: http://www.rampsplus.com/ada-ramp.html)

Silver Cross: Recycler and New HealthCare: http://www.silvercross.com/stairlifts.html/

Education

Road Scholar: Elderhostel Programs, Adventures in Lifelong Learning: http://www.roadscholar.org/

Emergency Call Services

LifeFone Personal Response System: http://www.lifefone.com/index.html

LifeStation: http://www1.lifestation.com/

MobileHelp: http://www.mobilehelpnow.com/ (no landline required)

Philipps Lifeline Medical Alert Service: http://www.philips.lifelinesystems.com/content/home

Rescue Alert: http://www.rescuealert.com/

Senior Medical Alarm System: http://www.senioralarm.com/

Employment and Volunteer Opportunities

Bureau of Land Management Seasonal Employment: http://www.blm.gov/wo/st/en/res/blm_jobs.html

Caretakers Gazette: http://www.caretaker.org

Dinosaur Exchange: http://www.dinosaur-exchange.com/index.php

Experience Works: http:www.experienceworks.org

Forest Fire Lookout Association: http://www.firelookout.org/

JobsOver50.com: http://www.jobsover50.com/student/

National Older Worker Career Center (NOWCC): http://www.nowcc.org/

National Park Service: http://www.nps.gov/search/index.htm?page=1&query=campground+host+jobs

National Park Service Temporary and Seasonal Employment: http://www.nps.gov/personnel/seasonal.htm

Recreation Resource Management: http://www.camprrm.com/

RetiredBrains.com: http://www.retiredbrains.com/Home/default.aspx

Retirement Jobs.com: http://www.retirementjobs.com/

Workampers: http://www.workamper.com/

United States Department of Agriculture: http://www.fs.usda.gov/ volunteer

Working Couples: http://www.WorkingCouples.com,

Workforce50.com: http://www.workforce50.com/

Freighters

The Cruise People, Ltd: http://www.cruisepeople.co.uk/freighters.htm and http://thecruisepeople.wordpress.com/tag/rickmers-pearl-string/

FreighterCruises.com: https://www.freightercruises.com/

Internet Guide to Freighter Travel: http://www.geocities.com/ freighterman.geo/mainmenu.html

Geriatric Care Managers and Social Workers

The National Association of Professional Geriatric Care Managers: http://www.caremanager.org/

The National Association of Social Workers: http://www.HelpStartsHere. org

Healthcare Services

Affordable Care Act: http://www.whitehouse.gov/healthreform

Certified Urgent Care Centers: http://www.ucaoa.org/recognition_ certification_certifiedsites.php

Coalition of Community Health Clinics: http://www.coalitionclinics.org/

HealthCare.gov: http://www.heathcare.gov/index.html

Healing Touch: http://www.healingtouchprogram.com/

Health Insurance Portability and Accountability Act (HIPAA): http:// www.hipaasurvivalguide.com/

MedCottage: http://www.medcottage.com/

NeedyMeds.com: http://www.needymeds.org/index.htm

Organ Donation: http://organdonor.gov/about.asp

Physician Orders for Life-Sustaining Treatment (POLST): http://www. ohsu.edu/emergency/research/polst/

Home HealthCare and Hospice

American Cancer Society: http://www.cancer.org/treatment/ findingandpayingfortreatment/choosingyourtreatmentteam/hospicecare/ hospice-care-toc

Home Healthcare Directory: http://www.homehealthcareagencies.com/ directory/

National Association for Home Care and Hospice: http://www.nahc.org

International Association for Hospice and Palliative Care: http://www. hospicecare.com/home/

Medicare comparison of Home Healthcare Agencies: http://www. medicare.gov/HomeHealthCompare/search.aspx

MedlinePlus: http://www.nlm.nih.gov/medlineplus/hospicecare.html

National Hospice & Palliative Care Organization (NHPCO): http://www. nhpco.org

Original Medicare Part B Home Healthcare Services: http://www. medicare.gov/coverage/home-health-services.html

Houseboats, Eco-sea cottages, and Floating Homes

Eco-Sea Cottages: http://www.eco-seacottage.com/

Floating Homes Association in Sausalito, CA: http://www.floatinghomes. org

Gangplank on the Potomac: http://www.gangplank.com/

Lakefront Marina, Port Clinton, Ohio: http://www.lakefrontmarina.com/ Amenities/FloatingHomes/tabid/910/Default.aspx

Our Sausalito.com: http://www.oursausalito.com/houseboats-in-sausalito.html

Seattle Floating Homes Association: http://www.seattlefloatinghomes. org/

SeattleCondo.com: http://www.seattlecondo.com/houseboats

Seattle Afloat: http://www.seattleafloat.com/

On-line Yachting Magazine with Yacht Forums: http://www.yachtforums.com/forums/

The World, a Residential Condominium Ship: http://www.aboardtheworld.com/

Yacht Clubs of the World: http://www.yachtclub.com/

Yacht Club of America: http://www.ycaol.com/

Yachting Magazine.com: http://www.yachtingmagazine.com/

Information and Referral Resources

A Place for Mom: http://www.aplaceformom.com

Administration on Aging: http://www.aoa.gov

American Association of Retired Persons (AARP): http://www.aarp.org/

The Administration for Community Living (ACL): http://www.acl.gov/Get_Help/Help_Older_Adults/Index.aspx

Elder Care Link: http://www.eldercarelink.com/

Eldercare Locator: http://www.eldercare.gov/Eldercare.NET/Public/Index.aspx

National Association of Area Agencies on Aging: http://www.n4a.org

National Citizens Coalition for Nursing Home Reform: http://www.nccnhr.org

National Council on Aging:http://www.ncoa.org/ and http://www.benefitscheckup.org/ (for low-income seniors)

Ombudsman Resource Center: http://www.ltcombudsman.org

Pioneer Network: http://www.pioneernetwork.net

Senior Resources: http://www.seniorresource.com/

Transitional Assistance and Design: http://www.helpseniorsmove.com/

Yellow pages: http://www.yellowpages.com

Insurance

> **AARP International Health Insurance**: http://ww.aarp.org/intl

> **BUPA International Health Insurance**: http://ww.bupainternational.com

> **Floating Home Insurance article by Ron Moreland, (2010) insurance coverage comparison chart:** http://www.floatinghomes.org/insarticle.htm

> **National Association of Insurance Commissioners (NAIC), "A Shopper's Guide to Long-Term Care Insurance:"** http://www.naic.org/index.htm

Internal Revenue Service

> **Energy Tax Credits:** http://www.irs.gov/uac/Energy-Incentives-for-Individuals-in-the-American-Recovery-and-Reinvestment-Act

> **Internal Revenue Service Tax information:** http://www.irs.gov/ and http://www.irs.gov/businesses/small/international/index.html

International Driver Permit

> **American Automobile Association (AAA):** http://www.aaa.com/vacation/idpf.html

> **National Automobile Club:** http://www.thenac.com/idp_faqs.htm

International Living

> **American Association of Americans Residents Overseas (AARO):** http://www.aaro.org/
> **International Living:** http://www.internationalliving.com

> **The Moon Guide Living Abroad Series:** http://www.moon.com/books/moon-living-abroad

> **Newspapers Worldwide**: http://www.onlinenewspapers.com

> **Peace Corps Application:** http://www.peacecorps.gov/learn/howvol/stepstoapply/

> **Peace Corps Overseas Positions for U.S. Citizens:** http://pcoverseasjobs.avuedigital.us/overseas-recruitment-process

> **Peace Corps Employment:** http://www.peacecorps.gov/jobs/workingpc/fedemp/

Peace Corps Federal Retirement Benefits: http://www.peacecorps.gov/index.cfm?shell=resources.returned.benefits.fedretire

Retired Expat: http://www.retiredexpat.com

Working Overseas Guide: A Guide for Staff and their Families: http://www.peacecorps.gov/jobs/overseasop/countrydir/

World Newspapers: http://www.world-newspapers.com

Language Programs

Pimsleur Language Program: http://www.pimsleur.com/

Rosetta Stone: http://www.rosettastone.com

Legal Services

National Academy of Elder Law Attorneys, Inc.: http://www.naela.org/public/

National Committee for the Prevention of Elder Abuse (NCPEA): http://www.preventelderabuse.org/elderabuse/

National Senior Citizens Law Center (NSCLC): http://www.nsclc.org/

Piecing Together Quality Long-term Care," A Consumer's Guide to Choices and Advocacy, state advance directive forms: http://www.caringinfo.org/stateaddownload.

Medicare

Centers for Medicare and Medicaid, 2014: Medicare and You: http://www.medicare.gov/pubs/pdf/10050.pdf

Medicare Assistance Programs: http://www.medicare.gov/navigation/medicare-basics/medical-and-drug-costs.aspx

Medicare Consumer Guide: http://www.medicareconsumerguide.com/?&allid=160163

U.S. Department of Health and Human Services LIHEAP Clearinghouse http://liheap.ncat.org/profiles/povertytables/FY2014/popstate.htm

Medicare.gov–Part A–Hospital Insurance Deductibles & Coinsurance, 2014:

http://www.medicare.gov/your-medicare-costs/costs-at-a-glance/costs-at-glance.html

Medicare enrollment on-line: http://www.socialsecurity.gov/medicareonly/

Medicare navigation: http://www.medicare.gov/navigation/help-and-support/contact-medicare.aspx

Mobile Home Parks

MobileHomeParkStore.com: http://www.mobilehomeparkstore.com/directory/listoregon.htm

Recreational Vehicles

CampClub USA: http://www.campclubusa.com/

Changin' Gears, Trading City Lights for the RV Lifestyle: http://changingears.com/rv-sec-state-rv-license.shtml

Cruise America: http://www.cruiseamerica.com/

Escapees RV Club: http://www.escapees.com

Escapees CARE, Inc.: http://www.escapeescare.org/

Family Motor Coach Association: http://www.fmca.com/

Good Sam VIP Insurance: http://www.goodsamvip.com/

Motor Home International: http://www.motorhome-international.com/

RVers Online: http://www.rversonline.org/RV6.html

RV Dreams.com: http://www.rv-dreams.com/

RV.net: http://www.rv.net

RVers Online: http://www.rversonline.org/RV6.html

Senior Motor Home Rental in Australia: http://www.seniormotorhomerental.com.au

Trailer Life: http://www.trailerlife.com

USA RV Rental: http://www.usarvrentals.com/

Woodalls: http://www.woodalls.com

Rehabilitation Facilities

Commission on Accreditation of Rehabilitation Facilities: http://www. carf.org/providersearch.aspx and http://www.carf.org/aging/

Relocation Services

Direct Express: http://www.shipdei.com/householdgoodshipping.html

DAS Car shipping and auto transport services: http://www. dasautoshippers.com/

FreightCenter.com: http://www.freightcenter.com/landing/shipping_ costs/landing/shipping_cost.aspx?gclid=CKvly43nuLMCFUdxQgod1isAuw

National Association of Senior Move Managers: http://www.nasmm.org.

USA International Shipping: http://www.usainternationalshipping.org/

USAC International Shipping: http://www.usacintl.com/

Retirement Communities

Aging musicians: http://www.activelifestylecommunities.com/community/ the%20crescendo/the-crescendo-at-westhaven/

Best Retirement Destinations: http://www.bestretirementdestinations. com/ and http://www.bestguide-retirementcommunities.com/ Collegelinkedretirementcommunities.html

BOOM: http://www.boompalmsprings.com/

Burbank Senior Artist's Colony: http://www.seniorartistscolony.com/

Catholic Retirement Communities: http://seniors.lovetoknow.com/ Catholic_Retirement_Communities

Cultural-based retirement: http://www.aegisliving.com/

Episcopal Ministries to the Aging, Inc.: http://www.emaseniorcare.org/

Jewish Homes for the Aged: http://www.jche.org/Programs_Services.shtml

Mountain Meadows Retirement Community: http://www.mtmeadows. com/

NoLo Senior Arts Colony: http://www.apartments.com/California/North-Hollywood/NoHo-Senior-Arts-Colony/978606

Presbyterian Senior Services: http://www.pssusa.org/

Private Communities.com: http://www.privatecommunities.com/private-communities-with-equestrian-facilities.htm

Residences for Life-long Learners: http://www.campuscontinuum.com/resources.htm

Sunrise Senior Living: http://www.sunriseseniorliving.com/

Service Clubs

The American Legion: http://www.legion.org/services

The Elks Lodge Veteran Resource Center: http://www.elks.org/programs/vetsprograms.cfm

Skilled Nursing Facilities

SkilledNursingFacilities.org: http://www.skillednursingfacilities.org/blog/life-in-nursing-homes/federal-regulations-nursing-homes/ and http://www.skillednursingfacilities.org/articles/nursing-home-costs.php

State Ombudsman Programs: http://www.iqnursinghomes.com/

Social Security

Civil Service benefits: http://www.socialsecurity.gov/retire2/fedgovees.htm

Free Social Security Disability evaluation: http://www.socialsecurity-disability.org/

Online Social Security statement: http://www.socialsecurity.gov/mystatement/

Social Security, general information: http://www.socialsecurity.gov/

Social Security benefits and programs: http://www.ssa.gov

Social Security Handbook: http://www.ssa.gov/OP_Home/handbook/

Social Security Railroad Retirement Benefits: http://www.socialsecurity. gov/retire2/railroad.htm

Railroad Retirement Board (RRB): http://www.rrb.gov

Survivor's Benefits: http://www.ssa.gov/pubs/10084.html

Understanding the Benefits: http://www.ssa.gov/pubs/10024.html

What to Do When a Beneficiary Dies: http://www.ssa.gov/pubs/ deathbenefits.htm

State Agencies

SeniorsList: http://www.seniorslist.com/search/area-agency-on-aging-g. php

State Area Agency on Aging: http://www.aoa.gov/aoaroot/aoa_programs/ oaa/How_To_Find/Agencies/Find_Agencies.aspx?sc=OR

State Department of Motor Vehicles: http://www.dmvlocator.com/

United States Department of Housing and Urban Development (HUD): http://portal.hud.gov/hudportal/HUD?src=/program_offices/housing/sfh/ fharesourcectr and http://portal.hud.gov/portal/page/portal/HUD

United States Department of State Home Page: http://www.state.gov

United States Department of State Passports, Visas, immunizations, and travel in another country: http://www.travel.state.gov/

Tiny Houses, Eco-cottages, and Yurts

Blue Ridge Yurts: http://www.blueridgeyurts.com/index.php

Nationwide-Homes Eco-Cottages: http://www.nationwide-homes.com/ ecocottages/main.cfm?pagename=ecoMain /

Pacific Yurts Inc.: http://www.yurts.com /

Small Homes Oregon: Download plans for building your small home. http://www.smallhomeoregon.net/

Tiny Green Cabins: http://www.tinygreencabins.com/

Tumbleweed Tiny House Company: http://www.tumbleweedhouses.com/

Yurtinfo.org: http://www.yurtinfo.org/companies.php

Veteran Information

Comprehensive Veteran Information: http://www1.va.gov and http://www.va.gov

Locate nearest Veteran facilities: http://www2.va.gov/directory/guide/home.asp?isflash=1 and

http://www2.va.gov/directory/guide/division_flsh.asp?dnum=1

Military.com: http://www.military.com/veteran-jobs

Military Connection.com: http://www.militaryconnection.com/military-retirement-communities.html

Military Officers Association of America (MOAA): http://www.moaa.org/

My Army Benefits: http://myarmybenefits.us.army.mil/Home/Benefit_Library/Federal_Benefits_Page/Armed_Forces_Retirement_Home_.html?serv=148

United States Department of Veteran Affairs Caregiver Programs: http://www.caregiver.va.gov/

United States Department of Veteran Affairs Guide to Long-term Care: http://www.va.gov/geriatrics/guide/longtermcare/Adult_Family_Homes.asp

United States Department of Veteran Affairs - Veteran benefits: http://www.va.gov/healthbenefits/ and http://www.vba.va.gov/VBA/

VA National Computer Base: 1-800-827-1000.

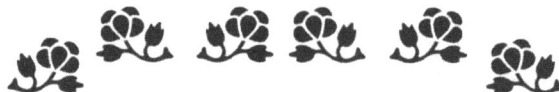

Appendix C

2013/2014 Federal Poverty Guidelines

Go to http://liheap.ncat.org/profiles/povertytables/FY2014/popstate.htm

48 Contiguous States and DC

Note: The 100% column shows the federal poverty level for each family size, and the percentage columns that follow represent income levels that are commonly used as guidelines for health programs.

Household Size	100%	133%	150%	200%	300%	400%
1	$11,490	$15,282	$17,235	$22,980	$34,470	$45,960
2	15,510	20,628	23,265	31,020	46,530	62,040
3	19,530	25,975	29,295	39,060	58,590	78,120
4	23,550	31,322	35,325	47,100	70,650	94,200
5	27,570	36,668	41,355	55,140	82,710	110,280
6	31,590	42,015	47,385	63,180	94,770	126,360
7	35,610	47,361	53,415	71,220	106,830	142,440
8	39,630	52,708	59,445	79,260	118,890	158,520
For each additional person, add	$4,020	$5,347	$6,030	$8,040	$12,060	$16,080

Alaska

Household Size	100%	133%	150%	200%	300%	400%
1	$14,350	$19,086	$21,525	$28,700	$43,050	$57,400
2	19,380	25,775	29,070	38,760	58,140	77,520
3	24,410	32,465	36,615	48,820	73,230	97,640
4	29,440	39,155	44,160	58,880	88,320	117,760
5	34,470	45,845	51,705	68,940	103,410	137,880
6	39,500	52,535	59,250	79,000	118,500	158,000
7	44,530	59,225	66,795	89,060	133,590	178,120
8	49,560	65,915	74,340	99,120	148,680	198,240
For each additional person, add	$5,030	$6,690	$7,545	$10,060	$15,090	$20,120

Hawaii

Household Size	100%	133%	150%	200%	300%	400%
1	$13,230	$17,596	$19,845	$26,460	$39,690	$52,920
2	17,850	23,741	26,775	35,700	53,550	71,400
3	22,470	29,885	33,705	44,940	67,410	89,880
4	27,090	36,030	40,635	54,180	81,270	108,360
5	31,710	42,174	47,565	63,420	95,130	126,840
6	36,330	48,319	54,495	72,660	108,990	145,320
7	40,950	54,464	61,425	81,900	122,850	163,800
8	45,570	60,608	68,355	91,140	136,710	182,280
For each additional person, add	$4,620	$6,145	$6,930	$9,240	$13,860	$18,480

Source: Calculations by Families USA based on data from the U.S. Department of Health and Human Services

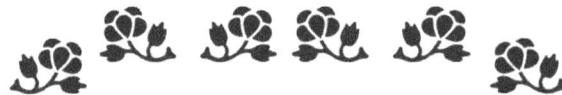

Appendix D

Bibliography

Newspapers

Abelson, Reed. "Hospitals Question Medicare Rules on Readmissions." New York Times: 29, March 2013

Alderman, Lesley. "Deciding on Care for elderly Parents in Declining Health." The New York Times: 2, November 2012

Andrews, Michelle. "Observation units may ease burdens of ER care, but benefits to patients come at a price." The Washington Post: 11, February 2013

Associated Press. "Are we prepared for aging baby boomers?" Mail Tribune: 25, March 2012

Brandon, Emily. "8 Tips for an Affordable Retirement Abroad." US News and World Report: 6, April 2009

Brody, Jane E. "Staying Independent in Old Age, with a Little Help." The New York Times: 24, December 2012

Brody, Jane E. "What to Do Now to Feel Better at 100." The New York Times: 10, November 2010

Carpenter, Dave. "What Those Birthdays Can Bring." Associated Press/Mail Tribune: 10, January 2010

Conrad, Chris. "Body, Mind, and Soul." Mail Tribune: 21, October 2012

Christie, Les. "Floating Homes: What it costs to live on the Water." CNN Money: 15, June 2012

Darling, John. "Aging Boomers Hitting Health Care System." Daily Tidings: 13, April 2012

Fram, Alan. "Recession becomes reality check for baby boomers, poll finds." The Mail Tribune: 10, April 2011

Gardner, Amanda. "Alzheimer's Cases could double with New Guidelines: Expert." Yahoo News: 19, April 2011

Gehrke-White, Donna. "Retirement: Success or Dread?" Sun Sentinel/ Mail Tribune: 25, March 2012

Greenhouse, Steven. "Pushing Back Retirement, and Not Always for Money." The New York Times: 12, March 2013

Gross, Jane. "When I Needed Help." The New York Times: 2, March 2012

Greene, Kelly. "Don't Grow Old Without It." The Wall Street Journal: 6, April 2012

Greene, Kelly. "The New Retirement Resorts: Forget Assisted Living Facilities. Some Intrepid Folks Are Venturing Out to Foreign Countries, Spas and Even Cruise Ships. Here's What You Need to Know." The Wall Street Journal: 18, March 2012

Gross, Jane. "When I Needed Help, Part 2." New York Times: 5, March 2012

Hambleton, Laura. "Now 75, Jane Fonda looks back – and ahead." The Washington Post: 7, January 2013

Hamilton, Walter. "Will you have enough cash? Study finds millions won't." Los Angeles Times/Mail Tribune: 25, March 2012

Hindman, Susan. "Aging in Place in the RV." The Silver Planet: 1, December 2009

Hunsberger, Brent. "Longevity casts a long shadow over retirement planning." Oregonian: 15, September 2012

Jacobs, Deborah L. "Leave the Children the House, Without a Hefty Tax Bill." The New York Times: 26, October 2010

Johnson, Avery. "More Health-Law changes coming in 2013." The Wall Street Journal: 21, October 2012

Johnson, Sharon. "Village Living Catches On." Daily Tidings: 27, March 2011

Johnson, Sharon. "It might be time to make your home 'age-friendly'." Daily Tidings: 15, September 2012

Jouvenao, Justin. "Guardianship case in McLean illustrates lack of regulation for those caring for the elderly." The Washington Post: 29, November 2012

Karp, Gregory. "Step Up to Seniority: The senior advantage discounts." Mail Tribune: 24, April 2011

Kellman, Laurie. "Poll: working boomers say age a plus at office." Yahoo News: 26, April 2011

Khazan, Olga. "As America grays, businesses help seniors age in place." The Washington Post: 23, March 2012

Kliff, Sarah. "Five ways your health care will change in 2013." The Washington Post: 26, December 2012

Konrad, Walecia. "Taking Care of Parents Also Means Taking Care of Finances." The New York Times: 19, September2009

Krantz, Matt. "Many have little or no savings as retirement looms." USA Today: 5, December 2011

Krupa, Carolyne. "Gerontologists outline how doctors can bridge communication gap with older patients." American Medical Association, amednews.com: 29, October 2012

Kunkle, Frederick. "Pioneering the granny pod: Fairfax County family adapts to high-tech dwelling that could change elder care." 25, November 2012

Leland, John. "Helping Elderly Leave Nursing Homes for a Home." The New York Times: 19, September 2009

Lloyd, Janice. "Something in the way they move seniors unloads stress." USA Today: 29, April 2013

Marchione, Marilyn. "New guidelines define pre-Alzheimer's disease." AP/Yahoo News: 19, April 2011

Neergaard, Lauran. "Report: 35 Million-plus worldwide have dementia." AP/Yahoo News: 21, September 2009

Powell, Robert. "Retirement Planning for Inflation." The Mail Tribune: 10, April 2011

Roberts, Cokie and Francis, Enjoli. "Person of the Week: Caregivers Allow for Dignified Living Situations for Aging Parents." 4, February 2011

Rudoren, Jodi. "A Quest for a Home, Put on Hold." The New York Times: 7, October 2009

Schlaerth, Katherine. "Early retirement may be hazardous to your health." Los Angeles Times: 22, April 2011

Seaman, Andrew/Reuters. "Baby boomers in worse health than their parents at the same life stage, study says." The Washington Post: 11, February 2013

Severeid, Susanne. "Words to say for sorrow." Daily Tidings: 9, January 2013

Span, Paula. "The Reluctant Caregiver." The New York Times: 20, February 2013

Span, Paula. "C.C.R.C. Fees: Prepare to be Bewildered." The New York Times: 3, December 2009

Strauss, Robert. "What Do You Want to Be, Now That You're Grown Up?" The New York Times: 12, March 2013

Wolfe, Warren. "Prevent Defense." Mail Tribune: 10, April 2011

Yoff, Emily. "Retirement Entrepreneurs." Slate: 24, March 2011

Magazines

Barovick, Harriet. "Niche Aging." Time: 12, March 2012

Klein, Joe. "The Long Goodbye." Time: 11, June 2012

Lippoff, Liz Rabiner. "What's a boomer to do?" Oregon Jewish Life: November 2012

Moon, Deborah. "Time of Growth, Time of Challenge." Jewish Review: March 2011

Pyati, Archana. "It takes a Village." Bethesda Magazine: May 2013

Website citation

2012, October. "2011 Boomer Housing survey." By Lampkin, Cheryl. AARP Research & Strategic Analysis:

http://www.aarp.org/home-family/livable-communities/info-10-2012/boomers-housing-livable-communities.html

2012, 10/24" "Medical Orders for Life-sustaining Treatment (MOLST)." www.health.ny.gov/p[rofessionals/patients/patient_rights/molst

2012,10/24. "Fact Sheet: The Affordable Care Act: Secure Health Coverage for the Middle Class." The White House: http://www.whitehouse.gov/the-press-office/2012/06/28/fact-sheet-affordable-care-act-secure-health-coverage-middle-class

2012, 10/26. "Ten Best States to Retire 2012." Money Rates: http://www.foxbusiness.com/personal-finance/2012/10/25/10-best-states-to-retire-2012/print

2012, 10/22. "Worst States to Retire 2012." By Barrington, Richard. Money Rates: http://www.money-rates.com/research-center/worst-states-for-retirement

2011, 12/21. "3 Questions to Ask About Assisted Living Memory Care Communities." Huffpost Healthy Living, retrieved 3/7/2013, www.huffingtonpost.com/marguerite-manteaurao/memory-care.

2011, June. "Baby Boomers Envision What's Next." AARP Research & Strategic Analysis, www.aarp.org/work/retirement-planning/info02011/boomers

2010, 10/29. Freakonomics. E-ZPass is a life-saver (literally) [Blog post]. Retrieved from http://freakonomics.blogs.nytimes.com/2010/10/29/e-zpass-is-a-life-saver-literally/

2009, 10/30. "Seniors finding that It does Take a Village." By Moeller, Philip. U.S. News Money: http://money.usnews.com/money/blogs/the-best-life/2009/10/30/seniors-finding-that-it-does-take-a-village

2009, 3/25. "Is a Naturally Occurring Retirement Community Right for You?" by By Moeller, Philip. U.S. News Money: http://money.usnews.com/money/blogs/the-best-life/2009/03/25/is-a-naturally-occurring-retirement-community-right-for-you

2009, 2/17. "Coops for Senior Citizens Offers Carefree Retirement." By Waggoner, Darren. Village Life News: http://www.villagelife.org/news/archives/3-14-97-seniorcoops.html

2009, 2/17. "America's Senior Boom: Where Will They Live?" By Simonette, Terry. Senior Coops.org: http://www.seniorcoops.org/cbj.html

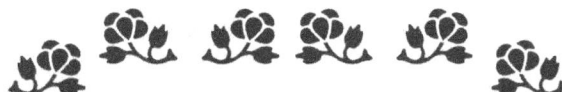

Appendix E

Glossary

Accreditation. Desirable standards for health care and administration, approved by the Joint Commission on Accreditation of Healthcare Organizations (JCAHO.)

Activities of daily living (ADL's.) The routine activities of everyday living , such as bed mobility, walking, eating , dressing, grooming, bathing, toileting, and personal care.

Adult care homes. (Also called board and care homes, adult foster care homes, family care homes, domiciliary homes, personal care homes, community residences or rest homes.) These homes provide basic personal care and limited medical care to seniors and the disabled. The amount of medical care may depend on the level of are provided in the home and the adult care home providers' skills and training.

Adult day care. A structured outpatient program for seniors or disabled people that provides activities, meals, healthcare, therapies, and supportive services.

Advanced directive. A legal form that allows a person to express her wishes and desires for medical treatment, care, and intervention in advance. A living will and a healthcare power of attorney are two types of advanced directives.

Age in place. The ability to remain in your home despite medical, physical, and/or emotional needs, with all the in-home services necessary to create a safe and secure home environment.

Alzheimer's disease. A disease of the brain in aging people characterized by progressive dementia and a loss over time of intellectual functioning.

Assisted living. A residence, usually for seniors or the disabled, that provides for independent living and helpful services, such as meals, transportation, laundry and housekeeping services, medication management, and general health and personal care.

At risk. When an elderly or disabled person places himself in danger of personal injury or harm.

Attending physician. Any doctor other than a primary care physician or hospitalist who provides your medical care in the hospital includes specialists, surgeons, and other physicians consulted about your medical care.

Base rate. An established charge.

Burnout. Strong feelings of physical and emotional exhaustion experienced by caregivers.

Caregiver. A person responsible for providing care and assistance to another person.

Care plan. An organized approach to medical treatment devised by healthcare professionals.

Caseworker. A professional social services worker, registered nurse, or healthcare professional who reviews, evaluates, coordinates, and directs services for seniors, the disabled, and others with healthcare issues.

Comfort care. To relieve the symptoms of a serious illness and to make a person as comfortable as possible.

Competent. Being qualified to understand information and make decisions on your own behalf. Legally qualified to perform an act.

Co-payment: a fixed fee for medical services provided by an insurance plan that subscribers pay when they receive medical care.

Conservatorship. A form of guardianship in which a court-appointed person is given legal right to manage specific or general authority for a person no longer able to manage this own affairs.

Continuing care retirement community. A seniors housing community that provides a wide range of residences, from independent homes and assisted living to skilled care nursing facilities.

Custodial care. General care and assistance with the activities of daily living, as well as supervision to prevent personal harm. This care can be provided by an unskilled person and is not considered medically necessary. It is not covered by Original Medicare, Medicare Advantage plans, or private insurance plans.

Deductible. A dollar amount paid by an individual before an insurance company will pay for benefits.

Depression. A decrease in physical and emotional energy, which can interfere with a person's normal daily functioning.

Discharge planners. Healthcare professionals responsible for organizing and arranging follow-up services for patients released from the hospital.

Disorientation. Inability to recognize and accurately relate to the time of day or familiar surroundings and people.

Durable medical equipment (DME). Medical equipment and supplies used during the treatment of an illness, injury, or disability necessary for a safe home environment.

Durable Power of Attorney. A legal document in which a person can appoint a legal representative to manage his affairs if he is no longer able to do so.

Electrotherapy. Electrical stimulation usually performed by a physical or occupational therapist.

Enteral nutrition. An essential source of nutrition that passes through a tube placed in the nose or stomach wall to be disintegrated in the intestines or stomach.

Guardianship. A person appointed by the court to make decisions on another person's behalf.

Healthcare power of attorney. A legal document in which a person appoints a family member, attorney, or other healthcare agent to make a healthcare decisions for him when he is no longer capable of making his own medical decisions.

Hidden charges. Fees which are not obvious.

Homebound. To be confined to the home and unable to leave without difficulty. A homebound person leaves the home only for a short time, infrequently, and primarily for medical reasons.

Homecare worker. A hired person who provides care and assistance in the home.

Home healthcare agency. A heath-oriented nonprofit or private business often affiliated with a medical facility that provides healthcare professionals to visit homebound people in the homes. These agencies can provide registered nurses, physical, occupational therapist, speech-communication therapists, social workers, and home health aides.

Home infusion therapy. Also known as home or outpatient intravenous (IV) therapy. Intravenous or therapy in which medication is administered through a peripheral, central, or PICC line or through a pump. A home infusion healthcare professional either administers the medications or teaches the patient or family how to do this.

Homemaker services. Homemaker services include the general maintenance and cleaning of a home, chore services, meal preparation, and grocery shopping.

Hospice. A health-oriented agency that provides healthcare professionals trained to evaluate, treat, counsel, and support people facing end-of-life issues in their home or in other settings, such as hospitals, assisted living facilities, adult care homes, and sometimes, skilled nursing facilities.

Hospitalist. A physician who specializes in hospital medicine.

Incompetent. Not legally qualified to handle specific legal rights.

Incontinence. Involuntary discharge of urine or stool.

Information and referral. To contact, send, or direct information to a person or place an order to receive aid, material, or treatment.

Intensivist. A physician, often a pulmonologist, who specializes in the care and treatment of critically ill or injured patients within the intensive care unit.

Intermediate care. A level of medical care in a hospital that is found between intensive and/or skilled care and basic personal care, usually provided to people with non-acute illnesses, the disabled, or elderly.

Levels of care. Different degrees of care designated by a healthcare or residential facility.

Living will. A type of advanced directive in which a person places in writing her wishes for medical treatment should she not be able to communicate this during a life-threatening situation. State law may limit the medical treatments stated in the living will.

Long-term care. Homes or institutions that provide nursing and personal care to people who are unable to care for themselves due to age, health, or disabilities.

Long-term care insurance. A supplemental healthcare insurance plan that provides benefits for people with chronic illness or disabilities, both medical and non-medical (custodial care), when they are no longer able to care for themselves. It can be provided at any age and used in the home, community, assisted living and in a nursing facility.

Medicaid. (Also known as medical assistance, welfare, public aid, or by specific names in some states.) The national insurance program administered by the states for low-income and disabled people, which provides health and long-term care. Eligibility and benefits vary widely from state-to-state.

Medically necessary. Medical care, services, and supplies essential to the treatment and diagnosis of an illness or injury.

Medically stable. To be in a state of unchanging health, that does not need immediate medical attention.

Medicare, Original or Traditional. The national healthcare insurance program available to most people older than age sixty-five and the disabled, which covers hospital care, outpatient medical care, tests and procedures, physician bills, and other medical expenses.

Medicare-certified. A certified or approved provider of care that meets federal regulations to provide Medicare services.

Medicare managed care. An option to the original or traditional Medicare healthcare program in which healthcare benefits are provided by an individual healthcare organization that has agreed to provide care to Medicare beneficiaries in exchange for a fixed amount of payment. These benefits may need to be pre-authorized and may be different from those provided under original Medicare.

Medication box. A small box designed to help people easily keep track of their medication schedule.

Medication management. The administration and supervision of medication by a qualified health care professional.

Medigap insurance. (Also known as Medicare supplemental insurance.) Private-pay insurance that supplements some the "gaps" in Medicare insurance benefits, including deductibles and coinsurance.

Memory care. Caregiver support in a facility designed to assist and supervise people with Alzheimer's disease and dementia with their activities of daily life

Non-service connected. To receive money or services not related to an injury received while in the military service.

Ombudsmen. Persons who investigate complaints and mediate disagreements and grievances. Ombudsmen plan an integral role in overseeing patient care in nursing facilities.

Palliative care. To relieve suffering and symptoms of a serious illness regardless of life expectancy.

Parenteral nutrition. A fluid medicinal preparation administered through the vein.

Personal care. Basic care given to an individual, which includes bathing, dressing, grooming, toileting, and eating

Physiatrist. A physician who specializes in physical medicine and rehabilitation.

Physical restoration. Skilled care and therapies provided to a patient after a lengthy or debilitating illness with a goal of improving a person's level of functioning.

Pre-authorization. Approval needed from the insurance company before medical treatment can be administered.

Premium: The amount paid or payable, for an insurance plan.

Primary-care physician. The doctor responsible for coordinating an individual's medical care with other physicians, hospitals and healthcare agencies.

Ramp. A walkway without steps that is easily accessible to people using walkers, wheelchairs, and power scooters or wheelchairs.

Reasonable and necessary care. The physical care and medical treatment deemed essential for management of a medical condition.

Referral. To contact, send, or direct information to a person or place in order to receive aid, material, or treatment.

Respite care. Break or rest time for a caregiver.

Service-connected disability. To receive money or services for an injury received while in military service.

Skilled nursing care. This is reasonable and necessary medical care provided by a skilled healthcare professional working under the orders of a physician. This care is required to assure the safety or to achieve the desired medical result requested by a physician.

Sliding scale or fee. A flexible charge dependent on income.

Stair glide. Durable medical equipment used to enable disabled or elderly people to ride up a stairway.

Supervision. Management by an individual who provides direction to another person to ensure safety of a disabled or older person.

Supportive services. Assistance from family, friends, and community that helps a person remain in their home.

Transfer training. To move from one place to another. For example, to move from a bed to a chair or from a chair to a toilet or bedside commode chair.

Usual, customary, and reasonable costs. This refers to the standard payment charges or the fixed rates of reimbursement set by the insurance company.

Workamping. A contraction of "work camping" is a form of RV camping involving singles, couples or families who work part-time or full-time.

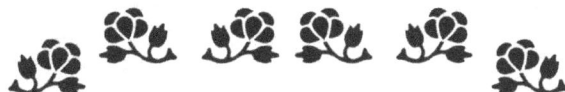

INDEX

State Area Agency on Aging (AAA), 49, 128, 133, 178, 195, 196, 198, 204, 205, 255, 278, 359
State Supplemental Payment (SSP), 197
Steiner, Hannah, 116
Stoppard, Tom, 274
sundowner's syndrome, 216
Supplemental Security Income (SSI), 192, 197
supportive services, 45, 47, 158, 282, 332, 373

T

taxi services, 130, 151
terminal care. *See hospice & end-of-life*
theme-based retirement communities. *See accommodations, retirement communities*
Todd, MPT, 273
transitional care units (TCU), 268-269
travel trailer, 63-64, 76
Tse, Lao, 33
Twain, Mark, 78

U

Ullman, Harvey, 139
United States Census Bureau, 10
United States Department of Commerce, 10
United States Department of Health and Human Services, 256, 355, 362
United States Department of Housing and Urban Development (HUD). *See also HUD*
United States Department of State, 58, 99, 359
United States Department of Veteran Affairs, 140, 195-196, 234, 254, 281, 284, 319, 360
U.S. Equal Employment Opportunity Commission, 13
United States National Institute of Aging, 13, 212

university-based retirement communities, 136, 139-141. *See also accommodations, retirement communities*
urgent care centers, 228-230, 351

V

verbal abuse, 192
veterans benefits, 20, 254, 280-281, 306, 319, 332, 360. *See also United States Department of Veteran Affairs*
village-to-village movement, 135-136. *See also community movements*
volunteering, 8, 13, 66, 72-77, 96-97, 105-110, 135, 146, 204, 276, 324, 342, 350-351

W

walk-in clinic. *See urgent care centers.*
warning signs, 120-121, 191-193, 170-171, 216
website resource guide, quick. *See Appendix B*
Western Unabridged Dictionary, 292
Wilson, Tom, 3
Wikipedia, 72, 83, 91, 96, 230, 234
wisdom of experience, 339-347. *See Appendix A*
worker's compensation (WC), 281
worksheet, getting to know you. *See Getting to Know You worksheet*

X

Y

yurt. *See accommodations, yurt*

Z

Zogby International, 39